Imaging in Particle Therapy

Current practice and future trends

Online at: https://doi.org/10.1088/978-0-7503-5117-1

About the Series

The Biophysical Society and IOP Publishing have forged a new publishing partnership in biophysics, bringing the world-leading expertise and domain knowledge of the Biophysical Society into the rapidly developing IOP ebooks program.

The program publishes textbooks, monographs, reviews, and handbooks covering all areas of biophysics research, applications, education, methods, computational tools, and techniques. Subjects of the collection will include: bioenergetics; bioengineering; biological fluorescence; biopolymers *in vivo*; cryo-electron microscopy; exocytosis and endocytosis; intrinsically disordered proteins; mechanobiology; membrane biophysics; membrane structure and assembly; molecular biophysics; motility and cytoskeleton; nanoscale biophysics; and permeation and transport.

A full list of titles published in this series can be found here: https://iopscience.iop.org/bookListInfo/iop-series-in-biophysical-society.

Imaging in Particle Therapy

Current practice and future trends

Edited by
Chiara Paganelli
Dipartimento di Elettronica, Informazione e Bioingegneria, Politecnico di Milano,
Milano, Italy

Chiara Gianoli
Department of Experimental Physics - Medical Physics of the Faculty for Physics at the
Ludwig-Maximilians-Universität München, Germany

Antje Knopf
Institute for Medical Engineering and Medical Informatics, School of Life Science,
University of Applied Sciences and Arts Northwestern Switzerland, Muttenz, Switzerland

IOP Publishing, Bristol, UK

ISBN   978-0-7503-5117-1 (ebook)
ISBN   978-0-7503-5115-7 (print)
ISBN   978-0-7503-5118-8 (myPrint)
ISBN   978-0-7503-5116-4 (mobi)

DOI   10.1088/978-0-7503-5117-1

Version: 20240601

IOP ebooks

British Library Cataloguing-in-Publication Data: A catalogue record for this book is available from the British Library.

Published by IOP Publishing, wholly owned by The Institute of Physics, London

IOP Publishing, No.2 The Distillery, Glassfields, Avon Street, Bristol, BS2 0GR, UK

US Office: IOP Publishing, Inc., 190 North Independence Mall West, Suite 601, Philadelphia, PA 19106, USA

Contents

13 Integration of imaging in clinical protocols of particle therapy   13-1
P Trnkova, A Bolsi, A Knopf and A Hoffmann

**14 Conclusions and future perspectives of imaging in particle   14-1
therapy**
C Paganelli, C Gianoli and A Knopf

Preface

The physical and radiobiological advantages of particle therapy (PT) require dedicated imaging technologies and methodologies to achieve accurate treatment planning and delivery. In this book we aim at providing the basis of imaging in PT as well as research and clinical trends on the role of imaging in PT. A focus is put on near-room, in-room and in-beam technologies clinically available and under development for treatment planning and delivery, as well as for treatment verification, to trigger off-line or online adaptation. At the same time, methodological solutions based on the described imaging modalities to accurately model range uncertainties, anatomo-pathological variations and biological properties are also reported and discussed.

Editor biographies

Chiara Paganelli

Chiara Paganelli, PhD, is Associate Professor at the Department of Electronics, Information and Bioengineering at Politecnico di Milano, Milano, Italy. She obtained her PhD in Bioengineering at Politecnico di Milano in 2016. Her main research is on image-guided radiotherapy and particle therapy with a focus on MRI-guidance and personalized radiotherapy.

Chiara Gianoli

Chiara Gianoli, PhD, is a scientist affiliated to the *Ludwig-Maximilians-Universität München* since October 2014 and currently in the *Habilitation* program. Since November 2017 she has been the principal investigator of the *Deutsche Forschungsgemeinschaft* project 'Hybrid imaging framework in hadron therapy for adaptive radiation therapy' at the Department of Experimental Physics—medical physics in the faculty for physics of the same university. Her interest is focused on imaging in medical physics, with particular reference to imaging technologies and methodologies, including approaches relying on the use of artificial intelligence, for ion beam therapy.

Antje Knopf

Antje Knopf, obtained her PhD degree in Physics in 2009 from the Ruperto Carola University Heidelberg, Germany, carrying out the related research at the Massachusetts General Hospital/Harvard Medical School in Boston, USA. Afterwards, she pursued an international academic career in medical physics with a focus on adaptive treatment approaches, image guidance, motion management and particle therapy. Since 2022, she has been a Full Professor for Medical Imaging and Medical Image Processing at the University of Applied Sciences and Arts Northwestern Switzerland.

List of contributors

Amstutz, Florian, PhD, Division of Medical Radiation Physics and Department of Radiation Oncology, Inselspital, Bern University Hospital, and University of Bern, Switzerland, florian.amstutz@insel.ch

Baroni, Guido, Prof., Dipartimento di Elettronica, Informazione e Bioingegneria, Politecnico di Milano, Milano, Italy, guido.baroni@polimi.it

Bolsi, Alessandra, MSc, Paul Scherrer Institute, Center for Proton Therapy, Villigen, Switzerland, alessandra.bolsi@psi.ch

Bortfeldt, Jonathan, PhD, Ludwig-Maximilians-Universität München (LMU Munich), Germany, jonathan.bortfeldt@lmu.de

Buizza, Giulia, PhD, Dipartimento di Elettronica, Informazione e Bioingegneria, Politecnico di Milano, Milano, Italy, giuliabuizza.gb@gmail.com

De Simoni, Micol, PhD, Istituto Superiore di Sanità (Italian National Institute of Health), National Center for Radiation Protection and Computational Physics, Milano, Italy, micol.desimoni@iss.it

Gianoli, Chiara, PhD, Ludwig-Maximilians-Universität München (LMU Munich), Germany, chiara.gianoli@physik.uni-muenchen.de

Hoffmann, Aswin, Prof., OncoRay – National Center for Radiation Research in Oncology, Faculty of Medicine and University Hospital Carl Gustav Carus, TUD Dresden University of Technology, Helmholtz-Zentrum Dresden-Rossendorf, Dresden, Germany aswin.hoffmann@uniklinikum-dresden.de

Hua, Chia-Ho, PhD, St. Jude Children's Research Hospital, Memphis, Tennessee, USA, chia-ho.hua@stjude.org

Knopf, Antje, Prof., University of Applied Sciences and Arts Northwestern Switzerland, antje.knopf@fhnw.ch

Kurz, Christopher, PhD, Department of Radiation Oncology, LMU University Hospital, LMU Munich, Munich, Germany christopher.kurz@med.uni-muenchen.de

Landry, Guillaume, Prof., Department of Radiation Oncology, LMU University Hospital, LMU Munich, Munich, Germany, guillaume.landry@med.uni-muenchen.de

Maspero, Matteo, PhD, Radiotherapy Department, University Medical Center Utrecht, Utrecht, The Netherlands, m.maspero@umcutrecht.nl

Meschini, Giorgia, PhD, Dipartimento di Elettronica, Informazione e Bioingegneria, Politecnico di Milano, Milano, Italy, giorgia.meschini@polimi.it

Molinelli, Silvia, PhD, Centro Nazionale di Adroterapia Oncologia, Pavia, Italy, silvia.molinelli@cnao.it

Morelli, Letizia, MSc, Dipartimento di Elettronica, Informazione e Bioingegneria, Politecnico di Milano, Milano, Italy letizia.morelli@polimi.it

Nakas, Anestis, MSc, Dipartimento di Elettronica, Informazione e Bioingegneria, Politecnico di Milano, Milano, Italy, anestis.nakas@polimi.it

Oborn, Bradley, PhD, Centre for Medical Radiation Physics, University of Wollongong, NSW, Australia, boborn@uow.edu.au

Paganelli, Chiara, Prof., Dipartimento di Elettronica, Informazione e Bioingegneria, Politecnico di Milano, Milano, Italy, chiara.paganelli@polimi.it

Parker, Geoff JM, Prof., Centre for Medical Image Computing, Department of Medical Physics & Biomedical Engineering, University College London, London, United Kingdom, geoff.parker@ucl.ac.uk

Parrella, Giovanni, MSc, Dipartimento di Elettronica, Informazione e Bioingegneria, Politecnico di Milano, Milano, Italy, giovanni.parrella@polimi.it

Peters, Nils, PhD, Harvard Medical School & Massachusetts General Hospital, Boston, USA, npeters8@mgh.harvard.edu

Riboldi, Marco, Prof., Ludwig-Maximilians-Universität München (LMU Munich), Germany, marco.riboldi@physik.uni-muenchen.de

Richter, Christian, Prof., OncoRay – National Center for Radiation Research in Oncology, Faculty of Medicine and University Hospital Carl Gustav Carus, TUD Dresden University of Technology, Helmholtz-Zentrum Dresden-Rossendorf, Dresden, Germany, christian.richter@oncoray.de

Schulte, Reinhard, Prof., Loma Linda University, Loma Linda, California, rschulte@llu.edu

Smolders, Andreas, MSc, Paul Scherrer Institute, Center for Proton Therapy, Villigen, Switzerland, andreas.smolders@psi.ch

Spadea, Maria Francesca, Prof., Institute of Biomedical Engineering, Karlsruhe Institute of Technology (KIT), Karlsruhe, Germany, mf.spadea@kit.edu

Thummerer, Adrian, PhD, LMU University Hospital, LMU Munich, Germany, adrian.thummerer@med.uni-muenchen.de

Trnkova, Petra, PhD, Department of Radiation Oncology, Medical University of Vienna, Vienna, Austria petra.trnkova@meduniwien.ac.at

Wohlfahrt, Patrick, PhD, Siemens Healthineers, mpwohlfahrt@gmail.com

Zaffino, Paolo, PhD, Università degli Studi Magna Graecia di Catanzaro, Catanzaro, Italy p.zaffino@unicz.it

Zampini, Marco Andrea, PhD, MR Solutions Americas LLC, marco.zampini@mrsolutions.com

Zhang, Ye, PhD, Paul Scherrer Institute, Center for Proton Therapy, Villigen, Switzerland ye.zhang@psi.ch

Glossary

^{18}F-FDG	fluorodeoxyglucose
4DCT	respiratory-correlated four dimensional CT
4DDC	4D dose calculation
4DMRI	respiratory-correlated four dimensional MRI
AAPM	american association of physicists in medicine
AD and RD	axial and radial diffusivity
ADC	apparent diffusion coefficient
AI	artificial intelligence
AP	anterior–posterior
APT	adaptive particle therapy
ART	adaptive radiotherapy
ASL-MRI	arterial spin labelling MRI
BEV	beams eye view
BH	breath-hold
BOLD	blood-oxygen-level-dependent
bSSFP	balanced steady state free precession
BTV	biological target volume
CA	contrast agent
CBCT	cone beam CT
CBF	cerebral blood flow
cGAN	conditional generative adversarial network
CNN	convolutional neural networks
CSA	cranio-spinal axis
CT	computed tomography
CTN	CT number
CTV	clinical target volume
DCE-MRI	dynamic contrast-enhanced MRI
DECT	dual-energy CT
DIR	deformable image registration
DL	deep learning
DOF	degrees of freedom
DPBC	dose painting by contours
DPBN	dose painting by numbers
DRR	digitally reconstructed radiography
DSC	Dice similarity coefficient
DSC-MRI	dynamic susceptibility contrast MRI
DTI	diffusion tensor imaging
DVF	displacement/deformable vector field
DVH	dose volume histogram
DWI	diffusion weighted MRI
EPID	electronic portal imaging devices
EPTN	European Particle Therapy Network
FA	fractional anisotropy
FDK	Feldkamp–Davis–Kress
FFE	fast field echo
FLASH-RT	FLASH radiotherapy (irradiation of tissue at ultra-high dose rates)
FOV	field of view

GAN	generative adversarial network
GTV	gross tumor volume
HLUT	Hounsfield look-up table
HU	Hounsfield unit
IR-GRE	inversion-recovery gradient echo
IGPT	image guided particle therapy
IGRT	image guided radiotherapy
IMTP	intensity modulated particle therapy
ITV	internal target volume
IVIM	intra-voxel incoherent motion
J	Jacobian
LASSO	least absolute shrinkage and selection operator regression
LEM	local effect model
LET	linear energy transfer
LET_d	dose-averaged LET
linac	linear accelerator
LOR	line of response
MAE	mean absolute error
MA-ROOSTER	motion-aware reconstruction method using spatial andc temporal regularization
MC	Monte Carlo
MD	mean diffusivity
MDA	mean distance to agreement
ME	mean error
MI	mutual information
MKM	microdosimetric kinetic model
ML	machine learning
ML-EM	maximum likelihood expectation maximization
MRI	magnetic resonance imaging
MRI-linac	MRI integrated with linear accelerator
MRS	magnetic resonance spectroscopy
NTCP	normal tissue complication probability
OARs	organs at risks
OE-MRI	oxygen-enhanced MRI
OER	oxygen enhancement ratio
PBS	pencil beam scanning
PCA	principal component analysis
PET	positron emission tomography
PG	prompt gamma
PGI	prompt gamma imaging
PGS	prompt gamma spectroscopy
PGT	prompt gamma timing
PGTI	prompt gamma timing imaging
POP ART PT	patterns of practice for adaptive and real-time particle therapy
PSNR	peak signal-to-noise ratio
PSPT	passive scanning PT
PT	particle therapy
PTCOG	particle therapy co-operative group
PTV	planning target volume
PWI	perfusion weighted MRI

QIB	quantitative imaging biomarker
Q-imaging	quantitative imaging
qMRI	quantitative MRI
RBE	radiobiological effectiveness
r-COX	cox proportional hazards model regularized with an elastic net penalty
RECIST	response evaluation criteria in solid tumours
RL	right–left
ROI	region of interest
ROS	reactive oxygen species
RQS	radiomics quality score
RRMM	realtime respiratory motion management
RSI	restriction spectrum imaging
RSNA	Radiological Society of North America
RT	radiation therapy
sCT	synthetic CT
SDD	source-to-detector
SECT	single-energy CT
SI	superior-inferior
SID	source-to-isocenter
SNR	signal to noise ratio
SPGR	spoiled gradient recalled acquisition in steady state
SPR	stopping-power ratio
SSD	sum of squared differences
SSIM	structural similarity index measure
TCP	tumor control probability
TOF	time of flight
TOLD	tumor oxygenation level dependent
TPS	treatment planning system
TRE	target registration error
US	ultra sound
v4DCT	virtual 4DCT
VB	voxel-based
vCT	virtual CT
VERDICT	vascular extracellular and restricted diffusion for cytometry in tumours
WED	water equivalent depth
WEL	water equivalent path length
WET	water equivalent thcikness
WHO	World Health Organization

IOP Publishing

Imaging in Particle Therapy
Current practice and future trends
Chiara Paganelli, Chiara Gianoli and Antje Knopf

Chapter 1

Introduction

C Paganelli, C Gianoli and A Knopf

1.1 Basic concepts of particle therapy

During the past decade, external beam radiotherapy has been established as best practice care in approximately 50% of all cancer cases and it has undergone major technological and methodological developments (Rosenblatt 2017).

External beam radiotherapy makes use of an external source to treat a target while trying to spare surrounding organs at risk (OARs). Photons (i.e. x-rays), produced by linear accelerators (linac), are the external source used in conventional radiotherapy (RT). Charged particles, including protons or heavy ions (typically carbon ions), produced by more complex machines (cyclotrons or synchrotrons), can be exploited in particle therapy (PT) (Linz 2011, Loeffler and Durante 2013, Durante 2017, Grau *et al* 2020). Out of the approximately two-thirds of patients with cancer treated with RT, most of them receive RT and less than 1% receive PT (Durante *et al* 2017), a proportion that is rapidly increasing thanks to physical and radiobiological advantages of PT with respect to RT.

The rationale for PT arises from their favorable dose deposition properties, described by the Bragg peak (figure 1.1). Unlike for x-ray irradiation, for PT the energy deposited per unit track increases with depth, reaching a sharp and narrow maximum peak close to the end of the range. This feature is characterized by the linear energy transfer (LET [keV μm^{-1}], i.e. the energy released by a charged particle, through its interaction with matter, per unit of the trace length), which inversely depends on the particle kinetic energy and directly on its effective charge. At the beam entrance, the relative dose shows an initial plateau, which is associated with low LET at high particle energies. At lower particle energies, i.e. at larger penetration depths, two phenomena occur: the LET tends to increase in accordance with its inverse dependency on energy, while the effective projectile charge rapidly decreases, as the projectile collects electrons from the traversed matter (Kraft 2000). The combination of these phenomena generates the sharp Bragg peak, located just before the end of the particle range, that is its maximum penetration depth.

doi:10.1088/978-0-7503-5117-1ch1

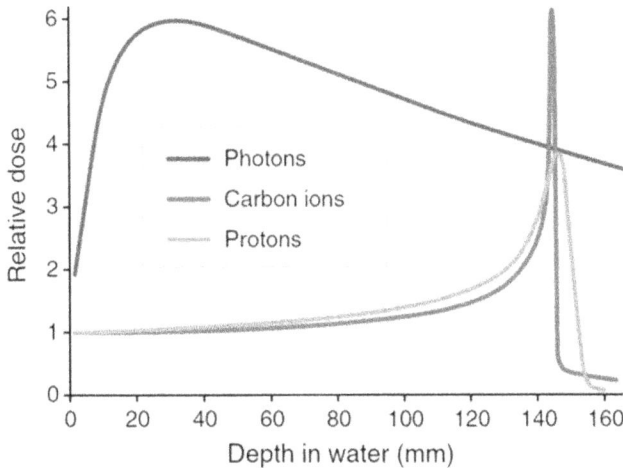

Figure 1.1. Depth dose profiles for conventional and particle beam radiation therapy. Reproduced from Grau *et al* (2020). CC BY 4.0.

The Bragg peak can be precisely adjusted by changing the initial energy of the particle beam, leading to a better dose conformation on the target volume and sparing of surrounding OARs than RT. This makes PT optimal for the treatment of deep-seated tumours or tumours in proximity to OARs. To cover the 3D geometry of the target, the Bragg peak has to be widened, creating a spread-out Bragg peak (SOBP). In the early days of PT, an SOBP was generally achieved through passively scattering a monoenergetic beam through absorbers and collimators. Nowadays, almost all newly opened particle therapy centers use pencil beam scanning (PBS) and intensity-modulated PT (IMPT), in which targets are scanned by small pencil beams in iso-energy slices, and those slices are reached in depth by actively changing the beam energy, for different particle beam fields (Fokas *et al* 2009, Linz 2011, Durante *et al* 2017).

An additional advantage of PT is the higher radiobiological effectiveness with respect to conventional RT, which allows for treating rare and radioresistant tumours. This is accounted for through the quantity relative biological effectiveness (RBE; Kraft 2000). The notion of RBE is typically used to compare the biological effect of different radiation species and is defined as the ratio between the x-rays dose and particle dose producing the same biological effect.

The RBE depends on several factors, such as the radiation type, the dose, the tissue radiosensitivity (i.e. α/β) and the LET, and it is estimated by means of dedicated radiobiological models of the interaction between the particle beam and the irradiated biological system (Karger and Peschke 2017). The dependence of RBE on LET implies that the biological effect is dependent on penetration depth into tissues and in particular, the RBE increases at the end of the particles' range, where the ionization density is highest (Kraft 2000). As such, the higher the ionization density of the radiation, the greater its biological efficacy: in the presence of a high ionization density, the probability of complex molecular effects (such as complex

DNA damage, inflammation and inter- and intra-cellular signaling and reactive oxygen species (ROS) production; Tinganelli and Durante 2020, Byun *et al* 2021, Kiseleva *et al* 2022) increases and the probability of repair is lower as their density increases. This is particularly evident in the case of heavy ions where LET is high (e.g. carbon ions), rather than in light particles where LET is lower (e.g. protons). Indeed, high-LET beams destroy cells by causing direct DNA damage and almost independently of oxygen levels, meaning that their RBE is negligibly affected by the oxygen enhancement ratio (OER), typically low in hypoxic tumour microenvironments (Byun *et al* 2021), and may elicit favorable responses such as an increased immune response, reduced angiogenesis and metastatic potential (Tinganelli and Durante 2020).

In proton therapy the radiobiological modelling uncertainty is comparable to RBE variations, and the RBE is assumed to be constantly 1.1. Although, how much the proton RBE variability impacts proton therapy treatment and, in particular, outcome, is still an open question (Paganetti *et al* 2002, Paganetti 2014). Carbon ion beams show instead a significantly higher variability in RBE than protons, ranging between 2 and 5 in the high dose region and exhibiting lower values at the beam entrance (Amaldi and Kraft 2005, Tinganelli and Durante 2020). To account for the variable RBE, radiobiological models are mainly derived based on the *in vitro* cell killing (Tinganelli and Durante 2020); for carbon ions, the RBE is estimated by the modified microdosimetric kinetic model (MKM; Hawkins 2003) in Japan while European centers apply the first version of the local effect model (LEM; Scholz *et al* 1997).

During treatment planning, the biological effectiveness of the particle beam has to be taken into account (Kraft 2000). For this reason, the biologically equivalent (or RBE-weighted) dose, measured in Gray Equivalent [Gy (RBE)], is defined as the physical dose corrected by the appropriate RBE value. This correction allows calculating the delivered physical dose that is required to obtain a uniform biological effect on the target, estimating the expected gain in Tumour Control Probability (TCP) to the risk of Normal Tissue Complication Probability (NTCP) to achieve optimal tumour coverage and sparing of surrounding OARs (Paganetti 2017, Nuraini and Widita 2019); the therapeutic window between TCP and NTCP is superior for PT than RT, owing to the physical and biological principles governing dose distribution (Durante *et al* 2017).

In recent years, to optimize tumour control and reduce toxicities, advanced PT treatment approaches are developed, which aim at making the most of the geometrical and biological advantages of PT. Proton arc therapy has already demonstrated potential clinical benefits for various disease sites (Chang *et al* 2020); here, the proton beam is continuously delivered as the gantry rotates around the patient and its energy and intensity are adjusted during rotation to confer higher conformality to the tumour, more efficient delivery and increased plan robustness. Minibeam RT is a novel therapeutic strategy that combines the normal tissue sparing of sub-millimetric, spatially fractionated beams with the improved ballistics of PT (Schneider 2022). This approach may allow a safe dose escalation in the target and has already been proven to provide a remarkable increase of the therapeutic index in animal experiments. And finally, FLASH technology, i.e., ultra-high dose rate irradiation (>40 Gy s^{-1}, in contrast to ~ 0.1 Gy s^{-1} of conventional delivery), is investigated (El Naqa *et al* 2022, Atkinson *et al* 2023), although most studies rely on simplistic irradiation scenarios and the mechanistic understanding of the biological characteristics is still in its infancy.

1.2 Rationale of imaging in a PT workflow

The PT workflow mainly reflects that of RT, which comprises a planning stage where a patient-specific model is built to define the optimal dose to deliver, a delivery stage and an assessment/verification stage, which can eventually trigger off-line or on-line treatment adaptation (with the so-called adaptive radiotherapy, ART, or adaptive particle therapy, APT (Paganetti *et al* 2021)) in a closed-loop fashion (figure 1.2).

However, the higher geometrical selectivity and radiobiological effectiveness of charged particles than x-rays is at the cost of a full realization of the potential clinical benefits of PT, which is currently hindered by the relatively high susceptibility of particle beams to uncertainties, e.g. patient setup, organ motion (i.e. anatomical–pathological changes) and range variations. Large target margins are often needed to compensate for the impact of such uncertainties on the delivered dose.

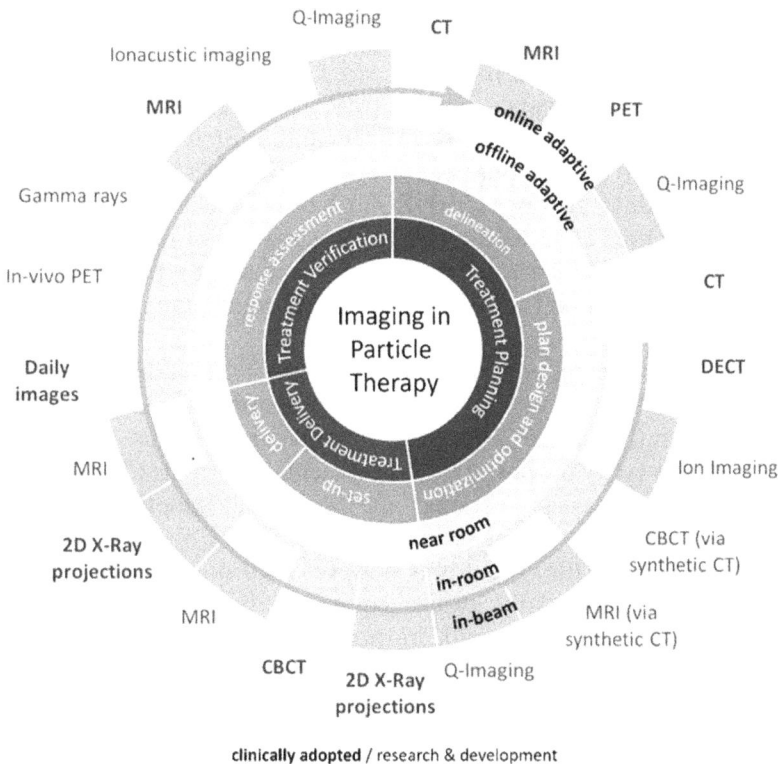

Figure 1.2. Imaging in particle therapy.

Imaging has been demonstrated to be a central pillar in RT (Jaffray 2012) and it is even more relevant for PT when dealing with the above-mentioned uncertainties. In the context of image-guided radiotherapy (IGRT), i.e. incorporating imaging tools that interface with the radiation delivery system and grant the improvement of treatment accuracy, imaging systems (figure 1.2) can be classified in (i) near-room, where the system is outside of the treatment room; (ii) in-room, when the system is within the treatment room and close to the treatment delivery system; and (iii) in-beam, when the imaging system provides images in treatment position (i.e. at the isocenter), thus allowing online adaptation.

In a conventional PT workflow, treatment planning is typically performed with near-room imaging systems. The main purpose of treatment planning is to build a patient-specific model relying on volumetric (3D) images of the patient acquired prior to treatment and to create the desired dose plan that will be delivered during the delivery stage. Specifically, imaging is exploited to delineate contours of the tumour and OARs. These structures are then used to derive the optimal dose distribution to be delivered, by typically relying on a treatment planning system (TPS) which optimize treatment parameters (e.g., radiation dose and beam geometry) in order to maximize TCP while minimizing NTCP. Computed tomography (CT) represents the clinical standard for RT/PT treatment planning as it provides high spatial resolution and information on relative electron density (in the case of photon therapy) or to stopping power ratio (SPR) of particles relative to water (in the case of PT) from the Hounsfield Units (HU), which is required for dose calculations. In some cases, CT can be supported in the clinical workflow by magnetic resonance imaging (MRI) or positron emission tomography (PET) for better organ delineation. As proper calibration is required to convert CT number (i.e. HU) into SPR, the use of two consecutive CT scans with different tube voltages through dual energy CT (DECT) has been clinically implemented in proton therapy (Peters *et al* 2022). The implementation of novel imaging systems that exploit ion beams to generate images (i.e. ion imaging) (Parodi 2014, Johnson 2017) is under investigation for direct in-room treatment planning, adaptation and verification.

The treatment is then delivered in different fractions (i.e. at different days), thus it is mandatory that the patient's condition at each treatment fraction reflects that of the planning as inter-fraction variations may occur. For this purpose, imaging systems are used to verify the position of the patients prior to irradiation. Up to now, in-room/in-beam 2D x-rays projections is the most widely adopted technique in most PT centers to correct for patient set-up errors by rigidly aligning bony structures with the planning CT. This modality is however inadequate for monitoring tissue changes along the beam paths (water equivalent length variations, WEL). In response, commercial or custom-made in-room 3D Cone Beam CT (CBCT) systems are emerging in PT (Landry and Hua 2018), although they are affected by a low image contrast and the usual uncertainty in HU-SPR conversion. Different methodological solutions have been proposed in the literature to overcome these issues, generating so-called virtual/synthetic CTs, for example by mapping the planning CT content on the anatomy of the day via image registration algorithms (Landry *et al* 2015) or by employing deep learning-based methods (Thummerer *et al* 2020). Indeed, if relevant anatomical–pathological changes are present between the planning CT and the in-room imaging, the off-line acquisition of re-evaluation CT is currently preferred, and the plan is adapted accordingly.

Significant changes in the position of the patient or the configuration of the internal organs in the treated area can also occur during a single fraction (intra-fraction), as for example in the presence of organs that move with respiration. In this scenario, it is important to account for respiratory motion during both treatment planning and delivery. Respiratory-correlated (4D) CT is the current imaging standard to depict the average breathing cycle of the patient in both RT and PT (Keall *et al* 2006, Mori *et al* 2018). Different medical imaging modalities to monitor the patient during the treatment have been introduced in RT (Bertholet *et al* 2019) with novel integrated MRI-linac systems (Paganelli *et al* 2018, Keall *et al* 2022) as effective RT treatment solutions for tracking of moving organs. No imaging solutions that enable time-resolved 3D information of the tumour location at all times during treatment are available up to now in PT (Mori *et al* 2018). In a research context, 4DMRI has shown potential to be utilized to verify treatment robustness against motion during planning as it can capture information on breathing variations contrary to 4DCT which only provides an average information (Paganelli *et al* 2018). Prototypes for in-beam MRI-guided proton therapy are currently under investigation (Hoffmann *et al* 2020), but still with limited real-time 3D imaging capabilities.

After treatment delivery, one should verify that the delivered dose has been correctly deposited in the target area. There exist different ways to accomplish this. One approach is to retrospectively accumulate the dose relying on the daily images acquired at different fractions in conjunction with beam information collected during treatment (Meijers *et al* 2019, Paganetti *et al* 2021). Alternatively, direct *in vivo* range verification can be performed by prospectively acquiring dedicated imaging modalities relying on PET or prompt gamma (Knopf and Lomax 2013). Follow-up images acquired after treatment (mainly MRI) are instead conventionally acquired in the clinical routine to evaluate radiological variations of the tumour or OARs, which may reflect radiation-induced changes.

In addition to the 'geometrical' use of 2D/3D/4D medical imaging for treatment planning, delivery and verification, recently interest arises to investigate and adopt quantitative imaging (Q-imaging) modalities (Gurney-Champion *et al* 2020), i.e., imaging techniques with the ability to display pathophysiological features by reporting or mapping quantitatively physical tissue or metabolic properties. Up to now, Q-imaging is rarely adopted in PT. Image modalities, such as PET and quantitative MRI, can provide quantitative imaging biomarkers (e.g. tumour hypoxia, cellularity and perfusion; O'Connor *et al* 2017) that, in conjunction with multi-scale modeling techniques can reveal macroscopic, microscopic and radio-biological properties, that could support patients' stratification and treatment outcome prediction. This would allow subsequent treatment optimization and personalization in PT.

1.3 Summary of the book structure

This book aims to provide a technological and methodological basis of imaging in PT as well as an overview on research and clinical trends concerning the role of imaging in PT.

After this chapter, introducing the aim of PT, its basic concepts related to physical and radiobiological properties, and the need for image-guidance in PT to plan, adapt and verify the treatment, chapter 2 provides a definition of organ motion in terms of inter- and intra-fraction variations that need to be accounted for. Furthermore, chapter 2 introduces several motion compensation techniques that demand imaging, including respiratory-correlated (4D) imaging. As images of the patients are acquired with different imaging modalities and at different time-points during a PT workflow, chapter 3 reports the notion and the current status of image registration in PT for contour propagation, dose warping, and accumulation. Rigid and non-rigid (i.e. deformable) image registration is outlined, with an emphasis on their validation.

CT represents the clinical standard to plan a PT treatment. In chapter 4, this state-of-the-art image modality is described to explain its current clinical usage. Limitations of CT in PT are presented, including uncertainties due to HU calibration to SPR of ions in tissue, and potential solutions are presented as for example the use of DECT. X-ray in-room imaging modalities including x-ray projections for patient positioning, C-arms, CBCT and in-room CT configurations with related challenges are described in chapter 5. Although no commercial system exists yet, several research groups worldwide pursue ion imaging technology and related methodologies to enable the measurement of the tissue SPR and to overcome the limitation of x-rays imaging calibration during treatment planning, adaptation and verification in PT. These efforts are described in chapter 6. Similarly, MRI has recently become successful in radiation oncology thanks to its exquisite soft tissue contrast, radiation free properties and dynamic sequences. In chapter 7, we review the current and potential future use of MRI in PT, with a specific section dedicated to the novel technology integrating MRI with proton units.

Methodological strategies which can support treatment planning and delivery are described in chapters 8 and 9. The former describes artificial intelligence (AI) methods for the generation of synthetic CTs from imaging modalities that do not provide correct electron density or stopping power information, with an overview of these methods for PT applications, including strategies to facilitate CBCT-based image-guided adaptive PT and to replace CT in MRI-based treatment planning. Chapter 9 instead provides the current state-of-the-art of respiratory motion modelling techniques, including conventional and AI methods, which enables the generation of time-resolved volumetric imaging to accurately predict the impact of irregular breathing motion on the dose distribution in PT treatment.

To make the most of the physical and biological potentials of PT, it is desirable to verify dose deposition *in vivo*, either prior to, during, or after therapy. Chapter 10 describes and compare state-of-the art *in vivo* range verification methods currently being proposed, developed or clinically implemented, including on-line and off-line

PET and prompt gamma imaging. In addition, the potential of ionoacustic imaging as well as MRI for treatment verification is cited.

Quantitative imaging (Q-imaging) and conventional quantitative imaging biomarkers (QIBs) that can be directly extracted from Q-imaging are discussed in chapter 12, with a focus on PET and quantitative MRI; high dimensional QIBs (e.g., as those derived with radiomics or deep learning) extracted from any image modality (anatomical, quantitative images or more in general volumetric maps, such as dose maps) and related multi-scale modelling revealing macroscopic and microscopic characteristics are reported in chapter 12.

Finally, an overview of the imaging systems currently adopted in the different PT centres is reported in chapter 13, whereas conclusions and different visions of the current research activities and future perspectives of imaging in PT are reported in chapter 14.

References

Amaldi U and Kraft G 2005 Radiotherapy with beams of carbon ions *Rep. Prog. Phys.* **68** 1861

Atkinson J, Bezak E, Le H and Kempson I 2023 The current status of FLASH particle therapy: a systematic review *Phys. Eng. Sci. Med.* **46** 1–32

Bertholet J, Knopf A, Eiben B, McClelland J, Grimwood A, Harris E, Menten M, Poulsen P, Nguyen D T and Keall P 2019 Real-time intrafraction motion monitoring in external beam radiotherapy *Phys. Med. Biol.* **64** 15TR01

Byun H K, Han M C, Yang K, Kim J S, Yoo G S, Koom W S and Kim Y B 2021 Physical and biological characteristics of particle therapy for oncologists *Cancer Res. Treat.: Off. J. Korean Cancer Assoc.* **53** 611–20

Chang S, Liu G, Zhao L, Dilworth J T, Zheng W, Jawad S, Yan D, Chen P, Stevens C and Kabolizadeh P 2020 Feasibility study: spot-scanning proton arc therapy (SPArc) for left-sided whole breast radiotherapy *Radiat. Oncol.* **15** 1–11

Durante M, Orecchia R and Loeffler J S 2017 Charged-particle therapy in cancer: clinical uses and future perspectives *Nat. Rev. Clin. Oncol.* **14** 483–95

El Naqa I, Pogue B W, Zhang R, Oraiqat I and Parodi K 2022 Image guidance for FLASH radiotherapy *Med. Phys.* **49** 4109–22

Fokas E, Kraft G, An H and Engenhart-Cabillic R 2009 Ion beam radiobiology and cancer: time to update ourselves *Biochim. Biophys. Acta Rev. Cancer* **1796** 216–29

Grau C, Durante M, Georg D, Langendijk J A and Weber D C 2020 Particle therapy in Europe *Mol. oncol.* **14** 1492–9

Gurney-Champion O J, Mahmood F, van Schie M, Julian R, George B, Philippens M E, van der Heide U A, Thorwarth D and Redalen K R 2020 Quantitative imaging for radiotherapy purposes *Radiother. Oncol.* **146** 66–75

Hawkins R B 2003 A microsimetric-kinetic model for the effect of non-Poisson distribution of lethal lesions on the variation of RBE with LET *Radiat. Res.* **160** 61–9

Hoffmann A, Oborn B, Moteabbed M, Yan S, Bortfeld T, Knopf A, Fuchs H, Georg D, Seco J and Spadea M F 2020 MR-guided proton therapy: a review and a preview *Radiat. Oncol.* **15** 1–13

Jaffray D A 2012 Image-guided radiotherapy: from current concept to future perspectives *Nat. Rev. Clin. Oncol.* **9** 688–99

Johnson R P 2017 Review of medical radiography and tomography with proton beams *Rep. Prog. Phys.* **81** 016701

Karger C P and Peschke P 2017 RBE and related modeling in carbon-ion therapy *Phys. Med. Biol.* **63** 01TR02

Keall P J, Brighi C, Glide-Hurst C, Liney G, Liu P Z, Lydiard S, Paganelli C, Pham T, Shan S and Tree A C 2022 Integrated MRI-guided radiotherapy—opportunities and challenges *Nat. Rev. Clin. Oncol.* **19** 1–13

Keall P J *et al* 2006 The management of respiratory motion in radiation oncology report of AAPM task group 76 a *Med. Phys.* **33** 3874–900

Kiseleva V, Gordon K, Vishnyakova P, Gantsova E, Elchaninov A and Fatkhudinov T 2022 Particle therapy: clinical applications and biological effects *Life* **12** 2071

Knopf A and Lomax T 2013 In vivo proton range verification: a review *Phys. Med. Biol.* **7** R131–60

Kraft G 2000 Tumour therapy with heavy charged particles *Prog. Part. Nucl. Phys.* **45** S473–544

Landry G and Hua C h 2018 Current state and future applications of radiological image guidance for particle therapy *Med. Phys.* **45** e1086–95

Landry G, Nijhuis R, Dedes G, Handrack J, Thieke C, Janssens G, Orban de Xivry J, Reiner M, Kamp F and Wilkens J J 2015 Investigating CT to CBCT image registration for head and neck proton therapy as a tool for daily dose recalculation *Med. Phys.* **42** 1354–66

Linz U 2011 *Ion Beam Therapy: Fundamentals, Technology, Clinical Applications* (Berlin: Springer Science & Business Media)

Loeffler J S and Durante M 2013 Charged particle therapy—optimization, challenges and future directions *Nat. Rev. Clin. Oncol.* **10** 411–24

Meijers A, Jakobi A, Stützer K, Guterres Marmitt G, Both S, Langendijk J, Richter C and Knopf A 2019 Log file-based dose reconstruction and accumulation for 4D adaptive pencil beam scanned proton therapy in a clinical treatment planning system: implementation and proof-of-concept *Med. Phys.* **46** 1140–9

Mori S, Knopf A C and Umegaki K 2018 Motion management in particle therapy *Med. Phys.* **45** e994–e1010

Nuraini R and Widita R 2019 Tumour control probability (TCP) and normal tissue complication probability (NTCP) with consideration of cell biological effect *J. Phys.: Conf. Ser.* **1245** 012092

O'Connor J P, Aboagye E O, Adams J E, Aerts H J, Barrington S F, Beer A J, Boellaard R, Bohndiek S E, Brady M and Brown G 2017 Imaging biomarker roadmap for cancer studies *Nat. Rev. Clin. Oncol.* **14** 169–86

Paganelli C, Whelan B, Peroni M, Summers P, Fast M, Van de Lindt T, McClelland J, Eiben B, Keall P and Lomax T 2018 MRI-guidance for motion management in external beam radiotherapy: current status and future challenges *Phys. Med. Biol.* **63** 22TR03

Paganetti H 2014 Relative biological effectiveness (RBE) values for proton beam therapy. Variations as a function of biological endpoint, dose, and linear energy transfer *Phys. Med. Biol.* **59** R419

Paganetti H 2017 Relating the proton relative biological effectiveness to tumour control and normal tissue complication probabilities assuming interpatient variability in α/β *Acta Oncol.* **56** 1379–86

Paganetti H, Botas P, Sharp G C and Winey B 2021 Adaptive proton therapy *Phys. Med. Biol.* **66** 22TR01

Paganetti H, Niemierko A, Ancukiewicz M, Gerweck L E, Goitein M, Loeffler J S and Suit H D 2002 Relative biological effectiveness (RBE) values for proton beam therapy *Int. J. Radiat. Oncol. Biol. Phys.* **53** 407–21

Parodi K 2014 Heavy ion radiography and tomography *Phys. Med.* **30** 539–43

Peters N, Wohlfahrt P, Hofmann C, Möhler C, Menkel S, Tschiche M, Krause M, Troost E G, Enghardt W and Richter C 2022 Reduction of clinical safety margins in proton therapy enabled by the clinical implementation of dual-energy CT for direct stopping-power prediction *Radiother. Oncol.* **166** 71–8

Rosenblatt E and Zubizarreta E 2017 *Radiotherapy in cancer care: facing the global challenge* (Vienna, IAEA)

Schneider T 2022 Technical aspects of proton minibeam radiation therapy: minibeam generation and delivery *Phys. Med.* **100** 64–71

Scholz M, Kraft G, Kraft-Weyrather W and Kellerer A 1997 Computation of cell survival in heavy ion beams for therapy: the model and its approximation *Radiat. Environ. Biophys.* **36** 59–66

Thummerer A, De Jong B A, Zaffino P, Meijers A, Marmitt G G, Seco J, Steenbakkers R J, Langendijk J A, Both S and Spadea M F 2020 Comparison of the suitability of CBCT- and MR-based synthetic CTs for daily adaptive proton therapy in head and neck patients *Phys. Med. Biol.* **65** 235036

Tinganelli W and Durante M 2020 Carbon ion radiobiology *Cancers* **12** 3022

Chapter 2

Organ motion in particle therapy and the role of imaging

C Paganelli, S Molinelli and A Knopf

2.1 Introduction

To make the most of the geometrical and radiobiological advantages of particle therapy (PT), the treatment should be delivered with high accuracy, i.e., assuring that the beam is precisely focused on the target throughout irradiation. Tumour control could not be achieved if such an accuracy is not guaranteed, and serious side effects could be caused by harming healthy organs surrounding the target. It is well known that organ motion, i.e., variations of the anatomo-pathological structures in the tumour site, introduces geometric uncertainties into this procedure, leading to potential underdosage of the target region, and/or overdosage in nearby organs at risks (OARs; Keall *et al* 2006, Bert and Durante 2011, Mori *et al* 2018, Pakela *et al* 2022).

The term 'organ motion' refers to all those patho-physiological processes that develop during a radiation therapy treatment on different timescales. Since radiation therapy is delivered over several fractions, there can be variabilities that can occur between two fractions or within the same fraction, namely inter- and intra-fraction organ motion. Inter-fraction organ motion develops from day to day, due to geometrical variation, tumour shrinking or growth, or weight gain or loss of the patient. Intra-fraction organ motion develops instead within minutes or seconds due to respiratory, muscular, cardiac and gastrointestinal motion (figure 2.1).

Among the different organs that move as a function of respiration, the lung is the most affected. Seppenwoolde and colleagues (Seppenwoolde *et al* 2002) performed an extensive analysis of organ motion in lung tumours. In the superior-inferior (SI) direction, tumours situated in the lower lobes and not attached to rigid structures, such as the chest wall or vertebrae, moved more than those in the upper lobe or attached to rigid structures: 12 ± 6 and 2 ± 2 mm (mean $\pm$ standard deviation), respectively. In left-right (LR) and anterior-posterior (AP) directions there was no

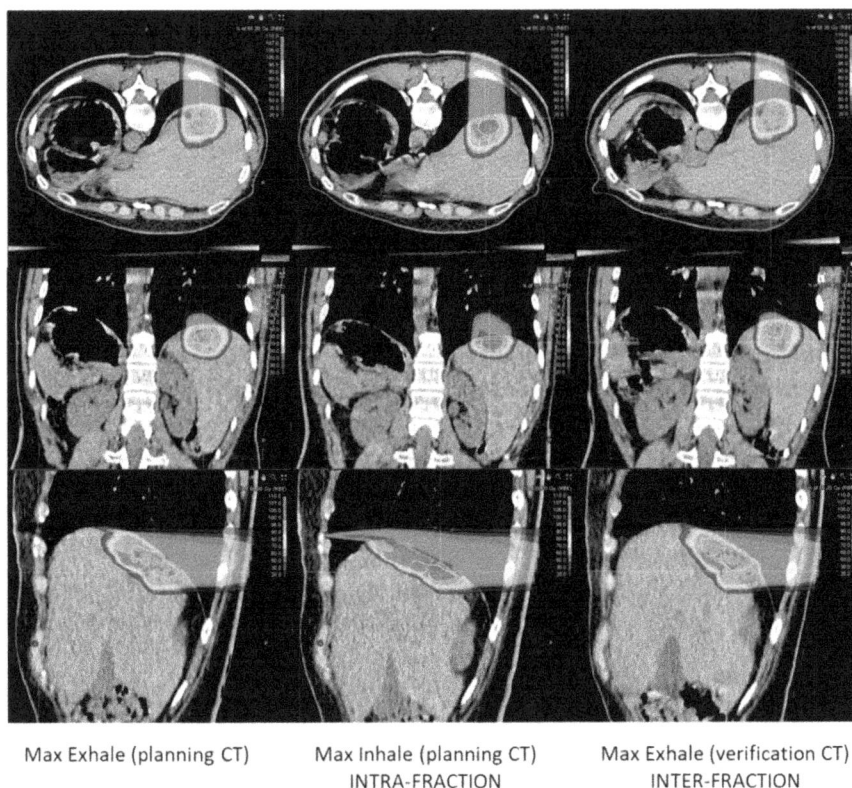

Max Exhale (planning CT)	Max Inhale (planning CT)	Max Exhale (verification CT)
	INTRA-FRACTION	INTER-FRACTION

Figure 2.1. Inter- and Intra-fraction motion in a liver patient. Maximum inhale (Max Inhale) and maximum exhale (Max Exhale) of a planning CT representing intra-fraction motion, and Max Exhale of a verification CT acquired X days after the planning CT representing inter-fraction motion.

difference in amplitude between upper- and lower-lobe tumours; in these directions the motion was small: 1.2 ± 0.9 mm (LR) and 2.2 ± 1.9 mm (AP). The heartbeat also influenced tumour motion, mainly in the LR direction (between 1 and 4 mm). Hysteresis, represented by a difference between the expiratory and the inspiratory trajectory and caused by a phase shift between different motion directions, was also observed in the AP-SI (sagittal) plane up to 5 mm and in the other planes up to 2 mm. Other studies (Sonke *et al* 2008) supported these results, highlighting that lung tumours show significant intra-fraction motion characterized by varying motion amplitudes depending on the specific site, baseline shifts and hysteretic non-linear trajectories, with also relevant inter-fraction baseline variations. Similarly in the liver, respiration-induced motion develops mainly in SI direction with range of motion of 15.5 mm in SI, 10.1 mm in AP, and 7.5 mm in LR directions (Kirilova *et al* 2008), whereas pancreas motion due to respiration is quantified in the range 7.3–27.3 mm in SI direction (Knybel *et al* 2014), with significant inter-fraction variations due to nearby bowel filling (Molinelli *et al* 2022).

Assessing motion in patients treated for lymphomas and receiving mediastinal irradiation is also of primary importance, to considerable reduce the dose to OARs, such as the heart and the lungs (Aznar *et al* 2021). This is valid also for accurate toxicity assessment in radiotherapy treatments of esophagus (Feng *et al* 2021a), prostatic (Su *et al* 2019) and gynecological (Gort *et al* 2021) tumours, and of all other organs that are not primarily affected by respiratory motion such as the head and neck (Park and Park 2016).

It should be noted that no standardized way to report motion is present, with different metrics being used, but recommendations for motion-assessment and motion-management techniques for PT has been recently reported in the AAPM Task Group Report 290 (Li *et al* 2022).

From a geometrical point of view, target motion results in blurring of the dose gradients. In addition to these geometrical effects, specifically for PT, the motion of organs in the target area and within the beam's path can change the radiological path length (i.e., the cumulated density of tissues traversed by the particle beam) and thus the distribution of the deposited dose (figure 2.2).

Radiological path length variations are caused by two concurrent phenomena: the motion of different structures in (or out of) the beam line (e.g., the interposition of a rib in the beam path during respiration) and the density variations of the traversed tissue (e.g., the lung density varying as a function of the respiratory phase).

An effective method to quantify these uncertainties is to compute the water equivalent path length (WEL) from a given beam direction (Mori and Chen 2008). The WEL calculation can be performed on a computed tomography (CT) volume by converting the Hounsfield Unit (HU) values into water-relative density and then integrating the density contribution of each voxel along a given beam line up to a specific plane (e.g., the distal edge of the target volume). This integral is known as water equivalent thickness (WET).

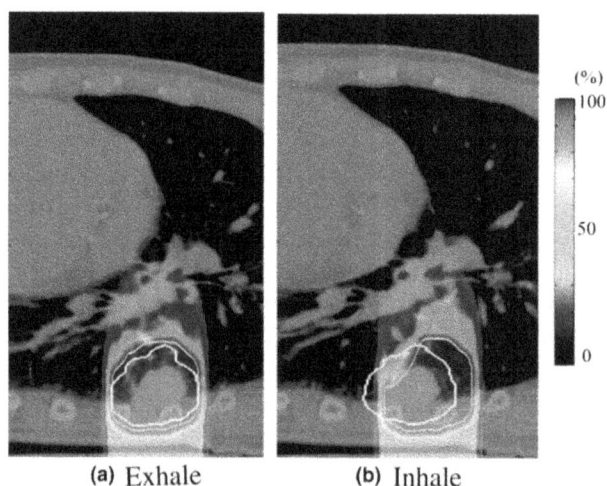

(a) Exhale   (b) Inhale

Figure 2.2. Carbon-ion beam dose distribution planned at the exhale phase. (a) The treatment beam was correctly delivered to the target at exhale. (b) Error due to intra-fraction motion (inhale) caused the position of the beam to shift relative to the actual target position. Reprinted from Mori *et al* (2013), Copyright (2013), with permission from Springer.

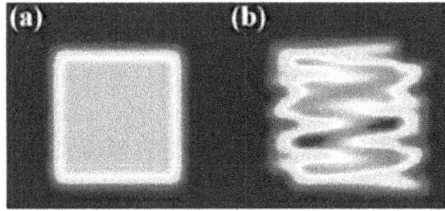

Figure 2.3. (a) Dose distribution delivered with a scanned beam to a static target. (b) Dose distribution delivered to a moving target: the interplay effect is clearly visible. Image from a simulation study by Furukawa *et al* (2010) John Wiley & Sons. © 2010 American Association of Physicists in Medicine.

For beam scanning, there are two additional interference sources: one is due to inter-field motion in intensity-modulated particle therapy (IMPT; Lomax 2008, Kooy and Grassberger 2015), which describes the motion of the patient, or an internal organ, between the delivery of the different fields of a fraction, but not necessarily within the delivery time of an individual field; the other is due to interference between scanning motion and intra-fractional (or intra-field) motion, which is often called interplay (Furukawa *et al* 2010, Bert and Durante 2011, Grassberger *et al* 2013, Mori *et al* 2018; see figure 2.3) and typically results in underdosage and over-dosage within the target volume.

Special protocols for motion monitoring and motion mitigation during treatment planning and delivery are therefore necessary to guarantee target dose coverage and compliance of dose constraints for close-by OARs. Among the different strategies to account and compensate for organ motion, imaging plays a crucial role, as it allows describing the internal anatomo-pathological configuration of the patient before, during and after treatment for plan optimization, treatment adaptation and verification. In this context, the concept of Image Guided Radiotherapy (IGRT) has emerged in both photon and particle therapy (Jaffray 2012, Mori *et al* 2013). It refers to the steps of patient setup, treatment planning and treatment delivery that incorporate imaging solutions which interface with the radiation delivery system and grant the improvement of treatment accuracy.

In the following sections, the current inter- and intra-fraction motion compensation techniques during planning, delivery and verification will be reported with a specific focus on those demanding for imaging.

2.2 Treatment simulation and plan optimization

The main purpose of treatment planning is to build a patient-specific model based on images of the patient where tumour and OARs are delineated, and to define the optimal treatment plan to be delivered to the patient. Computed tomography (CT) is the current standard to obtain the density information required for dose planning (chapter 4), and it is typically registered with other image modalities (e.g., magnetic resonance imaging (MRI)) for better tumour visualization and delineation. Traditionally, uncertainties in radiotherapy have been handled by adding margins to the tumour delineated on the CT (gross tumour volume, GTV, i.e., the macroscopic tumour with a radiological visible and measurable tumour; Hodapp 2012). The clinical target volume (CTV) is added to the GTV to cover neighboring sites that are at risk of harboring microscopic disease spread, which is then expanded to a larger planning target volume (PTV), which is irradiated with the prescribed dose (Newhauser 2009, Thomas 2006) and includes uncertainties that may occur due to set-up errors and tumour changes. Immobilization masks are also typically used during the whole treatment course (from simulation to treatment) to limit patient's motion. However, additional strategies have to be followed to make the plan robust against inter- and intra-fraction variations.

2.2.1 Organ motion management during image acquisition

Concerning intra-fraction variabilities, motion is primarily accounted for during image acquisition. Different motion compensation strategies specific for CT imaging have been developed to compensate for intra-fraction motion (e.g. breath hold and gating), with respiratory-correlated four dimensional CT (4DCT) (Keall *et al* 2006) being the current clinical standard for moving organs such as pancreas, liver and lung.

Among the different strategies to compensate for respiratory motion, slow 3D CT is performed with a reduced speed of gantry rotation and table motion, allowing for a CT acquisition in the duration of a breathing cycle (Shang *et al* 2014). This results in a blurred object as a rough estimation of the motion extent. Alternatively, in deep inhalation/exhalation breath-hold CT, 3D CT images are acquired at the extreme lung volume moments, requiring patient compliance (Baues *et al* 2018). In free-breathing protocols, instead, CT acquisition is correlated with continuous monitoring of the respiratory motion through external respiratory-related surrogates, such as respiratory belts (e.g., Anzai Medical Co. Ltd, Japan), optical systems (e.g. Real-time Position Management, RPM, Varian) or electromagnetic systems (Fattori *et al* 2017). The external surrogate is used either to trigger the scanning at the end-exhale phase in case of gating, or to continuously acquire CT slices that are then retrospectively sorted into 3D volumes at specific respiratory phases, thus depicting an average respiratory cycle of the patient (i.e. 4DCT; Keall *et al* 2006; figure 2.4).

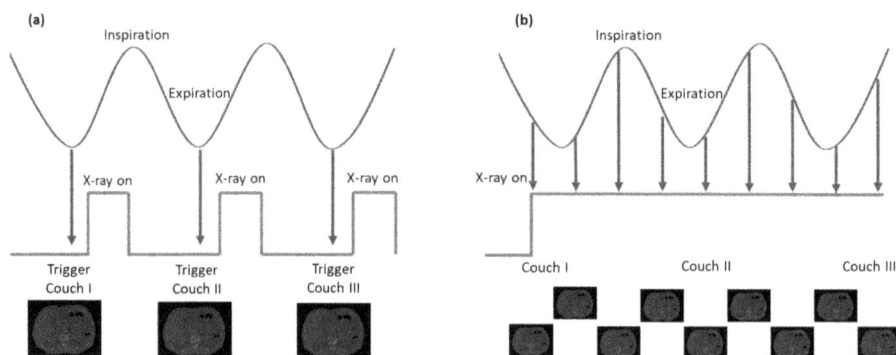

Figure 2.4. (a) Gated image acquisition; (b) respiratory-correlated 4DCT.

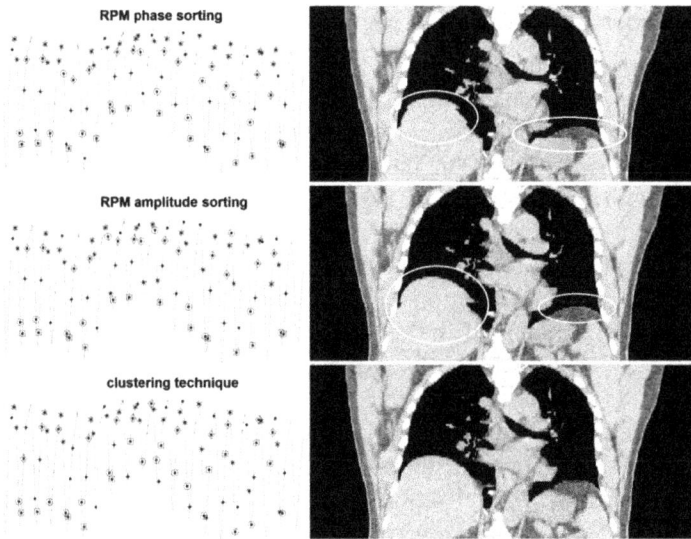

Figure 2.5. Qualitative comparison between the RPM phase sorting (upper panel), RPM amplitude sorting (central panel), and a multiple point clustering technique (lower panel). Artifacts in the reconstructed 4DCT are highlighted with a circle. With permission from Gianoli *et al* (2011) John Wiley & Sons. © 2011 American Association of Physicists in Medicine.

Retrospective sorting in respiratory-correlated 4DCT can be performed relying on the phase or the amplitude of the external respiratory surrogate.

Although 4DCT is considered the standard for moving organs (Mori *et al* 2018), it presents some limitations. Firstly, it relies on the assumption of a good correlation between the mono-dimensional external surrogate and the internal motion, which is not always guaranteed especially in the case of irregularly breathing patients (Gierga *et al* 2005). This assumption, when not satisfied, leads to artifacts in the reconstructed 4D volumes thus preventing an optimal motion description. It has been also demonstrated that the one-dimensional surrogate has limitations in describing the internal motion, with multiple markers used for 4DCT reconstruction improving motion description and reducing sorting artifacts (Gianoli *et al* 2011; figure 2.5). Finally, as 4DCT is an average description of the patient's respiratory cycle, it is not representative of each breathing cycle (intra-fraction variability) at each therapy fraction (inter-fraction variability; Riboldi *et al* 2012). When dealing with inter-fraction variabilities, instead, multiple re-evaluation CTs can be acquired before treatment delivery to check for compliance of dose constraints or, in case relevant anatomo-pathological variations are present, to create a new plan of the day (Chang *et al* 2017, Li *et al* 2022). Re-evaluation CTs can be supported (or substituted) by in-room volumetric imaging, typically based on cone beam CT (CBCT) acquisitions (Landry and Hua 2018; see chapter 5).

2.2.2 Organ motion management during plan optimization

When intra-fraction motion occurs, CTV variations in position, shape and size throughout all motion phases of the 4DCT can be considered during plan optimization using different concepts. The internal target volume (ITV; Knopf *et al* 2013) encompasses all motion and shape changes over the respiratory cycle and it can consider both geometric changes (gITV) and associated density variations (i.e. field-specific range adaptive ITV, rITV; Krieger *et al* 2020). Alternatively, one can also plan on an averaged 4DCT, by averaging the CT images of different respiratory phases; whereas the Mid Ventilation concept can be used to plan the treatment on a single frame of the 4DCT in which the tumour is closest to its time-average position (Wolthaus *et al* 2006). To allow disposing of a more robust 3DCT for planning (starting from a 4DCT) less susceptible to respiratory artifacts, the Mid Position approach has been also proposed, making use of deformable image registration (DIR) among 4DCT phases and then averaging the deformed frames to obtain a high-quality CT scan with fewer motion artifacts (Wolthaus *et al* 2006).

However, the geometrical margin approach, which assumes that dose is invariant for set-up uncertainties, has limitations, especially in scanned PT. Therefore, robust optimization methods have been developed to incorporate uncertainties directly into the treatment planning. Robust optimization refers to the optimization of the dose distribution where different uncertainty scenarios, due to anatomy variations, are considered via multiple image sets (e.g., different phases of the 4DCT; Unkelbach *et al* 2018, Knopf *et al* 2022) instead of optimizing the dose on just one 3D volume. A recent review published by Knopf *et al* (Knopf *et al* 2022) reports on the use of robust 4D multi-image-based optimization, highlighting the potential effectiveness of using multiple image sets to improve target coverage and dose homogeneity (figure 2.6), along with healthy tissues sparing. Up to now, the only image modality adopted in these studies and supported for particle dose calculation is CT, and the computational cost depends on the number of images considered in the optimization. Ideally, motion information derived from other image modalities could be incorporated in the optimization process, such as virtual 4DCTs derived from 4DCBCT or 4DMRI (Bernatowicz *et al* 2016, den Otter *et al* 2020, Meschini *et al* 2020, Meschini *et al* 2022b, Annunziata *et al* 2023).

Similarly, re-evaluation CTs accounting for inter-fraction motion can be incorporated as multiple image sets in the robust optimization process (Fracchiolla *et al* 2021, Molinelli *et al* 2022). In a study on head and neck patients treated with IMPT plans by Cubillos-Mesías and colleagues (Cubillos-Mesías *et al* 2019), planning CT and weekly control CTs were included in the optimization and compared with a classical robust plan using solely the planning CT, demonstrating that in 25% of the investigated cases, classical robust optimization was not sufficient to account for anatomical changes during the treatment. To avoid the acquisition of multiple repeated CTs, synthetic CT derived from other image modalities relying on deep learning strategies can be exploited to reduce the imaging dose to the patients (Spadea *et al* 2019, Thummerer *et al* 2020,). Details on generation of synthetic CT are reported in chapter 8.

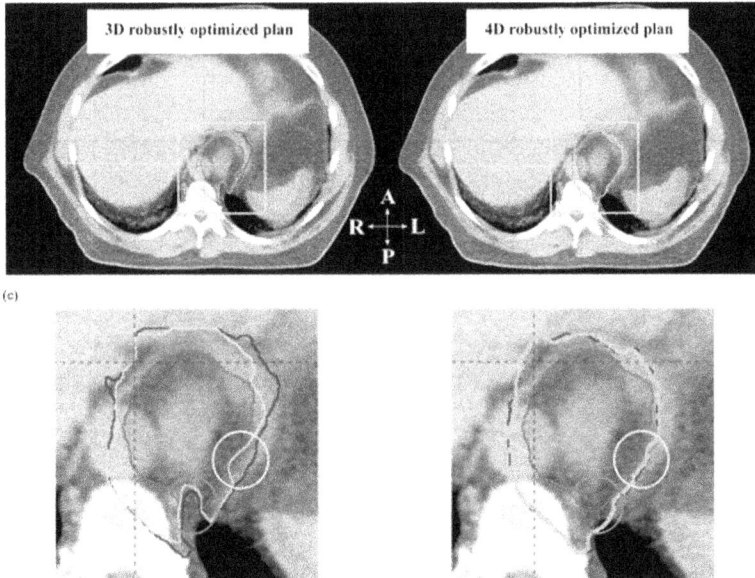

Figure 2.6. Dose distributions of a patient with esophageal carcinoma on a typical transverse plane from 3D robustly optimized plan and 4D robustly optimized plan (first row, left and right, respectively). Red contour is CTV, the iso-dose line of prescribed 5000cGy from 4D accumulated dose distribution is in blue, and the iso-dose line of prescribed 5000cGy from 4D dynamic dose distribution is in cyan. Zoom from the yellow boxes (second row). With permission from Feng *et al* (2021b) John Wiley & Sons. © 2021 American Association of Physicists in Medicine.

2.3 Treatment delivery

When delivering the dose to the patient, motion mitigation strategies should reflect the ones adopted for planning and account for inter- and intra-fraction variations.

2.3.1 Intra-fraction motion management during treatment delivery

As for CT acquisition, in the management of intra-fraction motion, a straightforward approach toward the reduction of tumour motion are Deep Inspiration Breath Hold-based (DIBH) treatments which implement the breath-hold technique (Boda-Heggemann *et al* 2016). The need for patient's compliance can be a drawback in the DIBH approach and the motion problem is frequently solved with gating and rescanning.

Beam gating provides irradiation of an intra-fractionally moving target only inside a specific time-respiratory window, which is defined during treatment planning. When the tumour is outside this window, beam delivery is interrupted. The same motion monitoring device used during image acquisition is used during delivery to gate the treatment by determining when the target is inside the gating window. Typically, the window comprises 30% of the respiratory cycle and is centered on the peak-exhale motion phase, which is the most stable and repeatable among different respiratory acts (Mori *et al* 2018). Gating allows one to partially compensate for dose degradation and prevents excessive dose to OARs by minimizing target motion and consequently the irradiated volume. On the other hand, however, it requires the minimization of latency time (i.e., delays in the turn on/off of the beam when opening/closing the gating window), determines treatment prolongation that can be uncomfortable for the patient and relies on the questionable assumption of a good correlation of the external surrogate with the internal motion.

Gating is also typically combined with rescanning, whose basic idea is to irradiate the target multiple times with a proportionally reduced dose (Mori *et al* 2018, Gut *et al* 2021). In this way, assuming that there is no phase correlation between the tumour motion period and the rescanning period and that a sufficient number of rescanning is applied, the interference effects are statistically averaged out and a uniform dose distribution is obtained, thus reducing the interplay effect.

Among all possible motion mitigation approaches, beam tracking has been considered as the optimal technique, since it should not lead to excessive treatment prolongation or target volume expansions (Grözinger *et al* 2006, Keall *et al* 2006, Riboldi *et al* 2012). In conventional radiotherapy, tumour tracking is already a clinical reality, with different commercial solutions available. Direct tumour tracking can be performed with 2D fluoroscopic acquisitions, which however increase the non-therapeutic dose to the patients and typically require implanted markers to identify the tumour position (Shirato *et al* 2004). Alternatively, local internal/external correlation models are used in commercial systems (e.g. CyberKnife and Vero), relying on inferring the position of the internal anatomy on the basis of the external surrogate (Kamino *et al* 2006, Kilby *et al* 2010). Also, the recent integration of MRI with accelerating units (i.e. MRI-linacs) (Paganelli *et al* 2018b, Keall *et al* 2022) are put towards the implementation of tumour tracking while directly imaging the patient with 2D dynamic images, but no clinical trials with tracking protocols have been implemented yet with these machines.

Despite the steps forward in implementing tumour tracking in x-ray radiotherapy and some attempts of fluoroscopic-based tumour tracking systems in PT (Mori *et al* 2019, Yoshimura *et al* 2020; REF), several limitations are still present in PT, as particle beams require not only lateral beam adjustments, but also energy adaptation for compensation of range changes resulting from motion induced density variations. Thus, tracking can only be effective if real-time 3D information on the tumour location is known at all times (Riboldi *et al* 2012, Zhang *et al* 2014, Mori *et al* 2018). However, current imaging capabilities still do not provide real-time 4D information and, so far, clinical implementation of tracking would rely on a combination of pre-acquired data and online surrogate information to estimate time-resolved 3D volumes (Zhang *et al* 2013, Zhang *et al* 2014, Fassi *et al* 2015, Meschini *et al* 2017; figure 2.7). These models are just at the research level and still present limitations in their validation and real-time implementation (chapter 9). In the future, a combined MR-proton machine (chapter 7) could potentially provide time-resolved 3D information (Hoffmann *et al* 2017).

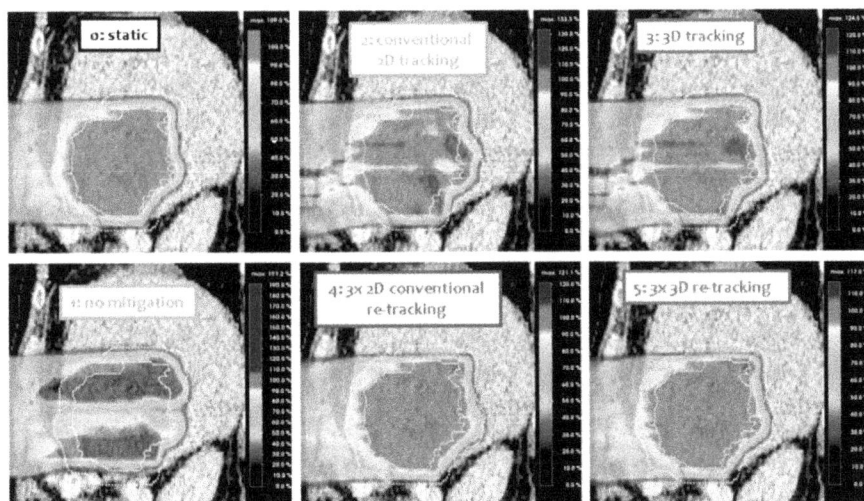

Figure 2.7. Comparison of dose distributions on an abdominal tumour with large motion (20 mm) with different motion mitigation strategies. 0: static plan; (1) No mitigation; (2) Conventional 2D tracking as those adopted in conventional radiotherapy (simple translational tracking of the projected center of mass of the tumour as a function of motion); (3) 3D tracking with the whole 3D information for tracking the tumour in all directions, including compensation for range changes due to the motion; 4/5: re-tracking, combination of tracking and rescanning. Reproduced from a simulation study by Zhang *et al* (2014). © 2014 Institute of Physics and Engineering in Medicine. All rights reserved.

2.3.2 Inter-fraction motion management during treatment delivery

It is well recognized that for most indications planning on a patient image acquired some time before the start of the therapy and using the same plan for the whole treatment is suboptimal, mainly because of inter-fraction variabilities (Müller *et al* 2015, Szeto *et al* 2016, Hoffmann *et al* 2017, Molinelli *et al* 2022). Therefore, it is recommended to regularly monitor the anatomy of the patient during the course of the treatment to trigger adaptation if necessary (Chang *et al* 2017, Li *et al* 2022). This can be achieved by acquiring imaging data just before treatment delivery with near-room and in-room systems (chapter 5), which allows for off-line and on-line adaptation, respectively (figure 2.8). Generally, the main idea of treatment adaptation consists in registering, either by a rigid or deformable registration (DIR) process, planning CT on the anatomy of the day (thus obtaining the so-called virtual CT) and verify if the plan satisfies the current patient's situation or not, and eventually adjust the plan. The impact of adaptive radiotherapy (ART) depends on the frequency of imaging (e.g. daily versus weekly), on the treatment schedule, because anatomical changes might be more pronounced during early fractions, and on the quality of the imaging, as in-room (online) imaging would potentially compromise it presenting, in some cases, lower image contrast. Among the imaging modalities near-room CT, in-room CT, cone beam CT (CBCT; Landry and Hua 2018) and potentially MR imaging (Keall *et al* 2022) can be exploited. Comprehensive reviews on adaptive proton therapy (APT) have been recently published in the literature by Albertini *et al* (2020) and Paganetti *et al* (2021).

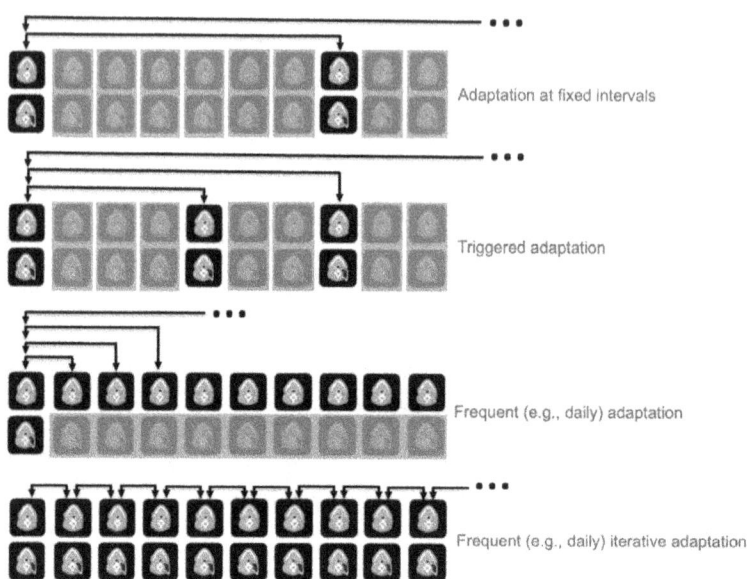

Figure 2.8. Adaptation workflow. (A) Adaptation at constant intervals using the initial plan assessed on the new image; (B) Adaptation triggered by on-line imaging based on the initial plan; (C) Daily adaptation using the initial plan assessed; (D) Frequent (e.g. daily) adaptation using the accumulated dose and previous day image and adapted plan as reference. Reproduced from Paganetti *et al* (2021). © 2021 Institute of Physics and Engineering in Medicine. All rights reserved.

Up to now, due to the complexity of the labor and time-intensive workflow, and the lack of automatization, for PT it is not yet possible to adapt the dose online. The APT process is therefore currently performed offline. Typically, it takes a few days from the acquisition of a new 3D image to the delivery of the clinically approved adapted plan. Such an adaptive approach, although improving the delivered dose especially in case of slow inter-fractional changes, such as weight gain or loss, is inadequate in the presence of faster changes (e.g. organs fillings). Indeed, to fully profit from the APT approach, the whole process needs to be established within the time span of the anatomy changes.

Therefore, an online daily plan adaptation is necessary to deal with daily inter-fractional changes, as for example variation of the nasal cavity- or rectal fillings. To implement adaptation, different aspects should be considered, ranging from the processing of the images acquired, the dose recalculation and the adaptation workflow. As regards imaging, the registration algorithm and the contour propagation strategy between the planning CT and the daily image need to be accurate and properly validated (Brock *et al* 2017, Paganelli *et al* 2018a). Similarly, dose calculation engines and adaptation workflows must be accurate and fast enough to implement online daily adaptation (Veiga *et al* 2016, Jagt *et al* 2018).

2.4 Dose reconstruction and accumulation for treatment verification

To verify treatment delivery, *in vivo* imaging modalities are available and will be discussed in detail in chapter 10. Alternative strategies for a retrospective dose evaluation, considering a specific motion and/or dose delivery scenario, consists in dose reconstruction and accumulation starting from imaging data and beam information collected during treatment (Meijers *et al* 2019, Albertini *et al* 2020, Meijers *et al* 2020, Paganetti *et al* 2021).

Specifically, to accurately record the treatment dose over the course of any fractionated radiotherapy, it is necessary to accumulate the daily delivered dose on a common anatomy. This is achieved by performing image registration (rigid or DIR) of the daily images to the reference anatomy (planning CT); the daily dose is then deformed by applying the same displacement vector field (DVF) generated during the image registration and then an average sum over all the delivered dose is performed (figure 2.9; chapter 3). It is worth mentioning that the accuracy of this procedure strongly depends on the accuracy of the registration and the dose warping (Brock *et al* 2017, Paganelli *et al* 2018a) and debates on the appropriateness of deforming dose along with deformable image registration are still ongoing (Chetty and Rosu-Bubulac 2019, Zhong and Chetty 2016). Nonetheless, Jaffray *et al* (2010) demonstrated that the use of deformable dose accumulation can support outcome analysis based on correlation of the treatment dose with tumour control, local recurrences and toxicities. Dose accumulation can also be supported by the availability of the so-called log-files, which are recorded during treatment and collect the beam parameters, like Bragg peak position and number of monitor units, to reconstruct the delivered dose in the patient (Meier *et al* 2015).

Dose reconstruction and accumulation are also adopted in organs that move as a function of respiration. In these cases, dose contributions to different motion states, represented by 4DCT phases, can be calculated and accumulated to obtain an estimate of the delivered dose to a moving anatomy, relying on log files and breathing pattern records depicted in the 4DCT (Richter *et al* 2014, Meijers *et al* 2019, Meijers *et al* 2020).

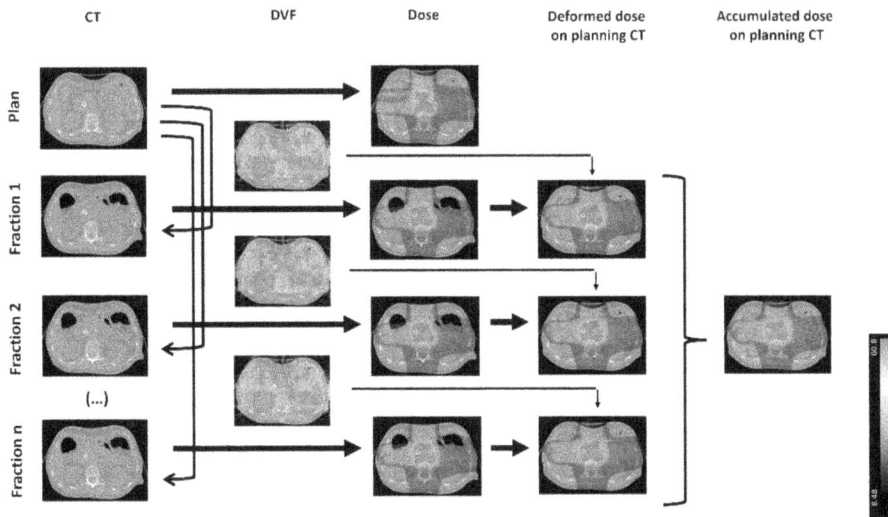

Figure 2.9. An example of the dose accumulation workflow, using the planning CT as reference image. Deformable vector fields for different fractions are displayed on the reference CT. DVF = displacement vector field.

As previously mentioned, however, the 4DCT is representative of just one breathing cycle of the patients; thus, in the future, online range estimates from prompt gamma emission, positron emission tomography or via proton radiography could be included into the reconstruction algorithm and/or online image data could be incorporated into 4D motion models to simulate time-resolved 3D CTs (Zhang *et al* 2013, Fassi *et al* 2015, Meschini *et al* 2019, 2022a, Knopf *et al* 2022).

2.5 Conclusions and future perspectives

Organ motion hinders treatment accuracy in PT, where the geometrical selectivity of particle beams cannot be effectively exploited in case of tumour position and radiological path length uncertainties. Image guidance is crucial to plan, adapt and verify the quality of the treatment, with CT and 4DCT being the current clinical standard for treatment planning in static and moving organs, respectively. However, CT and 4DCT present several limitations mainly related to the intrinsic nature in delivering additional non-therapeutical dose to the patients, the limited soft tissue contrast and the representation of a specific instant of the patient anatomo-pathological condition with a poor description of inter- and intra-fraction varia-tions. Different solutions have been put in place to deal with these aspects during image acquisition and plan optimization, along with treatment delivery, as described in this chapter.

Current in-room x-ray imaging systems, such as CT on rails or CBCT (Landry and Hua 2018), which allow describing the current patient situation directly in the treatment room, can further support the information provided by planning CT during treatment (robust) optimization and adaptation, but they present limitations of the same order (or even higher) of those of conventional CT. Indeed, 3D image information is required for treatment validation and adaptation, but 3D iso-centric imaging possibilities at particle facilities are still rare and need further development (Mori *et al* 2018).

The lack of 3D information is even more evident during treatment delivery, where imaging systems are not currently able to provide time-resolved 3D data required to account for geometry changes and density changes in the beam direction and perform tumour tracking. In this context, motion modelling approaches could play a role in the estimation of the missing 3D information by coupling the planning 4DCT with motion surrogates collected during treatment delivery (Zhang *et al* 2014, Fassi *et al* 2015, Meschini *et al* 2019), but they are still far from being adopted in the clinical routine. On the other side, with the development of combined MRI-linac machines for conventional radiotherapy (Keall *et al* 2022), it is believed that online MRI-guided radiotherapy can provide a feedback loop to enable gating and beam tracking in clinical routine. Since in a combined MRI-linac system time-resolved information of the patient geometry is provided online, these hybrid machines are especially suited to perform motion tracking. The combination of PT delivery and simultaneous MR imaging is under investigation (Hoffmann *et al* 2017), although the real clinical benefit of online MR data for particle radiotherapy remains to be shown.

References

Albertini F, Matter M, Nenoff L, Zhang Y and Lomax A 2020 Online daily adaptive proton therapy *Br. J. Radiol.* **93** 20190594

Annunziata S, Rabe M, Vai A, Molinelli S, Nakas A, Meschini G, Pella A, Vitolo V, Barcellini A and Imparato S 2023 Virtual 4DCT generated from 4DMRI in gated particle therapy: phantom validation and application to lung cancer patients *Phys. Med. Biol.* **68** 145004

Aznar M, Ntentas G, Enmark M, Flampouri S, Meidhal Petersen P, Ricardi U and Levis M 2021 The role of motion management and position verification in lymphoma radiotherapy *Br. J. Radiol.* **94** 20210618

Baues C, Marnitz S, Engert A, Baus W, Jablonska K, Fogliata A, Vásquez-Torres A, Scorsetti M and Cozzi L 2018 Proton versus photon deep inspiration breath hold technique in patients with hodgkin lymphoma and mediastinal radiation *Radiat. Oncol.* **13** 1–11

Bernatowicz K, Peroni M, Perrin R, Weber D C and Lomax A 2016 Four-dimensional dose reconstruction for scanned proton therapy using liver 4DCT-MRI *Int. J. Radiat. Oncol. Biol. Phys.* **95** 216–23

Bert C and Durante M 2011 Motion in radiotherapy: particle therapy *Phys. Med. Biol.* **56** R113

Boda-Heggemann J, Knopf A-C, Simeonova-Chergou A, Wertz H, Stieler F, Jahnke A, Jahnke L, Fleckenstein J, Vogel L and Arns A 2016 Deep inspiration breath hold—based radiation therapy: a clinical review *Int. J. Radiat. Oncol. Biol. Phys.* **94** 478–92

Brock K K, Mutic S, McNutt T R, Li H and Kessler M L 2017 Use of image registration and fusion algorithms and techniques in radiotherapy: report of the AAPM Radiation Therapy Committee Task Group No. 132 *Med. Phys.* **44** e43–76

Chang J Y, Zhang X, Knopf A, Li H, Mori S, Dong L, Lu H-M, Liu W, Badiyan S N and Both S 2017 Consensus guidelines for implementing pencil-beam scanning proton therapy for thoracic malignancies on behalf of the PTCOG thoracic and lymphoma subcommittee *Int. J. Radiat. Oncol. Biol. Phys.* **99** 41–50

Chetty I J and Rosu-Bubulac M 2019 Deformable registration for dose accumulation *Semin. Radiat. Oncol.* **29** 198–208

Cubillos-Mesías M, Troost E G, Lohaus F, Agolli L, Rehm M, Richter C and Stützer K 2019 Including anatomical variations in robust optimization for head and neck proton therapy can reduce the need of adaptation *Radiother. Oncol.* **131** 127–34

den Otter L A, Chen K, Janssens G, Meijers A, Both S, Langendijk J A, Rosen L R, Wu H T and Knopf A C 2020 4D cone-beam CT reconstruction from sparse-view CBCT data for daily motion assessment in pencil beam scanned proton therapy (PBS-PT) *Med. Phys.* **47** 6381–7

Fassi A, Seregni M, Riboldi M, Cerveri P, Sarrut D, Ivaldi G B, De Fatis P T, Liotta M and Baroni G 2015 Surrogate-driven deformable motion model for organ motion tracking in particle radiation therapy *Phys. Med. Biol.* **60** 1565

Fattori G, Safai S, Carmona P F, Peroni M, Perrin R, Weber D C and Lomax A J 2017 Monitoring of breathing motion in image-guided PBS proton therapy: comparative analysis of optical and electromagnetic technologies *Radiat. Oncol.* **12** 1–11

Feng A, Gu H, Chen H, Shao Y, Wang H, Duan Y, Huang Y, Zhou T and Xu Z 2021a Account for the full extent of esophagus motion in radiation therapy planning: a preliminary study of the IRV of the esophagus *Front. Oncol.* **11** 734552

Feng H, Shan J, Ashman J B, Rule W G, Bhangoo R S, Yu N Y, Chiang J, Fatyga M, Wong W W and Schild S E 2021b 4D robust optimization in small spot intensity-modulated proton therapy (IMPT) for distal esophageal carcinoma *Med. Phys.* **48** 4636–47

Fracchiolla F, Dionisi F, Righetto R, Widesott L, Giacomelli I, Cartechini G, Farace P, Bertolini M, Amichetti M and Schwarz M 2021 Clinical implementation of pencil beam scanning proton therapy for liver cancer with forced deep expiration breath hold *Radiother. Oncol.* **154** 137–44

Furukawa T, Inaniwa T, Sato S, Shirai T, Mori S, Takeshita E, Mizushima K, Himukai T and Noda K 2010 Moving target irradiation with fast rescanning and gating in particle therapy *Med. Phys.* **37** 4874–9

Gianoli C, Riboldi M, Spadea M F, Travaini L L, Ferrari M, Mei R, Orecchia R and Baroni G 2011 A multiple points method for 4D CT image sorting *Med. Phys.* **38** 656–67

Gierga D P, Brewer J, Sharp G C, Betke M, Willett C G and Chen G T 2005 The correlation between internal and external markers for abdominal tumours: implications for respiratory gating *Int. J. Radiat. Oncol. Biol. Phys.* **61** 1551–8

Gort E M, Beukema J C, Matysiak W, Sijtsema N M, Aluwini S, Langendijk J A, Both S and Brouwer C L 2021 Inter-fraction motion robustness and organ sparing potential of proton therapy for cervical cancer *Radiother. Oncol.* **154** 194–200

Grassberger C, Dowdell S, Lomax A, Sharp G, Shackleford J, Choi N, Willers H and Paganetti H 2013 Motion interplay as a function of patient parameters and spot size in spot scanning proton therapy for lung cancer *Int. J. Radiat. Oncol. Biol. Phys.* **86** 380–6

Grözinger S O, Rietzel E, Li Q, Bert C, Haberer T and Kraft G 2006 Simulations to design an online motion compensation system for scanned particle beams *Phys. Med. Biol.* **51** 3517

Gut P, Krieger M, Lomax T, Weber D C and Hrbacek J 2021 Combining rescanning and gating for a time-efficient treatment of mobile tumours using pencil beam scanning proton therapy *Radiother. Oncol.* **160** 82–9

Hodapp N 2012 The ICRU report 83: prescribing, recording and reporting photon-beam intensity-modulated radiation therapy (IMRT) *Strahlenther. Onkol.* **188** 97–9

Hoffmann L, Alber M, Jensen M F, Holt M I and Møller D S 2017 Adaptation is mandatory for intensity modulated proton therapy of advanced lung cancer to ensure target coverage *Radiother. Oncol.* **122** 400–5

Jaffray D A 2012 Image-guided radiotherapy: from current concept to future perspectives *Nat. Rev. Clin. Oncol.* **9** 688–99

Jaffray D A, Lindsay P E, Brock K K, Deasy J O and Tomé W A 2010 Accurate accumulation of dose for improved understanding of radiation effects in normal tissue *Int. J. Radiat. Oncol. Biol. Phys.* **76** S135–9

Jagt T, Breedveld S, Van Haveren R, Heijmen B and Hoogeman M 2018 An automated planning strategy for near real-time adaptive proton therapy in prostate cancer *Phys. Med. Biol.* **63** 135017

Kamino Y, Takayama K, Kokubo M, Narita Y, Hirai E, Kawawda N, Mizowaki T, Nagata Y, Nishidai T and Hiraoka M 2006 Development of a four-dimensional image-guided radiotherapy system with a gimbaled x-ray head *Int. J. Radiat. Oncol. Biol. Phys.* **66** 271–8

Keall P J, Brighi C, Glide-Hurst C, Liney G, Liu P Z, Lydiard S, Paganelli C, Pham T, Shan S and Tree A C 2022 Integrated MRI-guided radiotherapy—opportunities and challenges *Nat. Rev. Clin. Oncol.* **19** 458–70

Keall P J, Mageras G S, Balter J M, Emery R S, Forster K M, Jiang S B, Kapatoes J M, Low D A, Murphy M J and Murray B R 2006 The management of respiratory motion in radiation oncology report of AAPM task group 76 a *Med. Phys.* **33** 3874–900

Kilby W, Dooley J, Kuduvalli G, Sayeh S and Maurer C 2010 The CyberKnife® robotic radiosurgery system in 2010 *Technol. Cancer Res. Treat.* **9** 433–52

Kirilova A, Lockwood G, Choi P, Bana N, Haider M A, Brock K K, Eccles C and Dawson L A 2008 Three-dimensional motion of liver tumours using cine-magnetic resonance imaging *Int. J. Radiat. Oncol. Biol. Phys.* **71** 1189–95

Knopf A-C, Boye D, Lomax A and Mori S 2013 Adequate margin definition for scanned particle therapy in the incidence of intrafractional motion *Phys. Med. Biol.* **58** 6079

Knopf A-C, Czerska K, Fracchiolla F, Graeff C, Molinelli S, Rinaldi I, Rucincki A, Sterpin E, Stützer K and Trnkova P 2022 Clinical necessity of multi-image based (4DMIB) optimization for targets affected by respiratory motion and treated with scanned particle therapy—a comprehensive review *Radiother. Oncol.* **169** 77–85

Knybel L, Cvek J, Otahal B, Jonszta T, Molenda L, Czerny D, Skacelikova E, Rybar M, Dvorak P and Feltl D 2014 The analysis of respiration-induced pancreatic tumour motion based on reference measurement *Radiat. Oncol.* **9** 192

Kooy H and Grassberger C 2015 Intensity modulated proton therapy *Br. J. Radiol.* **88** 20150195

Krieger M, Giger A, Salomir R, Bieri O, Celicanin Z, Cattin P C, Lomax A J, Weber D C and Zhang Y 2020 Impact of internal target volume definition for pencil beam scanned proton treatment planning in the presence of respiratory motion variability for lung cancer: a proof of concept *Radiother. Oncol.* **145** 154–61

Landry G and Hua C h 2018 Current state and future applications of radiological image guidance for particle therapy *Med. Phys.* **45** e1086–95

Li H, Dong L, Bert C, Chang J, Flampouri S, Jee K W, Lin L, Moyers M, Mori S and Rottmann J 2022 AAPM task group report 290: respiratory motion management for particle therapy *Med. Phys.* **49** e50–81

Lomax A 2008 Intensity modulated proton therapy and its sensitivity to treatment uncertainties 1: the potential effects of calculational uncertainties *Phys. Med. Biol.* **53** 1027

Meier G, Besson R, Nanz A, Safai S and Lomax A J 2015 Independent dose calculations for commissioning, quality assurance and dose reconstruction of PBS proton therapy *Phys. Med. Biol.* **60** 2819

Meijers A, Jakobi A, Stützer K, Guterres Marmitt G, Both S, Langendijk J, Richter C and Knopf A 2019 Log file-based dose reconstruction and accumulation for 4D adaptive pencil beam scanned proton therapy in a clinical treatment planning system: implementation and proof-of-concept *Med. Phys.* **46** 1140–9

Meijers A, Knopf A-C, Crijns A P, Ubbels J F, Niezink A G, Langendijk J A, Wijsman R and Both S 2020 Evaluation of interplay and organ motion effects by means of 4D dose reconstruction and accumulation *Radiother. Oncol.* **150** 268–74

Meschini G, Seregni M, Molinelli S, Vai A, Phillips J, Sharp G C, Pella A, Valvo F, Ciocca M and Riboldi M 2019 Validation of a model for physical dose variations in irregularly moving targets treated with carbon ion beams *Med. Phys.* **46** 3663–73

Meschini G, Seregni M, Pella A, Ciocca M, Fossati P, Valvo F, Riboldi M and Baroni G 2017 Evaluation of residual abdominal tumour motion in carbon ion gated treatments through respiratory motion modelling *Phys. Med.* **34** 28–37

Meschini G, Vai A, Barcellini A, Fontana G, Molinelli S, Mastella E, Pella A, Vitolo V, Imparato S and Orlandi E 2022a Time-resolved MRI for off-line treatment robustness evaluation in carbon-ion radiotherapy of pancreatic cancer *Med. Phys.* **49** 2386–95

Meschini G, Vai A, Paganelli C, Molinelli S, Fontana G, Pella A, Preda L, Vitolo V, Valvo F and Ciocca M 2020 Virtual 4DCT from 4DMRI for the management of respiratory motion in carbon ion therapy of abdominal tumours *Med. Phys.* **47** 909–16

Meschini G, Vai A, Paganelli C, Molinelli S, Maestri D, Fontana G, Pella A, Vitolo V, Valvo F and Ciocca M 2022b Investigating the use of virtual 4DCT from 4DMRI in gated carbon ion radiation therapy of abdominal tumours *Z. Med. Phys.* **32** 98–108

Molinelli S, Vai A, Russo S, Loap P, Meschini G, Paganelli C, Barcellini A, Vitolo V, Orlandi E and Ciocca M 2022 The role of multiple anatomical scenarios in plan optimization for carbon ion radiotherapy of pancreatic cancer *Radiother. Oncol.* **176** 1–8

Mori S and Chen G T 2008 Quantification and visualization of charged particle range variations *Int. J. Radiat. Oncol. Biol. Phys.* **72** 268–77

Mori S, Knopf A C and Umegaki K 2018 Motion management in particle therapy *Med. Phys.* **45** e994–e1010

Mori S, Sakata Y, Hirai R, Furuichi W, Shimabukuro K, Kohno R, Koom W S, Kasai S, Okaya K and Iseki Y 2019 Commissioning of a fluoroscopic-based real-time markerless tumour tracking system in a superconducting rotating gantry for carbon-ion pencil beam scanning treatment *Med. Phys.* **46** 1561–74

Mori S, Zenklusen S and Knopf A-C 2013 Current status and future prospects of multi-dimensional image-guided particle therapy *Radiol. Phys. Technol.* **6** 249–72

Müller B S, Duma M N, Kampfer S, Nill S, Oelfke U, Geinitz H and Wilkens J J 2015 Impact of interfractional changes in head and neck cancer patients on the delivered dose in intensity modulated radiotherapy with protons and photons *Phys. Med.* **31** 266–72

Newhauser W 2009 *International Commission on Radiation Units and Measurements Report 78: Prescribing, Recording and Reporting Proton-Beam Therapy* (Oxford: Oxford University Press)

Paganelli C, Meschini G, Molinelli S, Riboldi M and Baroni G 2018a Patient-specific validation of deformable image registration in radiation therapy: overview and caveats *Med. Phys.* **45** e908–22

Paganelli C, Whelan B, Peroni M, Summers P, Fast M, Van de Lindt T, McClelland J, Eiben B, Keall P and Lomax T 2018b MRI-guidance for motion management in external beam radiotherapy: current status and future challenges *Phys. Med. Biol.* **63** 22TR03

Paganetti H, Botas P, Sharp G C and Winey B 2021 Adaptive proton therapy *Phys. Med. Biol.* **66** 22TR01

Pakela J M, Knopf A, Dong L, Rucinski A and Zou W 2022 Management of motion and anatomical variations in charged particle therapy: past, present, and into the future *Front. Oncol.* **12** 806153

Park E-T and Park S K 2016 Setup uncertainties for inter-fractional head and neck cancer in radiotherapy *Oncotarget* **7** 46662

Riboldi M, Orecchia R and Baroni G 2012 Real-time tumour tracking in particle therapy: technological developments and future perspectives *Lancet Oncol.* **13** e383–91

Richter D, Saito N, Chaudhri N, Härtig M, Ellerbrock M, Jäkel O, Combs S E, Habermehl D, Herfarth K and Durante M 2014 Four-dimensional patient dose reconstruction for scanned ion beam therapy of moving liver tumours *Int. J. Radiat. Oncol. Biol. Phys.* **89** 175–81

Seppenwoolde *et al* 2002 Precise and real-time measurement of 3D tumour motion in lung due to breathing and heartbeat, measured during radiotherapy *Int. J. Radiat. Oncol. Biol. Phys.* **53** 822–34

Shang D-p, Liu C-x and Yin Y 2014 A comparison of the different 3D CT scanning modes on the GTV delineation for the solitary pulmonary lesion *Radiat. Oncol.* **9** 1–6

Shirato H, Oita M, Fujita K, Watanabe Y and Miyasaka K 2004 Feasibility of synchronization of real-time tumour-tracking radiotherapy and intensity-modulated radiotherapy from viewpoint of excessive dose from fluoroscopy *Int. J. Radiat. Oncol. Biol. Phys.* **60** 335–41

Sonke J J, Lebesque J and van Herk M 2008 Variability of four-dimensional computed tomography patient models *Int. J. Radiat. Oncol., Biol. Phys.* **70** 590–8

Spadea M F, Pileggi G, Zaffino P, Salome P, Catana C, Izquierdo-Garcia D, Amato F and Seco J 2019 Deep convolution neural network (DCNN) multiplane approach to synthetic CT generation from MR images—application in brain proton therapy *Int. J. Radiat. Oncol. Biol. Phys.* **105** 495–503

Su Z, Slopsema R, Flampouri S and Li Z 2019 Impact of intrafraction prostate motion on clinical target coverage in proton therapy: a simulation study of dosimetric differences in two delivery techniques *J. Appl. Clin. Med. Phys.* **20** 67–73

Szeto Y Z, Witte M G, van Kranen S R, Sonke J-J, Belderbos J and van Herk M 2016 Effects of anatomical changes on pencil beam scanning proton plans in locally advanced NSCLC patients *Radiother. Oncol.* **120** 286–92

Thomas S J 2006 Margins for treatment planning of proton therapy *Phys. Med. Biol.* **51** 1491

Thummerer A, Zaffino P, Meijers A, Marmitt G G, Seco J, Steenbakkers R J, Langendijk J A, Both S, Spadea M F and Knopf A C 2020 Comparison of CBCT based synthetic CT methods suitable for proton dose calculations in adaptive proton therapy *Phys. Med. Biol.* **65** 095002

Unkelbach J, Alber M, Bangert M, Bokrantz R, Chan T C, Deasy J O, Fredriksson A, Gorissen B L, Van Herk M and Liu W 2018 Robust radiotherapy planning *Phys. Med. Biol.* **63** 22TR02

Veiga C, Janssens G, Teng C-L, Baudier T, Hotoiu L, McClelland J R, Royle G, Lin L, Yin L and Metz J 2016 First clinical investigation of cone beam computed tomography and deformable registration for adaptive proton therapy for lung cancer *Int. J. Radiat. Oncol. Biol. Phys.* **95** 549–59

Wolthaus J W, Schneider C, Sonke J-J, van Herk M, Belderbos J S, Rossi M M, Lebesque J V and Damen E M 2006 Mid-ventilation CT scan construction from four-dimensional respiration-correlated CT scans for radiotherapy planning of lung cancer patients *Int. J. Radiat. Oncol. Biol. Phys.* **65** 1560–71

Yoshimura T, Shimizu S, Hashimoto T, Nishioka K, Katoh N, Inoue T, Taguchi H, Yasuda K, Matsuura T and Takao S 2020 Analysis of treatment process time for real-time-image gated-spot-scanning proton-beam therapy (RGPT) system *J. Appl. Clin. Med. Phys.* **21** 38–49

Zhang Y, Knopf A, Tanner C, Boye D and Lomax A J 2013 Deformable motion reconstruction for scanned proton beam therapy using on-line x-ray imaging *Phys. Med. Biol.* **58** 8621

Zhang Y, Knopf A, Tanner C and Lomax A J 2014 Online image guided tumour tracking with scanned proton beams: a comprehensive simulation study *Phys. Med. Biol.* **59** 7793

Zhong H and Chetty I J 2016 Caution must be exercised when performing deformable dose accumulation for tumours undergoing mass changes during fractionated radiation therapy *Int. J. Radiat. Oncol., Biol., Phys.* **97** 182–3

Chapter 3

Image registration in particle therapy

Y Zhang, F Amstutz, A Smolders and C Paganelli

3.1 Rationale of image registration in radiotherapy

Medical imaging techniques have played an essential role in modern radiation therapy (RT) development to achieve personalised treatments. Image guidance is more critical for particle therapy (PT) than for conventional radiotherapy because the superior dose conformation of particle beams by the sharp dose gradients is intrinsically associated with higher dosimetric sensitivity. Therefore, the acquisition of relevant medical images is suggested at different RT/PT treatment stages to quantify the patient-specific information and to ensure the planned delivery quality (Jaffray 2012, Bolsi *et al* 2018, MacKay 2018). For instance, computer tomography (CT), magnetic resonance imaging (MRI) and occasionally positron emission tomography (PET) are routinely acquired during the planning phase. In addition, dynamic imaging, such as respiratory-correlated 4DCT or 4DMRI, is mandatory for motion assessment when treating moving tumours. Moreover, daily imaging assists and verifies patient positioning of each fractional delivery using either in-room imaging systems (e.g. cone-beam CT) and more frequently acquired images are emerging to evaluate geometric changes towards the implementation of daily or real-time adaptive PT (Albertini *et al* 2020). Obviously, RT/PT is associated with the above multi-dimensional knowledge, in the format of different images, by different modalities and at different times. Therefore, establishing the necessary correlation between these pieces of information is a natural prerequisite for information integration and comparison. Image registration is the elementary technique to achieve this goal (Maintz and Viergever 1998, Viergever *et al* 2016, Rigaud *et al* 2019). Furthermore, as most of the patient anatomy changes in the long process of fractional treatment exhibit non-rigid characteristics, deformable image registration (DIR) is employed to improve the accuracy of the geometrical correlation.

In this chapter, the basic knowledge of image registration is first introduced. Then, clinical applications of image registration along the whole RT/PT workflow are elucidated in terms of treatment (re-)planning, intra-fractional image guidance and inter-fraction plan assessment. In the end, we exhaustively discussed the associated challenges of DIR regarding its validation in RT/PT applications and its inherent uncertainty, particularly for dose accumulation.

3.2 Basic framework of image registration

Image registration is an optimisation process to determine a spatial transformation that correlates the geometry of one image to the corresponding features in the other images. It is a thoroughly studied research question in biomedical image analysis. Here, we only cover the basic knowledge, which is compulsory to understand the remaining chapter and interpret the literature on image registration for RT. For more comprehensive overviews of the technique itself, the reader is kindly referred to the reviews (Hill *et al* 2001, Rueckert and Schnabel 2011) for general medical image registration (Sotiras *et al* 2013) for DIR and (Oh and Kim 2017, Rigaud *et al* 2019) for image registration in radiotherapy.

Registration algorithms primarily consist of four basic components: a transformation model, a similarity metric, an interpolation and an optimisation method that updates the transformation parameters to maximise the correspondence between the *fixed* and the transformed *moving image*, i.e. the *moved image* (figure 3.1).

3.2.1 Transformation model

The transformation model determines the space of transformations the registration algorithm can find. In order of complexity, the most commonly used transformations are rigid, affine and deformable. The selected transformation model should reflect the expected transformation between the image data. Increasing the model complexity requires more parameters to be optimised, making convergence more difficult and results less consistent. Therefore, if the transformation can be described with a simpler model, i.e. lower number of parameters, this is advised.

A rigid transformation consists of six parameters in three dimensions (3D): three rotations and three translations. It is commonly used because it is well defined, robust and fast. Especially for RT treatments in the skull region, the rigid

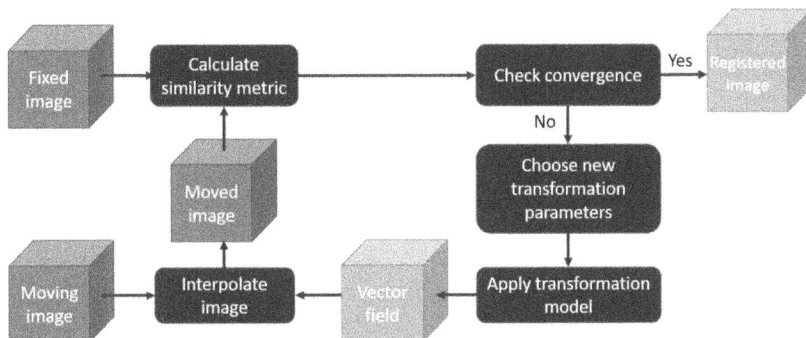

Figure 3.1. Basic workflow of image registration.

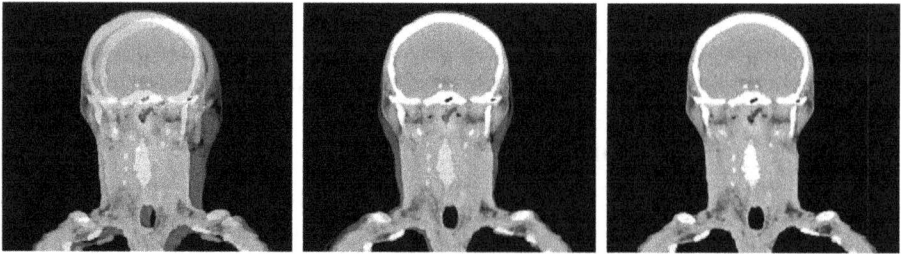

Figure 3.2. Visualisation of different transformation models in the head and neck region. Left: fixed (green) and moving (purple) images. Middle: fixed and **rigidly** moved image. Right: fixed and **deformably** moved image.

assumption is frequently valid (figure 3.2). Further, it is used for patient setup correction in clinical practice in RT and PT. It is also often used before applying more complex transformation models as initial alignment. Another global transformation is the affine transformation. It extends the rigid registration, also allowing for scaling and shearing, by introducing six additional degrees of freedom. Affine registration is not commonly used alone but more frequently as an initial alignment step like rigid registration (Oliveira and Tavares 2014).

In rigid registration, the patient is assumed to be a rigid object, but this is generally not the reality, especially when anatomical sites are affected by inter- and intra-fractional variations. Therefore, the most common registration type is DIR (figure 3.2). To capture the possible deformations in space, such transformation models consist of many more parameters, making convergence difficult and optimisation execution longer. Generally, two non-rigid transformation models are formulated: parametric and non-parametric. Non-parametric models describe the deformation at every voxel by directly calculating a dense 3D deformable vector field (DVF), resulting in a vast number of parameters ($\sim$80 million for an image with $512\times512\times100$ voxels). Several methods formulate the registration as a motion problem and solve it as a fluid or elastic deformation (Horn and Schunck 1981, Bajcsy and Kovačič 1989, Beg *et al* 2005). It can also be considered as a diffusion process, better known as the demons algorithm (Thirion 1998). In contrast, the parametric deformation models use a parameterised deformation space. Thus, the algorithms predict the values for these parameters instead of directly calculating the deformation for each voxel. A typical parameterisation uses a limited set of basis functions, such as Fourier series, splines or thin plate splines (radial basis functions). The advantage of the parametric model is the fewer degrees of freedom (i.e. the weights of the basis functions), but it is also associated with lower flexibility. A trendy model is a free-form deformation with B-splines (Rueckert *et al* 1999). The deformation is estimated at a limited number of control points, and the deformation between the control points is calculated with B-splines. The advantage of this approach is the local support, i.e. the deformation of a control point only affects a local region around itself instead of the whole grid, making it a computationally efficient algorithm (Shackleford *et al* 2010). However, since the B-spline-based DVF is assumed to be continuous, it is difficult to estimate the correct displacement when anatomical regions slide against each other (Delmon *et al* 2013).

3.2.2 Similarity metric

The parameters of the transformation model need to be optimised with respect to an objective function, which represents the similarity between the fixed and the moving image.

For the feature-based registration, the calculated features, such as points, lines and surfaces, are extracted from both images. The distance between those features is minimised to find the optimal transformation (Guan *et al* 2018). However, feature extraction can be difficult, time-consuming and prone to manual identification error, which propagates into the registration result (Rueckert and Schnabel 2011).

Alternatively, intensity-based registration is more frequently used thanks to its robustness (Rueckert and Schnabel 2011). For monomodal image registration (i.e. images acquired with the same scanner type), the sum of squared differences (SSD, assuming voxel-wise intensity equivalence) and cross-correlation (assuming a linear relationship between the intensities in the images) are primarily used. Contrarily, for multi-modality registration (e.g. CT to MRI), a voxel-wise difference or correlation of intensity values describing different properties is not feasible. Therefore, other metrics are required, such as mutual information (MI), which maximises the statistical relationship between the intensities in the two images in the optimisation process (Maes *et al* 1997, Viola and Wells III 1997).

3.2.3 Optimization method

The transformation is calculated by optimising its parameters for maximising/ minimizing the similarity metric using an optimisation algorithm, e.g., methods based on gradient descent. However, such optimisation schemes suffer from local minima, i.e., the optimiser gets stuck at a set of suboptimal parameters because the gradient of the loss function becomes close to zero (figure 3.3). This is especially critical for deformable registration. Effective approaches to improve convergence to a more accurate deformation are initial rigid alignment (see section 2.1), regularisation terms and multi-resolution approaches.

Regularisation terms are incorporated into the similarity metric in the objective function and impose a set of desired properties on the transformation (Terzopoulos 1986). For example, these terms often penalise large gradients or second-order derivatives of the vector field for ensuring deformation smoothness (Lötjönen and Mäkelä 2001, Shen and Davatzikos 2002). Another standard metric is the Jacobian determinant $|J|$ of the vector field, which measures local compression ($0 < |J| < 1$) or expansion ($|J| > 1$), which can be enforced to be close to 1 in case of incompressibility, or larger than 0 to avoid folding voxels (Christensen *et al* 1997, Rohlfing *et al* 2003).

In a multi-resolution or pyramid framework, the deformation is performed in multiple steps from coarse to fine registrations (Studholme *et al* 1996, Rueckert *et al* 1999). In the first steps, only very smooth deformations are allowed, which leads to

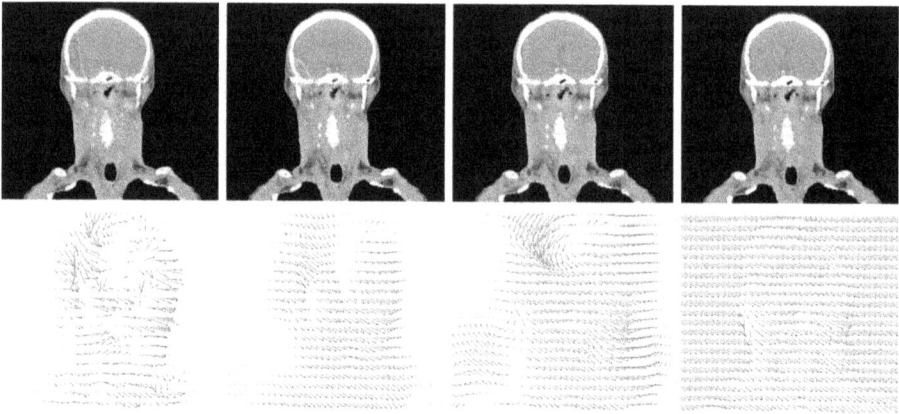

Figure 3.3. Effect of using different methods to improve convergence. The top row shows the overlay of the fixed (green) and moved (purple) images. The bottom row shows the resulting deformable vector field (DVF) of various transformation models. Without convergence improvement method (a). The DVF is not smooth and has more than 12% folding voxels. Regularisation improves smoothness (1% folding voxels), but the images do not match well yet (b). Multi-resolution also improves smoothness (2% folding voxels) and yields a better match (c). Initial rigid alignment leads to the smoothest transformation (<1% folding voxels) and a good image match (d).

an approximate matching of more relevant anatomical regions, after which the deformations are refined in subsequent steps.

3.2.4 Interpolation

After each optimisation step, the current transformation is applied to the *moving* image and the transformed image, i.e. the *moved* image, is subsequently compared to the fixed image for the next iteration of the optimisation. The transformation is applied by evaluating it for each voxel coordinate x of the fixed image, yielding corresponding coordinates $x' = T(x)$ in the moving image. Since the moving image is discretised and x' is continuous, the image intensity at x' has to be interpolated from the surrounding voxels. The linear or nearest neighbour interpolation is usually applied during the optimization iteration, thanks to its speed, while more expensive interpolation schemes can be used to improve the accuracy in the final image warping step (Hill *et al* 2001).

3.3 Image registration for treatment (re-)planning

The typical applications for registration in the planning phase are multimodal image fusion and atlas-based contouring (Rigaud *et al* 2019). In the emerging adaptive workflow, DIR is applied to evaluate the clinical necessity for re-planning, contour propagation, fractional plan calculation and re-optimization. Moreover, when treating moving tumours in the thoracic or upper abdomen regions, DIR is compulsory to extract and quantify the deformable motion between the phases of the 4D image.

3.3.1 Multi-modal image fusion

For most tumour indications, structure delineation has to be performed based on the multi-modality images at the pre-treatment phase. Due to the inferior soft-tissue contrast, tumours and OARs of certain types are not distinguishable on CT alone. Therefore, additional MRIs under various sequences and occasionally PET are complementarily obtained and fused to the planning CT to assist contouring (Fox *et al* 2005, Zhong *et al* 2015). To achieve this, the anatomic site and the time between successively acquired images are considered when defining the appropriate transformation models. If the time gap between images is short, rigid registration is probably sufficient to describe the transformation (Brock *et al* 2017). For the skull region, rigid registration is suitable as the deformations are often small, even if the time between the two scans is several days or weeks (Hill *et al* 2001). However, DIR is necessary for other anatomical sites (e.g. lung, liver and pancreas), which may introduce additional uncertainties.

3.3.2 Atlas-based contouring

Manual contouring is a labour-intensive process often sped up by an automatic contouring method. The most common automatic approaches are atlas-based and deep learning (DL)-based contouring (Vrtovec *et al* 2020). Although recent literature mostly favours DL because of its speed and accuracy (Lustberg *et al* 2018, Zabel *et al* 2021), atlas-based contouring is still the classical approach frequently used in clinical practice. This technique relies on a set of template images with annotated contours. When contouring a new image, the most representative atlas from the templates is chosen. DIR is used to map the template to it to account for differences between the template and the instant patient anatomy. Applying the same transformation on the template contours allows transferring the contours to the new anatomy (Han *et al* 2008, Bach Cuadra *et al* 2015). A standard extension is to use multiple atlases and majority voting, which further results in uncertainty estimates for the obtained contours (Warfield *et al* 2004).

3.3.3 Contour propagation for re-planning

Rapid plan adaptation is required when relevant anatomical changes occur during the fractionated treatment. Daily images, such as repeated CT or potential MRI, are acquired in such scenarios; thus, the associated contours on the new images must be re-defined. Although the general procedure of planning CT contouring can be repeatedly applied, it is more convenient and efficient to propagate the planning contours instead, since the planning CT is highly similar to the daily image (Kumarasiri *et al* 2014). This procedure can be considered a particular scenario of atlas-based contouring where the template is the planning CT instead of a generic one.

3.3.4 4D treatment planning

When treating tumours in the presence of respiration motion, 4D images (e.g. 4DCT or 4DMRI) are typically acquired to measure the respiratory-affected anatomic changes (Knopf *et al* 2022, Li *et al* 2022). As shown in figure 3.4, DIR is

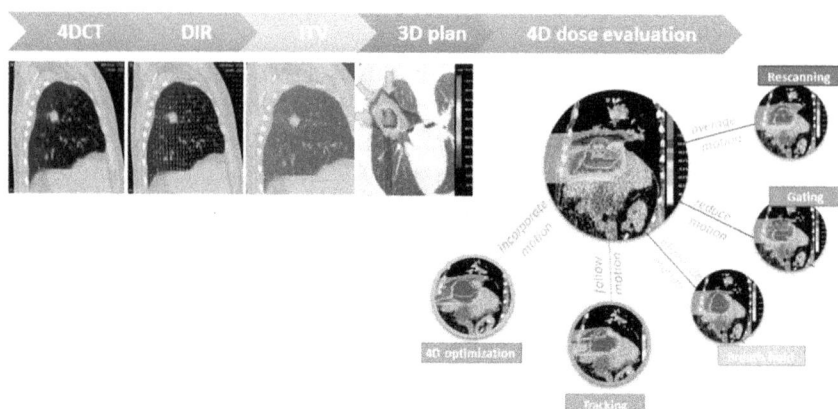

Figure 3.4. 4D dose calculations for motion effects evaluation and motion mitigation optimization based on 4D image and the derived deformable vector fields.

subsequently used to estimate the DVF between two image phases, giving the point-to-point geometric correlations, referred to as motion (Zhang *et al* 2012). Such dense 3D information not only provides an evaluation of the foreseen intra-fractional motion magnitude of the patient but also acts as an important input for various procedures in the 4D treatment workflow.

One classical example is to derive the planning margin based on the extracted DVFs. Geometric internal target volume (gITV) is defined by encapsulating target volumes at each of all motion phases. To avoid tedious manual work, those volumes are normally obtained by propagating the reference contours at the planning CT to all other image phases (Krieger *et al* 2020). For PT, besides considering the lateral blurring effect, further integrating the motion-induced density variation is essential. The field-specific range adaptive internal target volume (rITV) is derived by combining both geometric deformations with the associated density variation of the corresponding dose calculation grids given by the DVFs (Knopf *et al* 2013). Alternatively, a more robust 4D plan can be achieved if motion impact has been considered statistically, such as planning on the Mid Position CT instead of any of the 4D image phases (Wolthaus *et al* 2008). The Mid Position CT is a synthetic image generated by warping the reference CT using the averaged DVFs.

In addition to the applications in 4D plan generation, DIR is also an important component in the 4D dose calculation (4DDC; Dolde *et al* 2018, Meijers *et al* 2019, Smolders *et al* 2023), to evaluate the motion-induced dosimetric deterioration. Although motion effects have been partially considered in the treatment planning phase by defining a proper margin and effective density model, the optimized plan is still based on a static scenario. Particularly to the dynamic dose delivery using pencil beam scanned (PBS) technique, 4DDC is indispensable to assess the interplay effects (Grassberger *et al* 2014) and more importantly to determine the optimal motion mitigation strategy (Zhang *et al* 2016, 2018) for individual patients. 4DDC can be considered as a special dose recalculation process. By carefully considering the plan delivery timeline, the dosimetric contribution of the individual particle beams is calculated at different 4D image phases. The total 4D dose distribution is successively derived by warping the phase-specific dose distributions to the selected reference phases based on the pre-calculated DVFs of the 4D image.

3.4 Intra-fractional image registration

For a fractionated RT/PT treatment, it is vital to keep the geometric consistency of patient anatomy at each fraction to the initially optimized therapeutic radiation beam. To implement an accurate and reproducible patient setup for individual dose delivery days, online image guidance is undoubtedly the most indispensable and effective tool. Depending on the tumour type and affected anatomic site, the patient anatomy of each fraction is varied at different levels of magnitude, which consequently requires different image registration frameworks for corresponding purposes.

3.4.1 Patient positioning

The most straightforward and frequently used image registration application for online image guidance is for patient setup. This procedure is conducted after the pre-alignment of the patient with or without fixation devices (e.g. bite block, masks, moulage, etc). Depending on the capability for couch correction mechanically, the computation is based on either a rigid (6 degrees of freedom (DOF)) or only a translational (3 DOF) registration framework. The subsequently derived outputs are the executable parameter settings for couch position correction. Depending on the clinical protocol, one additional image is acquired after correcting the misalignment as verification (Landry and Hua 2018).

Subject to the integrated in-room imaging system, the input for the registration framework can be either a single/orthogonal 2D x-ray image(s) or a 3D image of the patient at the therapeutic position. Accordingly, the in-room imaging system can either be a gantry-mounted x-ray system (e.g., cone-beam CT (CBCT)) or a CT-on-rail system (Bolsi *et al* 2018; see chapter 5). Both can provide the projected 2D image (in cone-beam or fan-beam geometry) or a reconstructed volumetric image (CT or CBCT). Obviously, volumetric images have advantages by providing more comprehensive spatial information, promoting the 3D–3D image registration framework for a more accurate correction vector. Nevertheless, a single or pair of projection images is conventionally preferred due to consideration of extra imaging dose concerns for daily CT. When only a projection image is available as online information, the additional component for computing the digitally reconstructed radiography (DRR) is demanded in the 2D–3D registration framework. Hence, the DRRs were simulated using the geometric calibrated imaging system for different patient positioning scenarios (Palaniappan *et al* 2022). Nevertheless, given the trends of the daily adaptive regime, more and more PT clinics also start to implement volumetric images for daily patient positioning, by CBCT or by low-dose in-room CT, with the ultimate goal of daily plan evaluation or optimization either online or offline (Landry and Hua 2018).

3.4.2 Online plan adaptation

Besides using daily acquired images for verifying patient positioning, the updated anatomic information enables more advanced functions, such as offline or online plan adaptation (Albertini *et al* 2020). As triggers, the magnitude of patient changes can be quantified by directly registering daily and planning images. Additionally, with the derived deformation vector field, the dosimetric impact and the necessity for re-planning can be assessed by warping the recalculated plans on the new CTs to the planning CT. When daily imaging differs from the high-quality planning CT image, virtual CT can be generated by warping the planning CT to the daily image (e.g. in-room CBCT, offline MRI or eventually in-beam MRI). DIR is critical for such applications by enabling the dosimetric evaluation based on multi-modality daily imaging, real-time motion monitoring and plan adaptation.

To certain extents, the basic methods for achieving real-time motion tracking or plan adaptation have no fundamental difference than for online patient position or plan adaptation (Zhang *et al* 2013). The most important feature for real-time applications is clearly the computational time. The classic 2D–3D registration framework was shown to be able to achieve satisfying results within seconds when GPU programming techniques were used for implementation with several algorithmic refinements (Gendrin *et al* 2012). Nevertheless, the main challenge for online image guidance is to obtain the real-time image with entire dosimetric affected regions. As real-time volumetric imaging with a sufficiently large volume of interests is still technical demanding, only the motion of certain surrogates can be measured and monitored in real-time, such as surface motion, 2D images from in-room x-ray or 2D cine MRI (for MRI-linac only) (chapter 7). To tackle this problem, deformable motion models (McClelland *et al* 2013, Zhang *et al* 2013) have been demonstrated as an effective approach for bridging the gap, allowing prediction for dense motion field in 3D from sparse surrogate motion, which can be tracked during treatment. The dense motion fields extracted by DIR are the direct input for generating such motion models, which will be described in detail in chapter 9.

3.5 Inter-fractional and post-treatment image registration

Finally, next to the usage of image registration for treatment (re-)planning (section 3.3) and within a treatment fraction (section 3.4), image registration is also used for inter-fractional and post-treatment evaluations, mainly for summing, respectively assessing, the delivered dose of multiple fractions or the complete treatment. Knowledge of the delivered dose distribution in 3D is important for triggering plan adaptation, planning of re-irradiation, or follow-up evaluations (Veiga *et al* 2015, Landry *et al* 2015, Xu *et al* 2021, Palaniappan *et al* 2022), as described in more detail below. Of note, these image registration applications are not specific to PT but essential for the whole radiotherapy world. The principles are easily transferable between the different radiotherapy treatment modalities (Rigaud *et al* 2019).

3.5.1 Dose accumulation

Dose accumulation is the sum of delivered doses on different geometries to a common reference geometry. This common reference geometry is often the pre-treatment planning CT. However, other options for reference, such as the latest acquired CT, are considered sometimes (Heukelom and Fuller 2019). Furthermore, due to the time frame of days or weeks, one has to expect anatomo-pathological changes when accumulating the dose on a common geometry. Therefore, DIR is generally used for dose accumulation, often referred to as deformable dose accumulation. To accumulate the dose, the DVFs giving the correspondence between the fixed and the moving image in the radiotherapy context, planning CT and fraction CT are used to propagate the dose to the common reference geometry. After propagation to the same geometry, it is possible to sum up the doses (Chetty and Rosu-Bubulac 2019). The left panel in figure 3.5(A) illustrates the process of deformable dose accumulation. In the following, three typical applications of deformable dose accumulation are described.

3.5.2 Dose monitoring

During the treatment, summing the dose of the individual fractions can help to detect potential problems in reaching the initially set objectives in treatment planning. If the patient presents substantial anatomical changes, the delivered

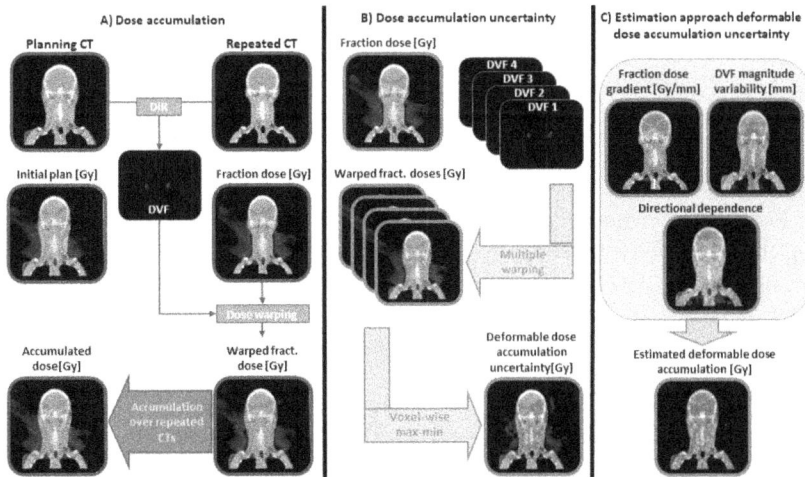

Figure 3.5. (A) For dose accumulation, the correspondence between the planning CT and the fraction CT is determined by DIR. The fraction dose is then warped with the resulting DVF to the planning CT. Repeating this step for each available fraction CT gives the possibility to accumulate the total dose. (B) One option to evaluate the range of possible deformable dose accumulation uncertainties is to apply for each fraction CT multiple different DIR algorithms and warp the fraction dose with each resulting DVF. The deformable dose accumulation uncertainty is determined by taking the voxel-wise range of the dose values (Nenoff *et al* 2020). (C) Another approach for estimating these uncertainties is by combining the fraction dose gradient with the DVF magnitude variability and their directional dependence. The DVF magnitude variability could be modelled in the first fraction, and multiple DIR applications for each fraction would not be necessary anymore (Amstutz *et al* 2021).

plan on the new anatomy can differ from the initial treatment plan. By accumulating the fraction doses on the planning CT, it is possible to monitor the delivered dose against the planned one (Rigaud *et al* 2019). If there is a discrepancy between the delivered and plan dose, this could trigger plan adaptation. In a fully adaptive treatment regime, one could even accumulate the dose after each treated fraction to adapt the treatment according to the treatment goals. This could lead to an even better total dose than initially possible on the planning CT.

3.5.3 Re-irradiation

Luckily, the time of survival for treated cancer patients is increasing. On the other side, this increases the probability that some patients will experience a cancer recurrence and require additional treatment. This may include re-irradiation of tissue that already received radiation in the primary treatment. To perform a safe re-irradiation, it is crucial to know the dose received by each OAR in the initial treatment. For this, one needs to accumulate the dose of the initial treatment. This task can be especially challenging due to the long period in which the anatomy can change drastically, e.g., due to weight gain/loss or surgical interventions. Finding the correspondence between the images is then tricky for DIRs (Dörr and Gabryś 2018, Seidensaal *et al* 2020, Munoz *et al* 2021, Hunter *et al* 2021).

3.5.4 Follow-up evaluation

One application for dose accumulation further down the road could also be to improve follow-up evaluations and outcome modelling. At the moment, outcome modelling is not based on accumulated doses, but strategies of dose spatial normalization based on DIR (such as voxel-based analysis) have been demonstrated useful to identify regions with significant correlations between a clinical outcome and the local dose release (Palma *et al* 2020) (chapter 12). Thus, it is supposed that knowing the total delivered dose to specific OARs through dose accumulation can help to improve models for toxicity or recurrences (Jaffray *et al* 2010, McCulloch *et al* 2018, Niebuhr *et al* 2021).

3.6 Challenges and opportunity

3.6.1 Caveats on validation of image registration

To adopt an image registration algorithm in a clinical workflow, proper verification and validation are required. However, while a rigid registration algorithm can be easily checked by quantifying the setup error with independent measures, the main drawback for DIR is the absence of a ground truth with respect to which the performance of the algorithm can be evaluated (i.e. the actual patient's deformation is unknown). This, combined with the variety of proposed DIR algorithms with different performance (Veiga *et al* 2015, Zhang *et al* 2018, Nenoff *et al* 2020), prevents a proper use of DIR in the clinical routine.

Recently, a task group (AAPM TG132) report (Brock *et al* 2017) was published outlining the essential aspects of DIR for image guidance in radiotherapy. In this report, several guidelines including adoption of known DVFs and quantitative geometric metrics to quantify DIR accuracy have been reported. Disposing of well-known deformations from physical or computational phantoms are essential for DIR quality assurance and commissioning of a registration algorithm; whereas quantitative control metrics can be adopted to provide evidence of a stable and well understood system. Among these latter, AAPM TG132 reports metrics based on landmarks or contours, such as target registration error (TRE), mean distance to agreement (MDA), Dice coefficient (DSC), as well as metrics based on the regularity of the DVF (i.e. Jacobian determinant and inverse consistency error). These metrics are strongly suggested to be computed for DIR assessment, but they present some limitations: TRE is time-consuming as landmarks, typically manually clicked, need to be available, DSC is strongly dependent on the volume of the structure and DVF metrics only provide information about tissue expansion and shrinkage without conveying any information on DIR uncertainties.

Therefore, an accurate and efficient patient-specific validation is not yet defined, and appropriate metrics should be identified to achieve the definition of both geometric and dosimetric accuracy, especially when dealing with PT where errors can be introduced notably in regions of steep dose gradients. This aspect is covered in depth in a review by Paganelli *et al* (2018), where the importance of a patient-specific validation of DIR in terms of both geometric and dosimetric paradigm is highlighted.

In this respect, the use of a dense set of anatomical landmarks, along with additional evaluations on contours or deformation field analysis, are likely to drive patient-specific DIR validation in clinical image-guided radiotherapy applications to account for geometric inaccuracies. Automatic and efficient strategies able to provide spatial information of DIR uncertainties and to evaluate monomodal and multimodal image registration, as well as to describe homogenous and un-contrasted regions, are believed to represent the future direction in DIR validation (Paganelli *et al* 2018). Some applications in PT towards this direction have been reported in the literature. In a study by Landry *et al* (2015) on the investigation of CT to CBCT image registration for head and neck proton therapy as a tool for daily dose recalculation, DIR accuracy was evaluated by automatically extracted landmarks (Paganelli *et al* 2013b, 2013a), reporting an error below 1.4 mm (maximum CT voxel resolution of 3 mm).

However, especially in the case of DIR applications for dose mapping and accumulation, the need of accurate patient-specific validation is not only limited to the evaluation of the geometric accuracy. In fact, the need to account for dosimetric inaccuracies due to DIR represents another important area in the field of adaptive treatments. Disposing of a dense set of landmarks on a voxel-by-voxel level to evaluate dose accumulation is not feasible in general. Different approaches are therefore currently being investigated to quantify the effect of DIR error on dose analysis. The adoption of repeatedly acquired respiratory-correlated (4D) MRI was used as ground truth by Ribeiro *et al* (2018) in liver cancer treated with protons, assuming that MRI can provide a more reliable DVF than x-ray imaging thanks to its improved soft-tissue contrast. If this in principle can be considered a potential countermeasure, DIR inaccuracies can be also found in the registration of well-contrasted images such as MRI.

An alternative approach to evaluate uncertainties in deformable dose accumulation in proton treatments was instead proposed by accounting for uncertainties produced by different DIRs algorithms (figure 3.5(B)). For this purpose, multiple DIRs are applied for the same image pairs, consisting of planning and repeated CTs. The fraction doses from the respective repeated CT are afterwards warped with each resulting DVF individually. A map of expected worst-case discrepancies can be determined by assessing the range between the different warped doses on a voxel level. This approach was investigated for non-small cell lung cancer (Nenoff *et al* 2020). By improving this approach, another work showed that it might be possible to estimate this discrepancy between different algorithms without applying multiple DIRs for every fraction and warping multiple times. The idea is to combine the fraction dose gradient (highlighting high-dose gradient regions where dose uncertainties are expected to be prominent) with the expected DVF magnitude variability to get the deformable dose accumulation uncertainty. The DVF magnitude variability can be determined in the first fraction by applying multiple DIRs and building a model for the later fractions (Amstutz *et al* 2021). An example of the combined factors and a resulting estimated deformable dose accumulation uncertainty is visualised in figure 3.5(C).

Considering the lack of a gold standard metric for DIR evaluation, quality assurance checks should be performed as suggested by AAPM TG132 and a multi-parametric analysis is preferable to quantify both geometric and dosimetric errors. In addition, novel research is required for the definition of dedicated and personalized measures capable of relating the geometric and dosimetric inaccuracies, thus bearing useful information for a safe use of DIR by clinical end-users especially when applied in PT.

3.6.2 Advanced registration based on artificial intelligence

In many computer vision tasks, such as classification, semantic segmentation and object detection, deep learning (DL) has achieved state-of-the-art performance. Accordingly, DL-based registration gained significant attention in recent years, primarily because of its large increase in speed (Yang *et al* 2017, Haskins *et al* 2020, Fu *et al* 2020). This is of interest in many applications, among which is adaptive radiotherapy.

However, DL has not yet overcome the performance of traditional, iterative registration algorithms. The main hurdle is the lack of ground truth data for training and evaluation. For any pair of two images, it is nearly impossible to obtain the true underlying transformation, and hence, it is challenging to learn. Therefore, supervised methods are often trained on artificial data (Eppenhof and Pluim 2019), the result of an iterative DIR (Yang *et al* 2017) or weak and sparse annotations, such as organ segmentations or anatomical landmarks (Hu *et al* 2018), each with its own limitations. Also, unsupervised methods have been proposed in which the loss function for training resembles the similarity metric in iterative registration (Beg *et al* 2005, de Vos *et al* 2019, 2017, Fu, *et al.* 2020b).

More recently, the combination of DL and iterative registration has shown excellent potential (Hansen *et al* 2022). The DL model provides an initial alignment, like rigid registration in conventional algorithms. From there, an iterative method is applied to further improve the alignment, which showed considerable improvements over an extensive range of registration tasks.

Finally, DL has also been used to support the registration, without solving the registration itself (Fu *et al* 2020a). Examples are DL-based auto segmentation to guide the registration, DL-based advanced similarity metrics, or even the use of DL to predict the uncertainty in the registration (Smolders *et al* 2023).

References

Albertini F, Matter M, Nenoff L, Zhang Y and Lomax A 2020 Online daily adaptive proton therapy *Br. J. Radiol.* **93** 20190594

Amstutz F, Nenoff L, Albertini F, Ribeiro C O, Knopf A-C, Unkelbach J, Weber D C, Lomax A J and Zhang Y 2021 An approach for estimating dosimetric uncertainties in deformable dose accumulation in pencil beam scanning proton therapy for lung cancer *Phys. Med. Biol.* **66** 105007

Bach Cuadra M, Duay V and Thiran J-P 2015 Atlas-based segmentation *Handbook of Biomedical Imaging: Methodologies and Clinical Research* ed N Paragios, J Duncan and N Ayache (Boston, MA: Springer) pp 221–44

Bajcsy R and Kovačič S 1989 Multiresolution elastic matching *Comput. Vis. Graph. Image Process.* **46** 1–21

Beg M F, Miller M I, Trouvé A and Younes L 2005 Computing large deformation metric mappings via Geodesic flows of diffeomorphisms *Int. J. Comput. Vis.* **61** 139–57

Bolsi A, Peroni M, Amelio D, Dasu A, Stock M, Toma-Dasu I, Nyström P W and Hoffmann A 2018 Practice patterns of image guided particle therapy in Europe: a 2016 survey of the European particle therapy network (EPTN) *Radiother. Oncol.* **128** 4–8

Brock K K, Mutic S, McNutt T R, Li H and Kessler M L 2017 Use of image registration and fusion algorithms and techniques in radiotherapy: report of the AAPM radiation therapy committee task group no. 132: report *Med. Phys.* **44** e43–76

Chetty I J and Rosu-Bubulac M 2019 Deformable registration for dose accumulation *Semin. Radiat. Oncol.* **29** 198–208

Christensen G E, Joshi S C and Miller M I 1997 Volumetric transformation of brain anatomy *IEEE Trans. Med. Imaging* **16** 864–77

Delmon V, Rit S, Pinho R and Sarrut D 2013 Registration of sliding objects using direction dependent B-splines decomposition *Phys. Med. Biol.* **58** 1303–14

Dolde K, Naumann P, Dávid C, Gnirs R, Kachelrieß M, Lomax A J, Saito N, Weber D C, Pfaffenberger A and Zhang Y 2018 4D dose calculation for pencil beam scanning proton therapy of pancreatic cancer using repeated 4DMRI datasets *Phys. Med. Biol.* **63** 165005

Dörr W and Gabryś D 2018 The principles and practice of re-irradiation in clinical oncology: an overview *Clin. Oncol.* **30** 67–72

Eppenhof K A J and Pluim J P W 2019 Pulmonary CT registration through supervised learning with convolutional neural networks *IEEE Trans. Med. Imaging.* **38** 1097–105

Fox J L, Rengan R, O'Meara W, Yorke E, Erdi Y, Nehmeh S, Leibel S A and Rosenzweig K E 2005 Does registration of PET and planning CT images decrease interobserver and intraobserver variation in delineating tumour volumes for non-small-cell lung cancer? *Int. J. Radiat. Oncol. Biol. Phys.* **62** 70–5

Fu Y, Lei Y, Wang T, Curran W J, Liu T and Yang X 2020a Deep learning in medical image registration: a review *Phys. Med. Biol.* **65** 20TR01

Fu Y, Lei Y, Wang T, Higgins K, Bradley J D, Curran W J, Liu T and Yang X 2020b LungRegNet: an unsupervised deformable image registration method for 4D-CT lung *Med. Phys.* **47** 1763–74

Gendrin C, Furtado H, Weber C, Bloch C, Figl M, Pawiro S A, Bergmann H *et al* 2012 Monitoring tumour motion by real time 2D/3D registration during radiotherapy *Radiother. Oncol.* **102** 274–80

Grassberger C, Daartz J, Dowdell S, Ruggieri T, Sharp G and Paganetti H 2014 Quantification of proton dose calculation accuracy in the lung *Int. J. Radiat. Oncol. Biol. Phys.* **89** 424–30

Guan S-Y, Wang T-M, Meng C and Wang J-C 2018 A review of point feature based medical image registration *Chin. J. Mech. Eng.* **31** 76

Han X, Hoogeman M S, Levendag P C, Hibbard L S, Teguh D N, Voet P, Cowen A C and Wolf T K 2008 Atlas-based auto-segmentation of head and neck CT images *Medical Image Computing and Computer-Assisted Intervention—MICCAI 2008* ed D Metaxas, L Axel, G Fichtinger and G Székely (Berlin: Springer) pp 434–41

Hansen L, Hering A, Großbröhmer C and Heinrich M P 2022 Continuous benchmarking in medical image registration-review of the current state of the Learn2Reg challenge, MIDL Short Paper, http://openreview.net/forum?id=6JdGvJhKZgp

Haskins G, Kruger U and Yan P 2020 Deep learning in medical image registration: a survey *Mach. Vis. Appl.* **31** 8

Heukelom J and Fuller C D 2019 Head and neck cancer adaptive radiation therapy (ART): conceptual considerations for the informed clinician *Semin. Radiat. Oncol.* **29** 258–73

Hill D L G, Batchelor P G, Holden M and Hawkes D J 2001 Medical image registration *Phys. Med. Biol.* **46** R1–45

Horn B K P and Schunck B G 1981 Determining optical flow *Artif. Intell.* **17** 185–203

Hu Y, Modat M, Gibson E, Li W, Ghavami N, Bonmati E, Wang G *et al* 2018 Weakly-supervised convolutional neural networks for multimodal image registration *Med. Image Anal.* **49** 1–13

Hunter B, Crockett C, Faivre-Finn C, Hiley C and Salem A 2021 Re-irradiation of recurrent non-small cell lung cancer *Semin. Radiat. Oncol.* **31** 124–32

Jaffray D A 2012 Image-guided radiotherapy: from current concept to future perspectives *Nat. Rev. Clin. Oncol.* **9** 688–99

Jaffray D A, Lindsay P E, Brock K K, Deasy J O and Tomé W A 2010 Accurate accumulation of Dose for improved understanding of radiation effects in normal tissue *Int. J. Radiat. Oncol. Biol. Phys.* **76** 135–39

Knopf A C, Boye D, Lomax A and Mori S 2013 Adequate margin definition for scanned particle therapy in the incidence of intrafractional motion *Phys. Med. Biol.* **58** 6079–94

Knopf A C, Czerska K, Fracchiolla F, Graeff C, Molinelli S, Rinaldi I, Rucincki A *et al* 2022 Clinical necessity of multi-image based (4DMIB) optimization for targets affected by respiratory motion and treated with scanned particle therapy—a comprehensive review *Radiother. Oncol.* **169** 77–85

Krieger M, Giger A, Salomir R, Bieri O, Celicanin Z, Cattin P C, Lomax A J, Weber D C and Zhang Y 2020 Impact of internal target volume definition for pencil beam scanned proton treatment planning in the presence of respiratory motion variability for Lung cancer: a proof of concept *Radiother. Oncol.* **145** 154–61

Kumarasiri A, Siddiqui F, Liu C, Yechieli R, Shah M, Pradhan D, Zhong H, Chetty I J and Kim J 2014 Deformable image registration based automatic CT-to-CT contour propagation for head and neck adaptive radiotherapy in the routine clinical setting *Med. Phys.* **41** 121712

Landry G and Hua C ho 2018 Current state and future applications of radiological image guidance for particle therapy *Med. Phys.* **45** e1086–95

Landry G, Nijhuis R, Dedes G, Handrack J, Thieke C, Janssens G, Orban De Xivry J *et al* 2015 Investigating CT to CBCT image registration for head and neck proton therapy as a tool for daily dose recalculation *Med. Phys.* **42** 1354–66

Li H, Dong L, Bert C, Chang J, Flampouri S, Jee K W, Lin L *et al* 2022 AAPM task group report 290: respiratory motion management for particle therapy *Med. Phys.* **49** e50–81

Lötjönen J and Mäkelä T 2001 Elastic matching using a deformation sphere *Medical Image Computing and Computer-Assisted Intervention—MICCAI 2001* ed W J Niessen and M A Viergever (Berlin: Springer) pp 541–48

Lustberg T, van Soest J, Gooding M, Peressutti D, Aljabar P, van der Stoep J, van Elmpt W and Dekker A 2018 Clinical evaluation of atlas and deep learning based automatic contouring for lung cancer *Radiother. Oncol.* **126** 312–17

MacKay R I 2018 Image guidance for proton therapy *Clin. Oncol.* **30** 293–98

Maes F, Collignon A, Vandermeulen D, Marchal G and Suetens P 1997 Multimodality image registration by maximization of mutual information *IEEE Trans. Med. Imaging* **16** 187–98

Maintz J B A and Viergever M A 1998 A survey of medical image registration *Med. Image Anal.* **2** 1–36

McClelland J R, Hawkes D J, Schaeffter T and King A P 2013 Respiratory motion models: a review *Med. Image Anal.* **17** 19–42

McCulloch M M, Muenz D G, Schipper M J, Velec M, Dawson L A and Brock K K 2018 A simulation study to assess the potential impact of developing normal tissue complication probability models with accumulated dose *Adv. Radiat. Oncol.* **3** 662–72

Meijers A, Jakobi A, Stützer K, Guterres Marmitt G, Both S, Langendijk J A, Richter C and Knopf A 2019 Log file-based dose reconstruction and accumulation for 4D adaptive pencil beam scanned proton therapy in a clinical treatment planning system: implementation and proof-of-concept *Med. Phys.* **46** 1140–49

Munoz F, Fiorica F, Caravatta L, Rosa C, Ferella L, Boldrini L, Fionda B *et al* 2021 Outcomes and toxicities of re-irradiation for prostate cancer: a systematic review on behalf of the re-irradiation working group of the Italian association of radiotherapy and clinical oncology (AIRO) *Cancer Treat. Rev.* **95** 102176

Nenoff L, Ribeiro C O, Matter M, Hafner L, Josipovic M, Langendijk J A, Persson G F *et al* 2020 Deformable image registration uncertainty for inter-fractional dose accumulation of lung cancer proton therapy *Radiother. Oncol.: J. Europ. Soc. Ther. Radiol. Oncol.* **147** 174–85

Niebuhr N I, Splinter M, Bostel T, Seco J, Hentschke C M, Floca R O, Hörner-Rieber J *et al* 2021 Biologically consistent dose accumulation using daily patient imaging *Radiat. Oncol.* **16** 1–16

Oh S and Kim S 2017 Deformable image registration in radiation therapy *Radiat. Oncol. J.* **35** 101

Oliveira F P M and Tavares J M R S 2014 Medical image registration: a review *Comput. Meth. Biomech. Biomed. Eng.* **17** 73–93

Paganelli C, Meschini G, Molinelli S, Riboldi M and Baroni G 2018 Patient-specific validation of deformable image registration in radiation therapy: overview and caveats *Med. Phys.* **45** e908–22

Paganelli C, Peroni M, Baroni G and Riboldi M 2013a Quantification of organ motion based on an adaptive image-based scale invariant feature method *Med. Phys.* **40** 111701

Paganelli C, Peroni M, Riboldi M, Sharp G C, Ciardo D, Alterio D, Orecchia R and Baroni G 2013b Scale invariant feature transform in adaptive radiation therapy: a tool for deformable image registration assessment and re-planning indication *Phys. Med. Biol.* **58** 287–99

Palma G, Monti S and Cella L 2020 Voxel-based analysis in radiation oncology: A methodological cookbook *Physica Medica* **69** 192–204

Palaniappan P, Meyer S, Rädler M, Kamp F, Belka C, Riboldi M, Parodi K and Gianoli C 2022 X-ray CT adaptation based on a 2D–3D deformable image registration framework using simulated in-room proton radiographies *Phys. Med. Biol.* **67** 045003

Ribeiro C O, Knopf A, Langendijk J A, Weber D C, Lomax A J and Zhang Y 2018 Assessment of dosimetric errors induced by deformable image registration methods in 4d pencil beam scanned proton treatment planning for liver tumours *Radiother. Oncol.* **128** 174–81

Rigaud B, Simon A, Castelli J, Lafond C, Acosta O, Haigron P, Cazoulat G and de Crevoisier R 2019 Deformable image registration for radiation therapy: principle, methods, applications and evaluation *Acta Oncol.* **58** 1225–37

Rohlfing T, Maurer C R, Bluemke D A and Jacobs M A 2003 Volume-preserving nonrigid registration of MR breast images using free-form deformation with an incompressibility constraint *IEEE Trans. Med. Imaging* **22** 730–41

Rueckert D, Sonoda L I, Hayes C, Hill D L G, Leach M O and Hawkes D J 1999 Nonrigid registration using free-form deformations: application to breast MR images *IEEE Trans. Med. Imaging* **18** 712–21

Rueckert D and Schnabel J A 2011 Medical image registration *Biomedical Image Processing* ed T M Deserno (Berlin: Springer) 131–54

Seidensaal K, Harrabi S B, Uhl M and Debus J 2020 Re-irradiation with protons or heavy ions with focus on head and neck, skull base and brain malignancies *Br. J. Radiol.* **93** 20190516

Shackleford J A, Kandasamy N and Sharp G C 2010 On developing B-Spline registration algorithms for multi-core processors *Phys. Med. Biol.* **55** 6329–51

Shen D and Davatzikos C 2002 HAMMER: hierarchical attribute matching mechanism for elastic registration *IEEE Trans. Med. Imaging* **21** 1421–39

Smolders A, Hengeveld A C, Both S, Wijsman R, Langendijk J A, Weber D C, Lomax T, Albertini F and Guterres Marmitt G 2023 Inter- and intrafractional 4D dose accumulation for evaluating ΔNTCP robustness in lung cancer *Radiother. Oncol.* **182** 109488

Smolders A, Lomax T, Weber D C and Albertini F 2023 Deep learning based uncertainty prediction of deformable image registration for contour propagation and dose accumulation in online adaptive radiotherapy *Phys. Med. Biol.* **68** 245027

Sotiras A, Davatzikos C and Paragios N 2013 Deformable medical image registration: a survey *IEEE Trans. Med. Imaging* **32** 1153–90

Studholme C, Hill D L G and Hawkes D J 1996 Automated 3-D registration of MR and CT images of the head *Med. Image Anal.* **1** 163–75

Terzopoulos D 1986 Regularization of inverse visual problems involving discontinuities *IEEE Trans. Pattern Anal. Mach. Intell.* **8** 413–24

Thirion J P 1998 Image matching as a diffusion process: an analogy with Maxwell's Demons *Med. Image Anal.* **2** 243–60

Veiga C, Lourenço A M, Mouinuddin S, Van Herk M, Modat M, Ourselin S, Royle G and McClelland J R 2015 Toward adaptive radiotherapy for head and neck patients: uncertainties in dose warping due to the choice of deformable registration algorithm *Med. Phys.* **42** 760–69

Viergever M A, Antoine Maintz J B, Klein S, Murphy K, Staring M and Pluim J P W 2016 A survey of medical image registration—under review *Med. Image Anal.* **33** 140–44

Viola P and Wells III W M 1997 Alignment by maximization of mutual information *Int. J. Comput. Vis.* **24** 137–54

de Vos B D, Berendsen F F, Viergever M A, Sokooti H, Staring M and Išgum I 2019 A deep learning framework for unsupervised affine and deformable image registration *Med. Image Anal.* **52** 128–43

de Vos B D, Berendsen F F, Viergever M A, Staring M and Išgum I 2017 End-to-end unsupervised deformable image registration with a convolutional neural network *Deep Learning in Medical Image Analysis and Multimodal Learning for Clinical Decision Support* ed M Jorge Cardoso, T Arbel, G Carneiro, T Syeda-Mahmood, J M R S Tavares, M Moradi, A Bradley *et al* (Cham: Springer International) pp 204–12

Vrtovec T, Močnik D, Strojan P, Pernuš F and Ibragimov B 2020 Auto-segmentation of organs at risk for head and neck radiotherapy planning: from atlas-based to deep learning methods *Med. Phys.* **47** e929–50

Warfield S K, Zou K H and Wells W M 2004 Simultaneous truth and performance level estimation (STAPLE): an algorithm for the validation of image segmentation *IEEE Trans. Med. Imaging* **23** 903–21

Wolthaus J W H, Sonke J J, Van Herk M and Damen E M F 2008 Reconstruction of a time-averaged midposition CT scan for radiotherapy planning of lung cancer patients using deformable registrationa *Med. Phys.* **35** 3998–4011

Xu Y, Diwanji T, Brovold N, Butkus M, Padgett K R, Schmidt R M, King A *et al* 2021 Assessment of daily dose accumulation for robustly optimized intensity modulated proton therapy treatment of prostate cancer *Phys. Med.* **81** 77–85

Yang X, Kwitt R, Styner M and Niethammer M 2017 Quicksilver: fast predictive image registration—a deep learning approach *NeuroImage* **158** 378–96

Zabel W J, Conway J L, Gladwish A, Skliarenko J, Didiodato G, Goorts-Matthews L, Michalak A *et al* 2021 Clinical evaluation of deep learning and atlas-based auto-contouring of bladder and rectum for prostate radiation therapy *Pract. Radiat. Oncol.* **11** e80–89

Zhang L, Wang Z, Shi C, Long T and Xu X G 2018 The impact of robustness of deformable image registration on contour propagation and dose accumulation for head and neck adaptive radiotherapy *J. Appl. Clin. Med. Phys.* **19** 185–94

Zhang Y, Boye D, Tanner C, Lomax A J and Knopf A 2012 Respiratory liver motion estimation and its effect on scanned proton beam therapy *Phys. Med. Biol.* **57** 1779–95

Zhang Y, Huth I, Weber D C and Lomax A J 2018 A statistical comparison of motion mitigation performances and robustness of various pencil beam scanned proton systems for liver tumour treatments *Radiother. Oncol.* **128** 182–88

Zhang Y, Huth I, Wegner M, Weber D C and Lomax A J 2016 An evaluation of rescanning technique for liver tumour treatments using a commercial PBS proton therapy system *Radiother. Oncol.* **121** 281–87

Zhang Y, Knopf A, Tanner C, Boye D and Lomax A J 2013 Deformable motion reconstruction for scanned proton beam therapy using on-line x-ray imaging *Phys. Med. Biol.* **58** 8621–45

Zhong H, Wen N, Gordon J J, Elshaikh M A, Movsas B and Chetty I J 2015 An adaptive MR-CT registration method for MRI-guided prostate cancer radiotherapy *Phys. Med. Biol.* **60** 2837–51

IOP Publishing

Imaging in Particle Therapy
Current practice and future trends
Chiara Paganelli, Chiara Gianoli and Antje Knopf

Chapter 4

X-ray computed tomography for treatment planning: current status and innovations

N Peters, P Wohlfahrt and C Richter

4.1 Introduction

X-ray computed tomography (CT) is the undisputed primary imaging modality for treatment planning in particle therapy (PT), specifically for dose calculation (Richter and Wohlfahrt 2022). Due to the steep dose gradient at the end of the particle range, dose distributions are extremely sensitive to changes or uncertainties in the tissue composition along the particle track. Hence, the exact knowledge of tissue parameters is crucial to accurately predict the particles' stopping behaviour from CT. The conventional approach converts each CT number (CTN) derived from single-energy CT (SECT) into a quantity relevant for dose calculation in PT (usually the stopping-power ratio, SPR) using a heuristic stepwise linear conversion function, the so-called Hounsfield look-up table (HLUT). Despite this being unchanged since the pioneering years of PT (Hounsfield 1973, Goitein 1977), challenges still exist, which make the process error-prone and demand special attention as well as quality assurance. This concerns the optimisation and commissioning of the CT scan protocol, the settings and algorithms for image reconstruction, and lastly the HLUT specification itself (Peters *et al* 2023). This is especially true for PT centres in the pre-clinical preparation phase, where resources are often difficult to allocate for such, at first glance, sideline tasks. Notably, CT imaging and CTN-to-SPR conversion protocols vary largely between PT centres, introducing severe inter-centre variations in dose calculation (Peters *et al* 2021), potentially interfering with outcomes of multi-centric clinical trials.

In the past decades, innovative hardware and software developments in CT imaging improved the dose efficiency and overall image quality by, e.g., an automatic tube-voltage selection and tube current adaptation during CT acquisition with respect to the patients' anatomy as well as by iterative reconstruction techniques, to reduce image noise and artefacts (Wohlfahrt and Richter 2020).

doi:10.1088/978-0-7503-5117-1ch4

Recently, the application of dual-energy CT (DECT) for PT treatment planning has gained a lot of interest, as it offers several benefits compared to conventional SECT. However, the idea of using DECT in radiotherapy is anything but new. In his epoch-making publication introducing the first clinical x-ray CT scanner in 1973 (Hounsfield 1973), Godfrey Hounsfield already sketched the basic concept of DECT using two consecutive CT scans with different tube voltages. Only four years later, Michael Goitein, a Boston-based pioneer in proton therapy, saw its potential for improved PT treatment planning (Goitein 1977). Due to the physical difference in x-ray attenuation of tissues between the two CT scans, the impact of the two main interaction processes of kilovoltage (kV) x-rays, namely the photoelectric effect and incoherent scattering, can be separated for a better material classification. Despite its conceptual benefit, DECT was first used for clinical PT treatment planning in 2015, roughly 40 years after its invention (Wohlfahrt, *et al* 2017a). Nowadays, the direct SPR prediction from DECT is commercially available and finds its way into broad clinical application.

In this chapter, an overview of the use of x-ray computed tomography for PT treatment planning is given by summarising the basic principles of CT imaging, highlighting its benefits for quantitative imaging as well as its limitations, explaining the conversion from CT numbers to particle stopping power and discussing the potential of DECT and spectral CT imaging enabled by photon-counting CT using a semiconductor as detector instead of a scintillator as in conventional CT.

4.2 Principles of x-ray computed tomography

X-ray CT is a highly quantitative imaging technique with accurate geometrical fidelity enabled by a three-dimensional (3D) image reconstruction based on straightforward measurements of x-ray transmission through a scan object from different directions. The x-ray tube and the opposing detector are mounted on a rotating gantry and are combined with a patient couch for transversal movement of the scan object.

The information results from the partial absorption of x-rays in the scan object, which is described by the Beer–Lambert law:

$$N_D = N_0 \cdot e^{-\mu \cdot \Delta x},$$

with N_D and N_0 as number of photons reaching the detector with and without a scan object of thickness Δx, respectively. The detector is typically energy-integrating (EID), meaning that individual x-rays can't be detected, but the signal over time is assumed to be proportional to the number of photons. The parameter of interest is the attenuation coefficient μ, which depends on material properties, specifically the electron density ρ_e and atomic number Z, as well as on the x-ray energy E. It is the product of electron density and total electronic cross section σ_e:

$$\mu(E, Z) = \rho_e \cdot \sigma_e \ (E, Z) = \rho_e \cdot \left[\sigma_e^{ph}(E, Z) + \sigma_e^{coh}(E, Z) + \sigma_e^{inc}(E, Z) \right]$$

The total cross section is additive over all physical interaction processes, namely the photoelectric effect (σ_e^{ph}), coherent (σ_e^{coh}), and incoherent (σ_e^{inc}) scattering. This basic dependency of μ can be parameterised, taking into consideration the dependencies of the interactions from energy and atomic number, as done by Rutherford (Rutherford *et al* 1976):

$$\mu(E, Z) = \rho_e \cdot [A(E) + B_{ph}(E) \cdot Z^{3.62} + B_{coh}(E) \cdot Z^{1.86}]$$

Now, two layers of complexity are added. First, as the energy spectrum of an x-ray tube is polychromatic, the attenuation coefficient needs to be convoluted with the x-ray energy spectrum:

$$\widetilde{\mu}(Z) = \int_{E_{min}}^{E_{max}} S(E) \cdot \mu(E, Z) \quad dE$$

Second, for a heterogeneous scan object, the material composition and therefore its attenuation properties are different along the line of transmission. Therefore, the photon intensity measured behind the scan object describes the average attenuation of the tissue along the line between x-ray source and detector:

$$\overline{\mu} = \int_{x_1}^{x_2} \widetilde{\mu}(x, Z) \quad dx$$

During CT acquisition, $\overline{\mu}$ is measured from different angles φ and along different cranio-caudal positions z of the patient. The attenuation in every single voxel $\mu(x, y, z)$ can be derived from $\overline{\mu}(\varphi, z)$ by tomographic reconstruction—either analytical or using iterative algorithms.

For practical reasons, the CT number (CTN) in Hounsfield units (HU) has been introduced to describe the attenuation coefficient of the tissue μ_M relative to the attenuation of water μ_{H_2O}:

$$CTN = \frac{\mu_M - \mu_{H_2O}}{\mu_{H_2O}} \cdot 1000$$

The beauty of using CT imaging for particle therapy lies in the fact that CT numbers directly rely on the physical interaction of photons with matter. The underlying physical quantities, electron density and atomic number, are also relevant for describing the interaction of the therapeutic beam with matter.

Since x-ray CT scans in clinical scenarios are not as idealised as described above, several physical effects need to be considered. The **main challenges for accurate quantitative CT imaging** are:

- **Scattering:** The deflection of x-rays from the presumed straight line between source and detector, especially in the case of multiple scatter events, can deteriorate the image quality (Joseph and Spital 1982). In diagnostic fan-beam CT (in contrast to cone-beam CT), this effect is mitigated by two-dimensional anti-scatter grids to achieve a collimation in-plane and in the scan direction (Rührnschopf and Klingenbeck 2011).
- **Beam hardening:** Since low-energy x-rays are more likely to be absorbed due to a higher photon attenuation cross section, the energy spectrum is shifted towards higher energies with increasing penetration depth—the so-called

beam hardening (Brooks and Di Chiro 1976). This can lead to variations in CT numbers of materials. Based on physical assumptions, a beam hardening correction (BHC) can mitigate the impact on CT number stability and is thus implemented in the image reconstruction by default. It can either just correct the influence of water beam hardening (assuming the entire scan object to be water) or it differentiates between high-Z (e.g. bone, iodine, aluminium) and water-like materials in an iterative process (Kijewski and Bjärngard 1978, Van Gompel *et al* 2011).

- **Photon starvation:** If x-ray attenuation is too high, e.g. due to very dense bone structures or metal objects in the body, not enough photons or even none reach the detector. Hence, the tomographic reconstruction is missing information for these projections, which can result in so-called streak artefacts in the image. The selection of a higher tube voltage and/or beam filtration, an automatic tube current modulation (increased tube current for those projections) and iterative correction methods in image reconstruction can contribute to reducing image artefacts (Mori *et al* 2013, Chang *et al* 2017).

4.3 Practical considerations for CT-based stopping-power prediction

Various requirements on image quality at an 'As-Low-As-Reasonably-Achievable' (ALARA) x-ray dose need to be met to satisfy the accuracy demands of PT. Whereas a high image contrast is aimed for tissue differentiation in organ and tumour segmentation, quantitative material classifications impact the overall range uncertainty in dose calculation. Both characteristics need to be addressed in CT imaging protocols by optimising scan and reconstruction settings for different body regions, patient sizes and geometries. A harmonisation of CT scan protocols across treatment sites would ideally reduce the efforts for CT commissioning and quality assurance as well as the susceptibility to errors in the clinical workflow.

4.3.1 CT acquisition and reconstruction parameters

According to Wohlfahrt (2018), some scan and reconstruction settings like the selection of a sequential or spiral CT acquisition mode, pitch (in spiral mode) or reconstructed scan field of view (FOV) can be adjusted without relevant impact on image noise and absolute CT numbers, which are directly connected to the stopping-power prediction for dose calculation. The image noise is mainly influenced by the tube current, reconstructed slice thickness and sharpness of reconstruction kernels. Iterative image reconstruction can be applied to reduce either image noise (up to a factor of 1.5–1.6) at constant CT dose or to reduce the CT dose (up to 60%) at constant image noise while absolute CT numbers are kept unchanged (Wohlfahrt, *et al* 2017a). Since differences in absolute CT numbers are expected by varying the tube voltage (resulting in different x-ray spectra), slice collimation (accounting for the impact of x-ray scattering) as well as correction algorithms for beam hardening in image reconstruction, these parameters should be predefined. Guaranteeing stable CT numbers in image reconstruction for body regions with severe size

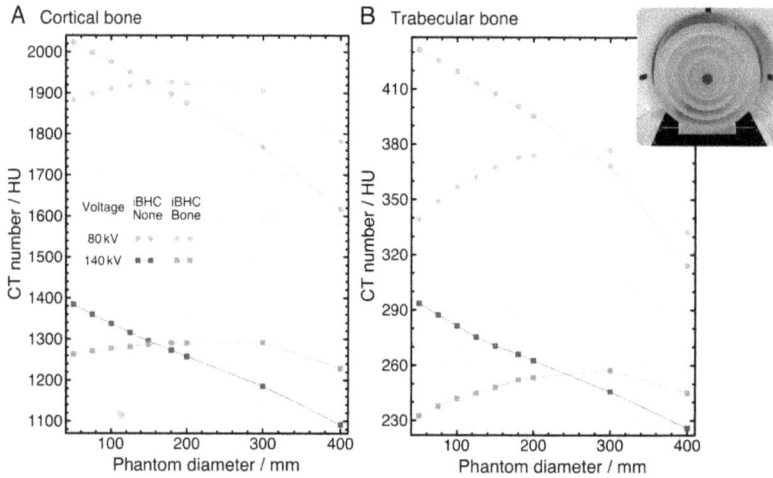

Figure 4.1. CT number stability for cortical (left) and trabecular bone (right) over a range of phantom diameters in an acrylic cylindrical phantom (shown in the top right) using water beam hardening correction only (iBHC None) or an iterative beam hardening correction for water and bone (iBHC Bone), respectively. Adapted from Wohlfahrt (2018).

variability in the scan field (e.g. head and neck) is an important prerequisite for SPR prediction.

This size-dependent decrease of material-specific CT numbers should therefore be mitigated by an iterative beam hardening correction considering high-Z materials like bones or iodine (figure 4.1). This cannot be easily achieved by individual CT scan protocols with dedicated calibration for SPR calculation.

The choice of the calibration phantom and materials is crucial for an accurate SPR prediction. The primary aim of the phantom is to match the x-ray attenuation and thus the beam hardening conditions of the patient as good as possible. Therefore, simple phantom geometries suffice (Siegel *et al* 2004), such as a round-shaped phantom for the head (water-equivalent thickness WET of 16–20 cm) and an oval one for the pelvis (WET of 30–40 cm). For scenarios diverging from those WET ranges (e.g. for paediatrics), additional phantoms are advisable.

The SPR calibration materials need to mimic human tissues regarding their interaction with x-rays and protons. Both interactions are dominated by the electron density. However, while x-ray interactions additionally depend on the effective atomic number, the SPR is affected by the mean excitation energy of the material. All three quantities follow from the mass density and chemical composition of the materials, for which reference values are comprehensively tabulated (Woodard and White 1986, Valentin 2002). Several commercial phantoms are tissue-equivalent for x-rays, but not sufficiently optimised for protons (Gomà *et al* 2018, Peters *et al* 2021).

4.3.2 Artefacts from high-density materials

Artefacts are substantially limiting the quantitative analysis of CT images. Special consideration is necessary for artefacts caused by high-density materials such as

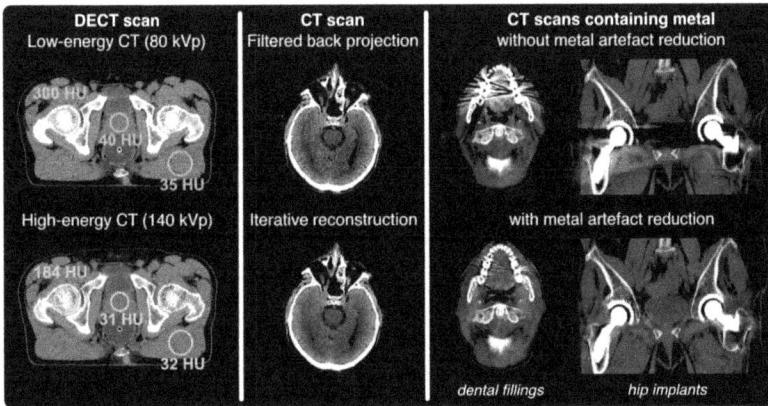

Figure 4.2. CT scan and reconstruction settings and their influence on image quality. From left to right: Influence of tube voltage, filtered back projection and iterative reconstruction as well as metal artefact reduction. Adapted from Wohlfahrt (2018).

metal implants (Giantsoudi *et al* 2017). The most common implants are dental fillings and hip prostheses, but also spinal rods, pacemakers and breast expanders after mastectomy cause relevant artefacts. Even for small metal implants, the x-ray attenuation is high enough that almost no x-rays reach the detector. Together with the additional scatter and noise induced by the implants, extensive image artefacts can superpose anatomical structures (figure 4.2).

Several strategies for the reduction of metal artefacts exist. For correction in the projection space (i.e. the sinogram), affected areas are identified and replaced with an estimation based on the surrounding data, either from the sinogram itself or in iterative steps from the reconstructed CT image (Kalender *et al* 1987, Meyer *et al* 2010). Artificial intelligence algorithms may increase image quality with corrections in the image space, i.e. in the reconstructed images (Zhang and Yu 2018). However, it should be noted that, while all algorithms to some extent improve image quality, they can also introduce new artefacts that are not distinctive in the image domain but relevant for PT. This concerns both the CT number accuracy and the depiction of small anatomical structures.

4.3.3 Artefacts from organ motion

As mentioned in chapter 2, organ motion due to respiration affects CT image acquisition, introducing artefacts in the reconstructed CT image. Respiratory-correlated 4DCT represents the current clinical standard to compensate for organ motion and limit respiratory-induced artefacts (Keall *et al* 2006, Mori *et al* 2018).

4.4 Conversion from x-ray attenuation to particle stopping power

The stopping power S is a material parameter that describes the energy loss per unit path length of the particle beam. Integrated along the beam path, it describes the maximum particle range within the patient and is thus the main quantity for dose calculation. It can be approximated by the Bethe equation (Bethe 1930, Berger *et al* 1993):

$$S = k_0 \rho_e \frac{z^2}{\beta^2} L(\beta) \approx k_0 \frac{z^2}{\beta^2} \rho_e \left[\ln\left(2m_e c^2 \frac{\beta^2}{1-\beta^2}\right) - \beta^2 - \ln I \right]$$

with the traversed material's electron density ρ_e and its stopping number L, the projectile charge z ($z=1$ for protons) and the velocity β relative to the speed of light c. The stopping number depends on the mean excitation energy I (often referred to as *I-value*) of the tissue; $k_0 = 5.1 \times 10^{-25}$ MeV cm^2 is a constant independent from the projectile or target; $m_e^2 c$ describes the electron rest energy. In PT, often the stopping power relative to water (SPR) is used.

Since particles differ in their interaction with tissue from photons, a conversion from CT number into SPR is necessary. This translation is performed voxelwise using a Hounsfield look-up table (HLUT), a stepwise function defined either by using tissue surrogates or information from real biological tissues (figure 4.3).

4.4.1 Hounsfield look-up table specification methods

The easiest way to obtain a HLUT is to scan different tissue-equivalent materials and perform fits of the materials' CT number and SPR. Because the elemental composition of different tissue types and thereby the relation between their CT number and SPR varies, the fit is performed individually for lung, adipose, soft and bone tissues (figure 4.3(A)). The SPRs are determined either experimentally (recommended) or analytically calculated from the respective elemental composition. The accuracy of correlating the CT number with the SPR this way, first introduced by Jäkel *et al* (2001), heavily depends on the number of used tissue surrogates and their respective tissue equivalency. To mitigate the influence of the tissue surrogates, the fit can also be performed with tabulated human tissue data. The most comprehensive database on human tissue was gathered by Woodard and White (Woodard and White 1986, White *et al* 1991), containing the elemental composition of 56 different tissues. For HLUT calibration, only a subset of those tissues is relevant, excluding those with a negligible volume or rare elemental compositions such as thyroid. In a so-called stoichiometric calibration, the scanner-specific CT numbers of those tabulated human tissues are predicted from their tissue composition (Schneider *et al* 1996, Schneider *et al* 2000). For this purpose, the x-ray attenuation needs to be modelled and calibrated for the individual scan setup using CT scans of tissue surrogates of known elemental composition. The accuracy of this calculation depends on the choice of the calibration materials (Gomà *et al* 2018) as well as the uncertainty of the I-value. The SPR prediction accuracy of the HLUT is increased by including both tissue surrogates and tabulated human tissue data in the fit (figure 4.3(A)). A comprehensive description of all calibration steps together with detailed recommendations is given in Peters *et al* (2023), summarising a consensus found within the European particle treatment community.

Lastly, the HLUT can be adapted by considering real tissues collected from humans or animals. However, due to the fast decay of tissue samples as well as their

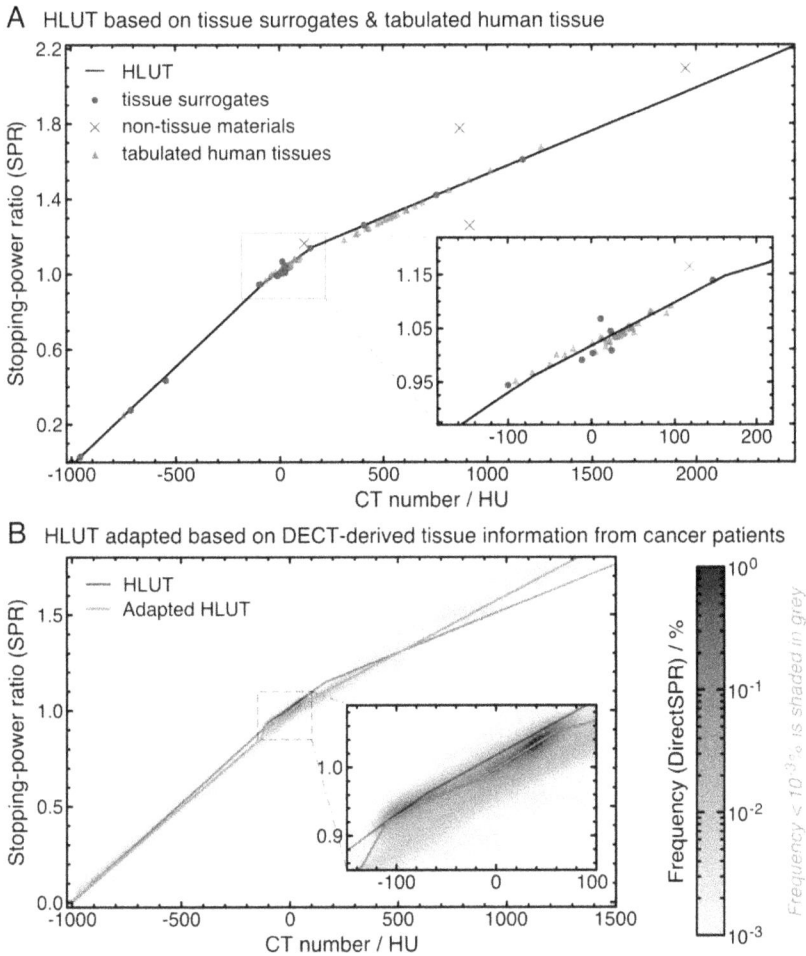

Figure 4.3. Hounsfield look-up table (HLUT) created using tissue surrogates and tabulated human tissues (A) or the frequency distribution of voxelwise correlations between CT number and stopping-power ratio derived from dual-energy CT (DECT) scans of cancer patients (B). Adapted from Wohlfahrt (2018).

heterogeneity, the accurate determination of CT numbers and SPR there is highly complex, limiting the benefit over using tissue surrogates. A different approach, first presented by Wohlfahrt *et al* (2020), is the adaptation of the HLUT based on tissue information obtained from dual-energy computed tomography (DECT). There, voxel-specific tissue parameters from clinical DECT scans are used to adjust the HLUT to better describe the SPR distribution found within the patient (figure 4.3(B)).

4.4.2 Consideration of non-tissue materials

Non-tissue materials are typically not considered in the HLUT specification, even though they can be present in the CT scan, e.g. as cushion and fixation devices around the patient as well as materials inside the patient, such as dental and prosthetic implants or silicone for breast reconstruction surgery. Special care is necessary to ensure a manageable effect on range prediction.

The most common strategy for metals is a segmentation of the implant as well as the areas affected by artefacts and a subsequent manual override with homogenous material parameters in the treatment planning system (TPS). While the application of metal artefact reduction algorithms can increase the accuracy of the segmentation, the non-consideration of heterogeneities as well as potential deviations between the tissue and the parameter used for the material override introduce relevant uncertainties (Stille *et al* 2013 Hansen *et al* 2017). Hence, avoiding the implant and regions affected by artefacts in the beam path whenever possible is the preferred choice (Giantsoudi *et al* 2017).

Silicone implants do not cause any artefacts, but have a much lower SPR than the HLUT would predict. Applying the HLUT would thus result in a range under-estimation of 11%–19% (Moyers *et al* 2014, Chacko *et al* 2021). For target volumes distal to the chest wall, this poses a high risk for irradiation of the heart and large parts of the lung. This can only be addressed with manual contouring and a volume override in the TPS. The accuracy of this material override depends on the knowledge of the silicone characteristics, which can vary between manufacturers.

4.4.3 Uncertainties in HLUT-based range prediction

The overall range uncertainty from the HLUT-based SPR prediction is on the level of 3.0%–3.5% of the particle range in water (Paganetti 2012, Yang *et al* 2012). This uncertainty is used by most European treatment facilities; some add an absolute uncertainty term of 1–2 mm (Taasti, *et al* 2018a). Factors contributing to this uncertainty can be separated into those affecting the CT number stability, directly impacting the input data for CTN-to-SPR conversion, and those affecting the SPR in the calibration.

As CT numbers might change with different beam hardening conditions, a discrepancy between the size of the patient and the calibration phantom introduces a deviation in SPR prediction. At sharp density gradients in the patient, such as between lung and muscle or muscle and bone, smoothing from the reconstruction kernel may result in an underestimation of the CT number for treatment beams crossing that gradient (Peters, *et al* 2022b). While the effect is small for individual gradients (about 0.2 mm at bone and 0.4 mm at lung edges), the overall uncertainty introduced by this can accumulate in inhomogeneous areas, such as the head and neck region, where the beam passes several of these gradient regions. This effect impacts every CT-based method to a varying degree (Wohlfahrt, *et al* 2018b, Polf *et al* 2019).

The main disadvantage of the HLUT approach is the non-consideration of the SPR variation for similar CT numbers (figure 4.3(B); Wohlfahrt *et al* 2020). Furthermore, both the tissue surrogates and the tabulated human tissues are based on data from a limited number of human tissue samples with insufficient consideration of the variation between patients (Peters, *et al* 2022a). In addition, in proton therapy, the SPR is typically calculated for a nominal beam energy between 100 and 200 MeV, which would introduce uncertainties for different proton energies, if not accounted for in modern TPS. The influence of the beam model and the proton beam range reproducibility introduces an absolute uncertainty term of about 1.5 mm (Peters, *et al* 2022b).

A study conducted within the European Particle Therapy Network (EPTN) evaluated the accuracy in range prediction of 17 European treatment facilities (Peters *et al* 2021). Inter-centre variations (2σ) of 8.7%, 6.3% and 1.5% relative to water were determined for SPR prediction in lung, soft tissue and bone, respectively. The uncertainties vary between different tissue types, with the deviations in bones being larger than in lung or soft tissue. By weighting them according to typical tissue distributions along the beam path, this translates into an inter-centre range prediction variation of 2.9%, 2.6% and 1.3% for the treatment of prostate- and lung cancer as well as of primary brain tumours. In multiple centres, the error in range prediction exceeded 2% (figure 4.4). Insufficient beam hardening correction as well as the lack of a clinical validation procedure were determined as the main contributor to these large deviations. In the aftermath of the study, one third of the treatment facilities reported to re-evaluate their clinical calibration or validation procedure.

For heavy ion therapy, all imaging-related effects and uncertainties are directly transferable, while at the same time the SPR energy dependency and the fragment tail need special consideration, specific to the ion choice (Pompos *et al* 2016).

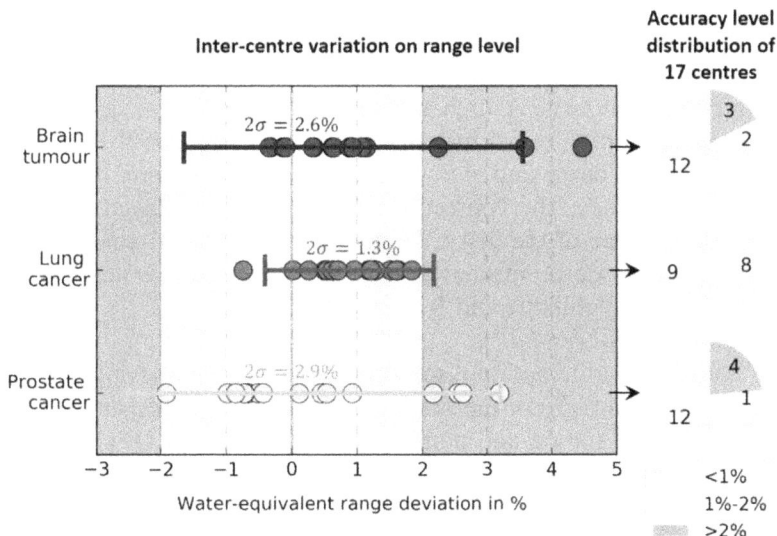

Figure 4.4. Inter-centre variation and absolute deviation in range prediction for representative beam paths and the respective quota for different shift levels. Reprint from Peters *et al* (2021), Copyright (2021), with permission from Elsevier.

4.5 From single-energy CT to dual-energy CT

4.5.1 Technological aspects

Various DECT acquisition techniques were implemented in dual-source and single-source CT scanners and have been steadily improved in the past two decades (Richter and Wohlfahrt 2022). Whereas DECT information in dual-source CT scanners are acquired with two independent x-ray tubes and detectors, DECT on single-source CT scanners is enabled by consecutive scan acquisition (dual-spiral mode), the use of a split-beam filter in scan direction (twin-beam mode), a dual-layer detector (dual-layer mode) or by slow/fast tube-voltage switching (slow/fast-kVp mode). The DECT image quality depends on the following technical criteria and needs to be assessed with respect to the type and range of clinical tasks in radiation oncology (Wohlfahrt and Richter 2020).

(a) *Spectral separation*

Material characterisation (e.g. for dose calculation) benefits from an increase in spectral separation. DECT modes with an independent adjustment of tube voltages (dual-source, dual-spiral, slow-kVp) achieve a high spectral separation. The spectral separation can be further increased by hardening the x-ray spectrum of the high-energy CT scan with an extra filter (dual-source, dual-spiral). In fast-kVp mode, a rectangular voltage modulation is technically challenging and thus the spectral separation decreases due to the partial mixture of the x-ray spectra in the transition period. A single tube voltage with two different filters in scan direction (twin-beam) or an energy discrimination at detector level (dual-layer) show an inferior spectral separation (McCollough *et al* 2020).

(b) *Temporal coherence*

A high temporal coherence reduces the impact of motion on DECT-based material differentiation. The dual-layer mode has an almost perfect temporal alignment. A high temporal coherence is achieved in fast-kVp (voltage alteration in 0.5 ms) and dual-source mode (90° offset). The time offset in twin-beam and slow-kVp mode is at least one rotation time. In dual-spiral mode, the consecutive CT scans are delayed by at least the acquisition time of the first CT scan. Motion-induced anatomical changes due to a temporal mismatch can be mitigated by deformable image registration (Wohlfahrt and Richter 2020).

(c) *Spatio-temporal resolution*

A high spatio-temporal resolution prevents edge blurring at high-density tissue transitions. Since the spatial resolution mainly depends on focal spot size, slice collimation and number of projections, all DECT modes except for fast-kVp (larger focal spot, distribution of projections per rotation) can utilise the full CT scanner capabilities.

(d) *Cross scattering*

The impact of cross-scatter radiation occurring in dual-source and dual-layer mode can be partly corrected during DECT post-processing (Petersilka *et al* 2010).

(e) *Imaging dose*

SECT and DECT scans can be performed at the same total dose without compromising on image quality (Wohlfahrt *et al* 2017a). Automatic tube current modulation works in all DECT modes except for fast-kVp due to restrictions in current tube technology. In dual-layer mode, the noise ratio between low- and high-energy CT data is set by the design of the detector layers.

(f) *Scan field of view*

All DECT modes except for current-generation dual-source provide DECT information in a scan field of view of at least 500 mm to allow for a proper coverage of immobilisation devices and body regions ranging from shoulder to pelvis.

(g) *Respiratory*

A 4D-DECT mode is not yet clinically available, but the general feasibility has been demonstrated in retrospective proof-of-concept studies (Ohira *et al* 2018, Wohlfahrt *et al* 2018a). So far, only conventional DECT acquisition in stable and static respiratory phases using a breath-hold technique is possible.

None of the recent DECT techniques satisfies the radiotherapeutic requirements for all possible clinical scenarios (table 4.1).

Table 4.1. Comparison of spectral CT imaging enabled by various dual-energy CT techniques and photon-counting CT with respect to technical criteria and clinical applications in radiation oncology. EID = energy-integrating detector. Reprinted from Richter and Wohlfahrt (2022). Copyright (2022), with permission from Springer.

		Dual-source CT with EID	Single-source CT with EID					Photon-counting CT
			dual-spiral	slow-kVp	fast-kVp	dual-layer	twin-beam	
Technical specification	Spectral separation	very high	very high	high	medium	low		high
	Temporal coherence	high	low	medium	high	perfect	medium	perfect
	Spatio-temporal resolution	full capabilities	full capabilities		limited capability *impaired spatial resolution*	full capabilities		full capabilities *superior spatial resolution*
	Cross scatter	yes	no			yes	no	no
	Imaging dose	individual tube current modulation	individual tube current modulation		no tube current modulation	tube current modulation		tube current modulation *less noise at same dose*
	Field of view	limited *up to 350 mm*	full					full
RO-relevant application	Time-resolved respiratory imaging	feasible with phase matching in post-processing	feasible with phase matching in post-processing			no limitation	feasible with phase matching in post-processing	no limitation
	Contrast-enhanced imaging	multi-phase (arterial & venous)	limited to late or delayed phase		multi-phase (arterial & venous)	limited to late or delayed phase		multi-phase (arterial & venous) *multiple contrast agents*
	Tissue segmentation	Improved compared to SECT	Improved compared to SECT					Superior spatial resolution, contrast and noise
	Projection-based material decomposition	no	no		yes	yes	no	yes

4.5.2 Methodological aspects

In addition to the various technical realisations of DECT, a multitude of algorithms for direct DECT-based SPR prediction (DirectSPR) have been proposed and thoroughly validated in the last decade (Wohlfahrt and Richter 2020). In general, many image-based algorithms for SPR prediction share the same physical principles and can be mathematically transferred into each other (Möhler *et al* 2018b). Most of them use the additional material information gathered by DECT to directly derive the electron density, as the dominating material parameter for SPR prediction, in a robust and accurate manner with a methodological uncertainty within 0.2% for biological tissue (Möhler *et al* 2017). Since the I-value in the Bethe equation cannot be directly obtained from DECT, many algorithms first calculate the effective atomic number from DECT and convert it into an I-value using a heuristic correlation. However, the impact of this empirical component on SPR accuracy is much smaller than in the HLUT approach (Möhler 2018).

A principal component analysis applied to DECT is another way to assign material compositions to each voxel based on predefined core materials (Lalonde and Bouchard 2016). This serves as input for voxelwise SPR calculation using the Bethe equation. In addition to these physics-based SPR algorithms, machine learning approaches to derive synthetic CT (Chapter 8) and completely empirical parametrisations have been introduced. Even though a comparison of projection- and image-based methods (Zhang *et al* 2018) as well as of various image-based methods (Bär *et al* 2017) did not yield relevant differences in SPR accuracy and precision, implementations differ regarding their robustness. Furthermore, the calibration of each method is crucial for the overall performance and robustness. It depends on various CT scan and reconstruction settings, such as the combination of low- and high-energy x-ray spectra, slice collimation and beam hardening correction. To avoid systematic SPR deviations due to noisy DECT datasets (Lee *et al* 2019), iterative image reconstruction and advanced noise suppression algorithms in DECT post-processing are highly recommended to obtain an image noise level within 1%, which is sufficient for precise dose calculation. A dedicated size-dependent calibration can cover remaining variations in CT numbers caused by beam hardening (Wohlfahrt 2018).

The reliability and superior accuracy of DECT-based SPR prediction compared to the conventional HLUT approach has been experimentally validated on several complexity levels. High-precision measurements in various homogeneous (Möhler, *et al* 2018a, Taasti, *et al* 2018b) and heterogeneous porcine and bovine tissue samples (Bär *et al* 2018) as well as in an anthropomorphic head phantom (Wohlfahrt, *et al* 2018b) confirmed the overall SPR accuracy. The clinical relevance of DECT-based DirectSPR has been demonstrated in large retrospective patient cohort studies by evaluating dose and range differences with respect to the conventional HLUT approach. Differences in water-equivalent proton range of 1.2%, 1.7% and 2.3% on average for brain-, prostate- and lung-cancer patients, respectively, confirmed the clinical impact (Wohlfahrt *et al* 2017b, Wohlfahrt *et al* 2018a). The accuracy of DirectSPR was further verified *in vivo* by prompt-gamma imaging during patient treatment (Berthold *et al* 2021).

It has been shown that with the use of DECT for treatment planning, the accuracy in range prediction can be improved from the previously mentioned 3.5% of the proton range to 2% or even 1.7% in specific treatment scenarios (Peters *et al* 2022b). This corresponds to a reduction of the safety margin by 35% and thus a relevantly decreased integral dose as well as dose to organs at risk, as shown in figure 4.5 for a representative patient case. Uncertainties in DECT-based range prediction can be classified as those related to the imaging process, the DirectSPR modelling and those unrelated to the previous two categories:

1. Relevant **imaging uncertainties** include the patient-specific beam hardening, the scan-field homogeneity, the noise level as well as the occurrence of sharp density gradients within the patient (such as between bone and soft tissue) where CT numbers are washed out. All these uncertainties also affect conventional SECT-based range prediction to a varying degree.

2. **Modelling uncertainties** originate from the methodology used for electron-density and stopping-number determination as well as from fitting procedures within the calibration process. Compared to SECT-based material parameter prediction, sophisticated DECT-based algorithms have the advantage that their uncertainties can be more comprehensively quantified.

3. **Other uncertainties** include the use of a nominal instead of an energy-specific SPR, the uncertainty in I-value determination as well as the proton beam reproducibility. All three factors again also affect conventional SECT-based range prediction.

In current DirectSPR implementations, the influence of beam hardening remains the dominating factor, contributing more than 1% to the overall uncertainty on the 2% level.

Monte Carlo dose calculation is steadily becoming the new standard in clinical routine. SPR datasets derived from DECT are also compatible with particle transport simulations of Monte Carlo algorithms by following a dedicated commissioning procedure (Permatasari *et al* 2020). Since Monte Carlo algorithms rely

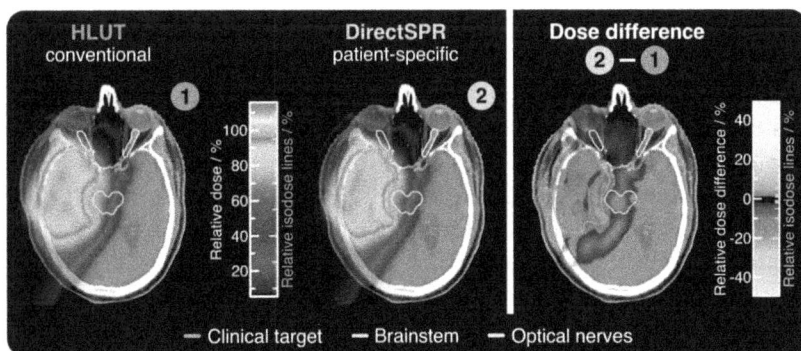

Figure 4.5. Exemplary differences in clinical proton dose distribution using the conventional Hounsfield look-up table (HLUT) with a relative range uncertainty of 3.5% of total proton range and a direct stopping-power prediction (DirectSPR) from dual-energy CT with a reduced range uncertainty of 1.7%. Critical anatomical structures such as the brainstem can be spared more effectively while increasing the tumour coverage close to the brainstem. Reprint from Richter and Wohlfahrt (2022). Copyright (2022), with permission from Springer.

on a voxelwise material assignment in terms of mass density and elemental composition, complimentary DECT results like electron density and effective atomic number or photon attenuation cross section could be used for a better material characterisation in a two-dimensional space to further improve the performance.

4.6 Conclusion and outlook

CT imaging will remain the gold-standard imaging modality for PT treatment planning and will continue to act as reference for other emerging technologies such as MR- or CBCT-based synthetic CT generation as well as proton CT. In recent years, the field of pre-treatment CT imaging for PT has seen substantial efforts in translational research, leading to relevant improvements. DECT enables a substantial reduction of range uncertainty and is currently on its way to broad clinical implementation, setting a new benchmark for other imaging techniques.

With photon-counting CT (PCCT) becoming clinically available in radiology after two decades of research and development, it becomes clear that further relevant innovations will find their way also in radio-oncological imaging. With new detector technologies, current limitations in CT imaging will likely be overcome (Richter and Wohlfahrt 2022). PCCT intrinsically allows for spectrally resolved multi-energy CT acquisitions in the full scan field of view with a high spectral separation, perfect temporal coherence, and high spatio-temporal resolution. Due to a threshold-based signal read-out of photon-counting detectors, electronic noise can be suppressed and thus a lower image noise or a further reduction of imaging dose as well as a higher CT number stability can be achieved. In combination with a near-constant detector sensitivity, even for low-energy x-rays, the soft tissue contrast as well as the contrast enhancement after contrast agent administration can be further improved (Flohr *et al* 2020). Since the energy discrimination is realised on the detector level, the spectral information is perfectly aligned, not hampered by motion-induced anatomical changes, and can thus be used for projection-based material decomposition and physics-based artefact correction, such as beam hardening. These advantages of photon-counting CT directly tackle current restrictions of the various DECT techniques. Therefore, photon-counting CT will potentially bring benefits for segmentation from tailored image contrasts and enable direct SPR prediction for a broader patient population (motion-influenced regions) and further decrease range uncertainties.

In conclusion, CT imaging is important for treatment planning in PT. It is an indispensable constituent to all parts of the workflow in radiation oncology, including diagnosis/staging and contouring of the target and organs at risk as well as for treatment control and follow-up.

References

Bär E *et al* 2017 The potential of dual-energy CT to reduce proton beam range uncertainties *Med. Phys.* **44** 2332–44

Bär E *et al* 2018 Experimental validation of two dual-energy CT methods for proton therapy using heterogeneous tissue samples *Med. Phys.* **45** 48–59

Berger M J *et al* 1993 6. Energy-loss straggling *J. Int. Comm. Radiat. Units Meas.* **os25** 61–8

Berthold J *et al* 2021 First-in-human validation of CT-based proton range prediction using prompt gamma imaging in prostate cancer treatments *Int. J. Radiat. Oncol. Biol. Phys.* **111** 1033–43

Bethe H 1930 Zur theorie des durchgangs schneller korpuskularstrahlen durch materie *Ann. Phys. (Berlin)* **397** 325–400

Brooks R A and Di Chiro G 1976 Beam hardening in x-ray reconstructive tomography *Phys. Med. Biol.* **21** 390–98

Chacko M S, Grewal H S, Wu D and Sonnad J R 2021 Accuracy of proton stopping power estimation of silicone breast implants with single and dual—energy CT calibration techniques *J. Appl. Clin. Med. Phys.* **22** 159–70

Chang Z *et al* 2017 Modeling and pre-treatment of photon-starved CT data for iterative reconstruction *IEEE Trans. Med. Imaging* **36** 277–87

Flohr T *et al* 2020 Photon-counting CT review *Physica Medica* **79** 126–36

Giantsoudi D *et al* 2017 Metal artifacts in computed tomography for radiation therapy planning: dosimetric effects and impact of metal artifact reduction *Phys. Med. Biol.* **62** R49–80

Goitein M 1977 The Measurement of tissue heterodensity to guide charged particle radiotherapy *Int. J. Radiat. Oncol. Biol. Phys.* **3** 27–33

Gomà C, Almeida I P and Verhaegen F 2018 Revisiting the single-energy CT calibration for proton therapy treatment planning: a critical look at the stoichiometric method *Phys. Med. Biol.* **63** 235011

Hansen C R *et al* 2017 Contouring and dose calculation in head and neck cancer radiotherapy after reduction of metal artifacts in CT images *Acta Oncol.* **56** 874–78

Hounsfield G N 1973 Computerized transverse axial scanning (tomography): part 1. description of system *Br. J. Radiol.* **46** 1016–22

Jäkel O *et al* 2001 Relation between carbon ion ranges and x-ray CT numbers *Med. Phys.* **28** 701–3

Joseph P M and Spital R D 1982 The effects of scatter in x-ray computed tomography *Med. Phys.* **9** 464–72

Kalender W A, Hebel R and Ebersberger J 1987 Reduction of CT artifacts caused by metallic implants *Radiology* **164** 576–77

Keall P J *et al* 2006 The management of respiratory motion in radiation oncology report of AAPM Task Group 76a *Med. Phys.* **33** 3874–900

Kijewski P K and Bjärngard B E 1978 Correction for beam hardening in computed tomography *Med. Phys.* **5** 209–14

Lalonde A and Bouchard H 2016 A general method to derive tissue parameters for monte carlo dose calculation with multi-energy CT *Phys. Med. Biol.* **61** 8044–69

Lee H H C *et al* 2019 Systematic analysis of the impact of imaging noise on dual-energy CT-based proton stopping power ratio estimation *Med. Phys.* **46** 2251–63

McCollough C H *et al* 2020 Principles and applications of multienergy CT: report of AAPM task group 291 *Med. Phys.* **47** e881–912

Meyer E *et al* 2010 Normalized metal artifact reduction (NMAR) in computed tomography *Med. Phys.* **37** 5482–93

Möhler C, Russ T *et al* 2018a Experimental verification of stopping-power prediction from single- and dual-energy computed tomography in biological tissues *Phys. Med. Biol.* **63** 025001

Möhler C 2018 Stopping-power prediction with dual-energy computed tomography. (http://ub.uni-heidelberg.de/archiv/24071)

Möhler C, Wohlfahrt P, Richter C and Greilich S 2017 Methodological accuracy of image-based electron density assessment using dual-energy computed tomography *Med. Phys.* **44** 2429–37

Möhler C, Wohlfahrt P, Richter C and Greilich S 2018b On the equivalence of image-based dual-energy CT methods for the determination of electron density and effective atomic number in radiotherapy *Phys. Imaging Radiat. Oncol.* **5** 108–10

Mori I, Machida Y, Osanai M and Iinuma K 2013 Photon starvation artifacts of x-ray CT: their true cause and a solution *Radiol. Phys. Technol.* **6** 130–41

Mori S, Knopf A-C and Umegaki K 2018 Motion management in particle therapy *Med. Phys.* **45** e994–1010

Moyers M F *et al* 2014 Medical dosimetry use of proton beams with breast prostheses and tissue expanders *Med. Dosim.* **39** 98–101

Ohira S *et al* 2018 Clinical implementation of contrast-enhanced four-dimensional dual-energy computed tomography for target delineation of pancreatic cancer *Radiother. Oncol.* **129** 105–11

Paganetti H 2012 Range uncertainties in proton therapy and the role of Monte Carlo simulations *Phys. Med. Biol.* **57** R99–117

Permatasari F F *et al* 2020 Material assignment for proton range prediction in Monte Carlo patient simulations using stopping-power datasets *Phys. Med. Biol.* **65** 185004

Peters N *et al* 2021 Experimental assessment of inter-centre variation in stopping-power and range prediction in particle therapy *Radiother. Oncol.* **163** 7–13

Peters N, Kieslich A *et al* 2022a *In vivo* assessment of tissue-specific radiological parameters with intra- and inter-patient variation using dual-energy computed tomography *Radiother. Oncol.* **175** 34–41

Peters N, Wohlfahrt P *et al* 2022b Reduction of clinical safety margins in proton therapy enabled by the clinical implementation of dual-energy CT for direct stopping-power prediction *Radiother. Oncol.* **166** 71–8

Peters N *et al* 2023 Consensus guide on CT-based prediction of stopping-power ratio using a Hounsfield look-up table for proton therapy *Radiother. Oncol.* **184** 109675

Petersilka M, Stierstorfer K, Bruder H and Flohr T 2010 Strategies for scatter correction in dual source CT *Med. Phys.* **37** 5971–92

Polf J C *et al* 2019 Determination of proton stopping power ratio with dual-energy CT in 3D-printed tissue/air cavity surrogates *Med. Phys.* **46** 3245–53

Pompos A, Durante M and Choy H 2016 Heavy ions in cancer therapy *JAMA Oncology* **2** 1539–40

Richter C and Wohlfahrt P 2022 Dual-energy CT in radiation oncology In *Spectral Imaging Dual-Energy, Multi-Energy and Photon-Counting CT* ed H Alkadhi, A Euler, D Maintz and D Sahani (Berlin: Springer) pp 333–46 https://link.springer.com/bookseries/174

Rührnschopf E-P and Klingenbeck K 2011 A general framework and review of scatter correction methods in cone beam CT. Part 2: scatter estimation approaches *Med. Phys.* **38** 5186–99

Rührnschopf E P and Klingenbeck K 2011 A general framework and review of scatter correction methods in x-ray cone-beam computerized tomography. part 1: scatter compensation approaches *Med. Phys.* **38** 4296–311

Rutherford R A, Pullan B R and Isherwood I 1976 Measurement of effective atomic number and electron density using an EMI scanner *Neuroradiology* **11** 15–21

Schneider U, Pedroni E and Lomax A 1996 The calibration of CT Hounsfield units for radiotherapy treatment planning *Phys. Med. Biol.* **41** 111–24

Schneider W, Bortfeld T and Schlegel W 2000 Correlation between CT numbers and tissue parameters needed for monte carlo simulations of clinical dose distributions *Phys. Med. Biol.* **45** 459–78

Siegel M J *et al* 2004 Radiation dose and image quality in pediatric CT: effect of technical factors and phantom size and shape *Radiology* **233** 515–22

Stille M *et al* 2013 Influence of metal segmentation on the quality of metal artifact reduction methods *Med. Imaging 2013: Phys. Med. Imaging* **8668** 86683C

Taasti V T, Bäumer C *et al* 2018a Inter-centre variability of CT-based stopping-power prediction in particle therapy: survey-based evaluation *Phys. Imaging Radiat. Oncol.* **6** 25–30

Taasti V T, Michalak G J *et al* 2018b Validation of proton stopping power ratio estimation based on dual energy CT using fresh tissue samples *Phys. Med. Biol.* **63** 15012

Van Gompel G *et al* 2011 Iterative correction of beam hardening artifacts in CT *Med. Phys.* **38** S36–49

Valentin J 2002 Basic anatomical and physiological data for use in radiological protection: reference values *Ann. ICRP* **32** 1–277

White D R, Widdowson E M, Woodard H Q and Dickerson J W T 1991 The composition of body tissues. (II) Fetus to young adult *Br. J. Radiol.* **64** 149–59

Wohlfahrt P, Möhler C, Hietschold V *et al* 2017a Clinical implementation of dual-energy CT for proton treatment planning on pseudo-monoenergetic CT scans *Int. J. Radiat. Oncol. Biol. Phys.* **97** 427–34

Wohlfahrt P, Möhler C, Stützer K *et al* 2017b Dual-energy CT based proton range prediction in head and pelvic tumour patients *Radiother. Oncol.* **125** 526–33

Wohlfahrt P, Troost E G C *et al* 2018a Clinical feasibility of single-source dual-spiral 4D dual-energy CT for proton treatment planning within the thoracic region *Int. J. Radiat. Oncol. Biol. Phys.* **102** 830–40

Wohlfahrt P 2018 *Dual-Energy Computed Tomography for Accurate Stopping-Power Prediction in Proton Treatment Planning [Dissertation Technische Universität Dresden]* Qucosa (http:// nbn-resolving.de/urn:nbn:de:bsz:14-qucosa2–317554)

Wohlfahrt P *et al* 2020 Refinement of the Hounsfield look-up table by retrospective application of patient-specific direct proton stopping-power prediction from dual-energy CT *Med. Phys.* **47** 1796–806

Wohlfahrt P, Möhler C, Richter C and Greilich S 2018b Evaluation of stopping-power prediction by dual- and single-energy computed tomography in an anthropomorphic ground-truth phantom *Int. J. Radiat. Oncol. Biol. Phys.* **100** 244–53

Wohlfahrt P and Richter C 2020 Status and innovations in pre-treatment CT imaging for proton therapy *Br. J. Radiol.* **93** 20190590

Woodard H Q and White D R 1986 The composition of body tissues *Br. J. Radiol.* **59** 1209–18

Yang M *et al* 2012 Comprehensive analysis of proton range uncertainties related to patient stopping-power-ratio estimation using the stoichiometric calibration *Phys. Med. Biol.* **57** 4095–115

Zhang S *et al* 2018 Impact of joint statistical dual-energy CT reconstruction of proton stopping power images: comparison to image- and sinogram-domain material decomposition approaches *Med. Phys.* **45** 2129–42

Zhang Y and Yu H 2018 convolutional neural network based metal artifact reduction in x-ray computed tomography *IEEE Trans. Med. Imaging* **37** 1370–81

IOP Publishing

Imaging in Particle Therapy
Current practice and future trends
Chiara Paganelli, Chiara Gianoli and Antje Knopf

Chapter 5

Conventional x-ray in-room imaging

C Kurz, C Hua and G Landry

5.1 Introduction

For several years, it was commonly understood that image guidance in particle therapy (PT) was more primitive than in linac-based photon therapy (Engelsman *et al* 2013). The developments in photon therapy were spurred by advancements in dose delivery techniques such as intensity-modulated radiation therapy (IMRT) or arc therapy, which allow ever more conformal sculpting of the dose distribution. This naturally makes positioning the target in three dimensions (3D) at the location assumed during treatment planning highly critical, since sharp dose gradients are unforgiving of geometric errors. By the 2010s image-guided radiation therapy (IGRT) was becoming commonplace in photon therapy (Bernier *et al* 2004, Ling *et al* 2006, Xing *et al* 2006, Balter and Kessler 2007, Dawson and Jaffray 2007, Verellen *et al* 2008). By now, linear accelerators are routinely equipped with on-board (in-room) cone-beam computed tomography (CBCT) scanners, which allow in-room imaging and bony anatomy alignment in 3D. For targets with sufficient contrast against background tissues, CBCT can be used to guide patient positioning as well. CBCT imaging is however neither the first nor last development in IGRT; early image guidance made use of two-dimensional (2D) images acquired using the treatment beam itself and radiographic films or electronic portal imaging devices (EPID) based on charge-coupled device (CCD) cameras (Leong 1986, Antonuk 2002). It was developments in EPID technology which led to the use of digital amorphous silicon flat-panel imagers for compact x-ray radiography systems, which were themselves precursors to modern CBCT scanners. Volumetric x-ray imaging is not only limited to classical gantry-mounted CBCT scanners; several devices with integrated image guidance capabilities have been developed, such as helical tomotherapy where a low energy MV fan beam can be detected as in a computed tomography (CT) scanner (Mackie *et al* 1993, Mackie *et al* 2003) or the now-defunct gimbal approach (Kamino *et al* 2006). Alternatives such as the Cyberknife exploit orthogonal 2D x-ray imaging to track targets in real time with a robotic arm, or the ExacTrac Dynamic system which additionally includes surface and thermal imaging (Chow *et al* 2022). Photon therapy has recently made yet another step ahead and embraced magnetic resonance (MR) image guidance (Corradini *et al* 2019, Kurz *et al* 2020), combining either 0.35 T or 1.5 T MR scanners with linear accelerators. These MRI-linacs have allowed the routine adoption of online adaptive radiotherapy (ART), where instead of only aligning the target at each fraction, a new treatment plan is re-optimized based on a delineated daily 3D MR image. Due to its larger user base, it is natural that photon therapy maintains a lead over PT in terms of image guidance technology, however as we see below the latter is catching up.

5.2 Image guidance in particle therapy

If modern photon therapy dose distributions require image guidance due to their highly conformal dose distributions, then it clearly is of importance for PT where conformity is the very reason for using this treatment modality, especially in the case of modern pencil-beam scanning intensity-modulated PT (IMPT). In fact, in-room image guidance using orthogonal x-rays, which has been standard equipment in PT centers for years (Slater *et al* 1992), was used very early on at the Massachusetts General Hospital (MGH) and the Lawrence Berkeley Laboratory (Gragoudas *et al* 1979, Verhey *et al* 1982). This was before the advent of linac-based image guidance (Biggs *et al* 1985). However, that early start did not translate into early adoption of volumetric image guidance such as CBCT; this is due to a few PT-specific reasons. The first reason is that PT dose distributions do not follow the shift invariance approximation used in photon therapy (McCarter and Beckham 2000, Booth and Zavgorodni 2001, van Herk *et al* 2002), meaning that it may not be sufficient to only align bony anatomy to ensure fidelity to the planning dose. Due to the dependence on the water equivalent thickness (WET) between the patient's skin and the target, which can be perturbed by bony structures, low density areas or changes in patient outline, the approximation rarely holds. This is illustrated in figure 5.1.

The second reason is that compared to linac-based facilities, historically there have been relatively few PT centres, and many were established before CBCT took off in photon therapy. Furthermore, these centres exhibited important heterogeneity in their design and important differences in their room layout compared to linac bunkers (requiring extended source to detector distances and higher source power for example), making retrofitting challenging. Nonetheless, the 2010s have seen the introduction of CBCT and other x-ray based volumetric image guidance in latest-generation particle therapy centres. This represents an important development given the high number of new centres that opened in that period, and it is safe to say that volumetric image guidance is becoming the norm in the field.

The next sections will go over the details of the different image-guidance approaches, including 2D x-ray and fluoroscopic imaging for patient positioning and tumour tracking, as well as in-room 3D imaging and its application in adaptive particle therapy (APT) workflows.

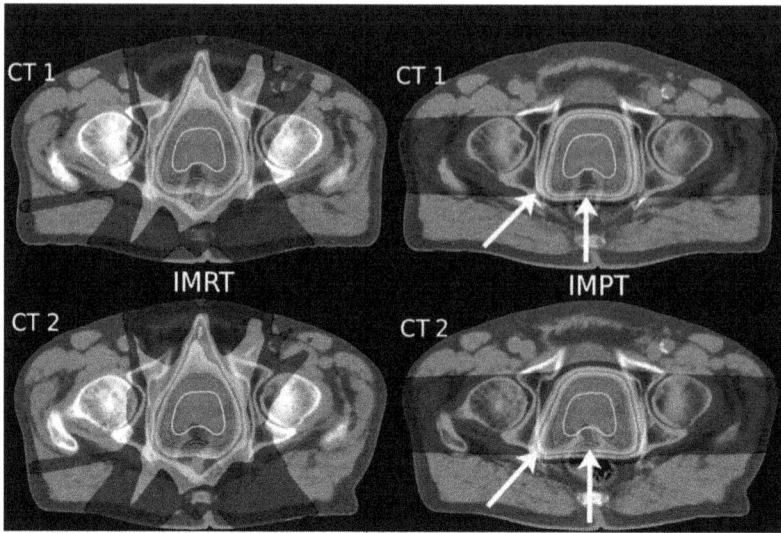

Figure 5.1. (Upper left) 8 field IMRT plan optimized on planning CT (CT 1) and (lower left) recalculated on a control CT image (CT 2) aligned to CT 1 by matching the target, which was delineated on both images. The IMRT dose distributions show little difference between CT 1 and CT 2. (Right panels) A two-field IMPT plan shows dose distribution degradation (marked by arrows) due to WET differences between (upper right) CT 1 and (lower right) CT 2. This illustrates the limitations of the shift invariance assumption for particle therapy. The CTV and PTV are shown as green and blue contours. Reproduced with permission from Landry and Hua (2018). John Wiley & Sons. © 2018 American Association of Physicists in Medicine.

5.3 2D and fluoroscopic x-ray for patient positioning and tumour tracking

Radiographic and fluoroscopic x-ray systems yielding 2D projection images of the patient anatomy are both utilized in PT. While the former are used for pre-treatment patient position verification and alignment and are widespread, the latter are exploited for intra-fractional tumour tracking and motion management in more specialized applications.

In-room 2D x-ray imaging, often implemented in an orthogonally oriented dual-source configuration, used to be the clinical standard for patient set-up in PT for many years and such systems are still in clinical use today (Schulte and Li 2006, Habermehl *et al* 2013, MacKay 2018). The systems typically consist of a standard x-ray source and an opposed flat-panel detector. These are either mounted on the gantry, the nozzle, the treatment room floor (x-ray source) and ceiling (flat panel) or on robotic C-arm systems, similar to those used for imaging during surgical interventions (Fattori *et al* 2015). The acquired pre-treatment x-ray images are then compared and registered to digitally reconstructed radiographs (DRRs) to facilitate accurate patient alignment. The DRRs are generated by forward projection of the initial planning CT according to the geometry of the in-room x-ray imaging system. On-the-fly generation of the DRRs allows for positioning the patient with up to 6 degrees of freedom (translation and rotation) by matching the generated DRRs and the acquired x-ray images. However, due to the 2D nature of these images and the unavoidable overlapping of structures in the acquired projections, alignment can typically only be performed based on bony anatomy or implanted fiducial markers. More accurate alignment can be achieved by tomographic 3D x-ray imaging, which is thus more and more replacing 2D x-ray imaging for patient alignment and is discussed in detail in the next section.

When it comes to tumour tracking during beam delivery, 2D in-beam x-ray imaging systems are still considered state-of-the art. The team at Hokkaido University in Japan has applied their development of a real time tumour tracking system for linear accelerator-based radiotherapy (Shirato *et al* 2000) to pencil-beam scanning proton therapy (Shimizu *et al* 2014). Disease sites that could benefit from such technique include the prostate, liver, pancreas, and lung. Fluoroscopic imaging is acquired with 1 or 10–30 frames per second for prostate and abdominal/lung tumours, respectively, using two orthogonal sets of x-ray sources and detector panels mounted in the rotating gantry and placed at ±45° relative to the proton beam direction. Imaging parameters are set for each patient based on anatomic site and the beam angle and kept as low as possible to reduce the radiation exposure from the fluoroscopic imaging. A 1.5 mm or 2.0 mm diameter gold fiducial marker is implanted near the tumour before radiotherapy simulation. The scanning proton beam is delivered only when the automatically recognized position of the fiducial marker is within ±2 mm of the planned position. The proton beam has a lag time of ∼0.05 s. The total treatment room time was reported to be on average 30 min (Yoshimura *et al* 2020).

Another fluoroscopy-based in-beam tumour tracking system for free-breathing thoracoabdominal treatment using carbon-ion scanning beams was reported by the National Institute of Radiological Sciences in Japan (Mori *et al* 2019). They employ a commercial markerless tracking technique originally developed for Cyberknife and now adapted for the compact superconducting rotating gantry, to which two orthogonal pairs of x-ray sources and flat-panel detectors are attached. To compensate the effect of gantry sag on source and detector positions as it rotates, a gantry flex map generated during the calibration process has to be applied. The auto calculation of the tumour position is achieved with machine learning after image processing and with multi-template matching. Tumour contours on 4D CT are projected onto DRRs for machine learning model training. The tracking accuracy achieved was reported to be <0.49 mm for imaging frame rates of 15 and 7.5 Hz but decreased to 1.84 mm for 30 Hz. For multi-template matching, staff can manually modify the tumour position on respective templates if needed and the tracking accuracy was found to be <0.52 mm for all imaging frame rates.

5.4 Approaches to volumetric image guidance

With the large number of PT centres established in the 2010s, we have seen the proliferation of several flavours of volumetric x-ray image guidance in treatment rooms. The solutions have often been supplied by the vendors of the PT equipment themselves, but also from third parties and have sometimes been implemented as

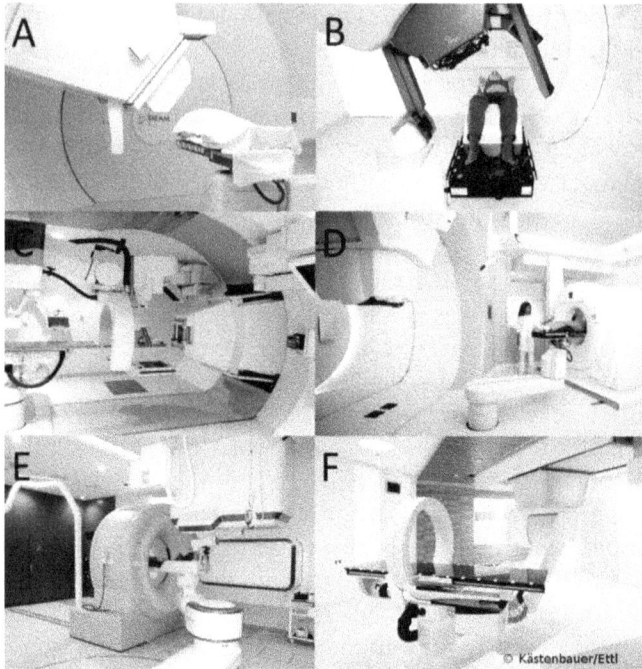

Figure 5.2. (A) Varian gantry-mounted CBCT at California Protons Cancer Therapy Center (former Scripps Proton Therapy Center; only one of the two flat-panel detectors is used for CBCT). (B) IBA nozzle-mounted CBCT. (C) C-arm mounted CBCT at St. Jude Children's Research Hospital. (D) Siemens in-room CT requiring couch rotation at an IBA gantry equipped facility. (E) Toshiba in-room CT with no couch rotation at the i-ROCK fixed beam line facility of the Kanagawa Cancer Center. (F) medPhoton couch-mounted CBCT. Reproduced with permission from Landry and Hua (2018). John Wiley & Sons. © 2018 American Association of Physicists in Medicine.

in-house solutions. The two main categories of devices are conventional diagnostic CT scanners and CBCT devices. In contrast to diagnostic fan-beam CT scanners, CBCT systems generally use a 3D cone-shaped x-ray beam for imaging. Instead of a multi- or single-line 1D detector array, CBCT employs 2D amorphous silicon flat-panel detectors to measure x-ray attenuation in the patient. The volumetric image is reconstructed from a set of a few hundred 2D projections acquired during a single rotation of the source and detector around the static patient (no table movement). Depending on the specific in-room CBCT design, source to isocenter and source to detector distance (SID and SSD) vary and can be substantially larger than in conventional CT scanners (Jaffray *et al* 2002). Figure 5.2 presents an overview of the approaches discussed below and additional details are provided in table 5.1.

5.4.1 CBCT scanners mounted on robotic arms

C-arm technology has been widely used to mount x-ray sources and detectors in hospital settings for applications such as fluoroscopic imaging. These devices have been adapted for CBCT scanning in PT centres by both commercial and in-house

Table 5.1. Comparison of radiological volumetric image guidance solutions in particle therapy. Reproduced with permission from Landry and Hua (2018). John Wiley & Sons. © 2018 American Association of Physicists in Medicine.

Type	Currently used for	Vendors	First clinical use	On- or off-isocenter imaging	Advantages	Current challenges
Gantry-mounted CBCT	360° gantry	Hitachi, IBA, Sumitomo, Varian	2014	On	Imaging at treatment isocenter, clearance with retracted imaging equipment, experience from more users	CT number accuracy, difficulty in retrofitting to existing facilities
Nozzle-mounted CBCT	Partial gantry	IBA	2015	On	Viable solution for partial gantry and treatment room with limited space	Physical clearance, large FOV with half fan mode, CT number accuracy
Robotic C-arm CBCT	Partial gantry	Hitachi	2015	Both	Viable solution for partial gantry, multiple imaging positions, high accuracy and precision robots, easier to upgrade with decoupling imaging system	Size of robot for occupying ceiling or floor space, collision avoidance, robot movement time, CT number accuracy
In-room CT on rails	Both	Siemens, Toshiba	1997	Off	Soft tissue image quality, larger radial and longitudinal FOV, 4D CT capability, automatic exposure control, dual energy CT potential	System integration, lack of imaging at treatment isocenter, longer overall image guidance time due to additional couch and CT movement
Couch-mounted CBCT	Both	medPhoton	2016	Both	Longitudinal FOV in helical mode, viable for both 360 and partial gantries, fan-beam CT possible with collimation	Impact of equipment weight on couch position accuracy, collision avoidance, CT number accuracy

solutions. Early efforts suffered from the lack of integration with the rest of the equipment and software present in the treatment room, making the calculation of rigid alignment cumbersome.

A leading example of this approach is the system developed at the Centro Nazionale di Adroterapia Oncologica (CNAO) using a six-joint robotic arm to hold the C-arm carrying the x-ray source and detector (Fattori *et al* 2015), which is capable of 220° rotation. At St. Jude Children's Research Hospital, a commercial Hitachi system combines a C-ring and a C-arm for 360° rotation and allows extended field-of-view (FOV) via laterally shifted detector panels (Hua *et al* 2017), and is mounted on ceiling rails.

5.4.2 CBCT scanners mounted on the couch

The leading example of couch-mounted systems is the ImagingRing from medPhoton where a ring is mounted directly to the treatment couch and allows independent rotation of x-ray source and detector for non-isocentric imaging (Rit *et al* 2016). Such systems can be found at the medAustron, MAASTRO and MGH (see figure in Bortfeld and Loeffler 2017) PT centers among others. This approach is one of the latest developments in CBCT imaging and allows extensive flexibility in terms of imaging trajectories (Albrecht *et al* 2022). Geometric calibration is critical given the large number of degrees of freedom and a dedicated procedure based on a proprietary ball bearing phantom allows determining the required geometric corrections (Zechner *et al* 2016). The vendor is also exploring several optical camera systems for further improved geometric fidelity for non-standard imaging trajectories.

5.4.3 CBCT scanners installed in the gantry

Gantry-mounted CBCT scanners have been mostly implemented by vendors of proton therapy equipment such as IBA, Varian, Hitachi or Sumitomo, and have generally been part of PT equipment since 2014. The vendors typically provide both CBCT scanner equipment and software for image reconstruction and position correction. There are important design differences from photon therapy, where the x-ray source and flat-panel detector are mounted in a perpendicular configuration to the main treatment beam with SDDs and SIDs of 150 and 100 cm. In PT these distances are typically in the range of 220–347 cm (SDD) and 160–288 cm (SID), which entails the use of more power when operating the x-ray source for a photon flux equivalent to that of photon therapy scanners. These differences in SDD and SID are due to the availability of mounting points for the x-ray source and flat-panel imager in PT gantries. Typically, the x-ray source will be mounted on the gantry below the rolling floor of the treatment room and the flat-panel detector will either unfold from the treatment nozzle or be mounted on an arm parallel to the rotation axis. A few recent systems have moved the x-ray source closer to the detector panel by using a retractable arm coming from behind the wall. The gantries have 360° rotation capabilities ensuring adequate angular coverage for the tomographic scan, and they typically allow a full rotation in 60 seconds, just as in photon therapy. Not all solutions offer the ability to shift the detector panel for extended FOV scans due to space and mechanical limitations. Although two pairs of source and detector are typically equipped in these 360° proton gantries, the ability to simultaneously acquire CBCT projections in significantly reduced time has yet to be implemented.

5.4.4 CBCT scanners installed on the nozzle

Some vendors offer more compact gantry and room designs (such as the Proteus One of IBA) which allow only partial rotation (up to 220° typically). Such a rotation range is sufficient to acquire the minimal number of tomographic projections (180° plus the fan angle) with a centred detector, and thus allows tomographic reconstruction as well. In these room designs, space is even more constrained, and the CBCT detector and x-ray source are both mounted on the nozzle on retractable arms, and they are only extended for CBCT scanning. Clearly in this configuration larger FOV scans with shifted detectors are challenging due to the limited rotation range. IBA currently acquires two 220° rotations, one clockwise and the other counter-clockwise with a detector offset and overlapping between them.

5.4.5 CT scanners on rail

An earlier alternative to the use of CBCT scanners is to use a conventional CT scanner directly in the treatment room. This scanner typically needs to be mounted on rails to allow moving it in and out of the imaging position, which allows space saving when the scanner is not in use, as well as reducing exposure to neutrons as much as possible. A special couch is needed to move the patient from treatment position to imaging position. The rail approach is the most common (Safai *et al* 2012, Li *et al* 2016, Oliver *et al* 2017), but is not the only option; horizontal CT scanners for seated patients are also found in treatment rooms, with an early example from the National Institute of Radiological Sciences in Japan at the end of the 1990s (Kamada *et al* 1999, Kress *et al* 1999). This approach is also found at the Northwestern Medicine Chicago Proton Center. Again, in this case the integration with the particle therapy equipment can be challenging, since the CT scanners are typically provided by third party vendors. The lack of isocentric imaging is compensated by the benefits of a fully-fledged CT scanner that allows automatic exposure control, beam hardening correction, limited scatter detection leading to accurate CT numbers for improved image quality, direct dose calculation and replanning, dual energy capability (see chapter 4), respiratory correlated or 4DCT (see chapter 9). An alternative solution can be found at the Heidelberg Ion-Beam Therapy Center, where a commercial mobile CT scanner (Brainlab Airo) is integrated in the horizontal beam lines and enables diagnostic quality imaging at the treatment isocenter.

5.5 In room imaging for adaptive particle therapy

As mentioned in the introduction of this chapter, WET changes between planning and beam delivery can substantially alter PT dose distributions. Unfortunately, in contrast to in-room CT scanners, CBCT-based in-room image guidance does not provide sufficiently accurate CT numbers to allow direct computation of the WET and thus recalculation and adaptation of the planned dose distribution according to the daily patient anatomy. Several factors contribute to the degradation of CT numbers in CBCT images, but the main culprit is commonly understood to be the detection of scattered photons from the patient by the large area flat-panel detector (Siewerdsen and Jaffray 2001). Other sources of image quality degradation are also important and include detector scatter (Poludniowski et al 2011), beam hardening (Herman 1979), detector lag (Siewerdsen and Jaffray 1999), and truncation of the field of view (Ohnesorge et al 2000). A good summary of these effects and their correction is presented by Thing et al, who used Monte Carlo simulation to estimate scatter (Thing et al 2016). Without correction, there will not be a bijective relation between CBCT and CT numbers (Kurz et al 2015). In parallel to the spread of CBCT scanners in PT centres, the 2010s and 2020s saw several studies investigating various CT number correction approaches specifically for PT (Giacometti et al 2020).

5.5.1 CBCT correction by virtual CT

Due to the increased sensitivity of protons and heavier ion species against CT number inaccuracies, simple phantom-, patient- or population-based look-up table-based rescaling or histogram matching approaches, as found in photon radiotherapy (Fotina et al 2012), are often not sufficiently accurate in the presence of pronounced CBCT artefacts (Kurz et al 2015, Arai et al 2017). Thus, the most common approach found in the literature to correct CBCT intensities relies on the idea of generating a so-called virtual CT (vCT; Peroni et al 2012), which allows exploiting the prior knowledge inherently available in the high-quality CT image used for treatment planning. By using deformable image registration (DIR), the diagnostic quality CT numbers from the planning image are mapped on the anatomy from the CBCT scan of the day. This allows bypassing lengthy Monte Carlo estimations of scatter. Given the longstanding availability of CBCT in that field, the approach was first applied to photon therapy (Veiga et al 2014). In proton therapy it was initially applied to head and neck cancer patients and evaluated in terms of dose calculation accuracy (Landry et al 2015), albeit using data from photon therapy CBCT scanners as a proof of principle. The approach showed good dose calculation accuracy when compared to replanning CT images acquired close in time to the CBCT scans, and was much better than using CBCT to CT look-up tables (Kurz et al 2015). As a by-product, the vector fields obtained from DIR could also be used to warp delineated structures used for treatment planning (Kurz et al 2016b). Good results were also reported when using virtual CTs for CBCT images of lung cancer patients reconstructed in 3D (without motion correlation) (Veiga et al 2016). However, for sites with pronounced anatomical changes difficult to model by DIR, such as the male pelvis, the virtual CT approach was found to lead to distorted anatomical structures (Kurz et al 2016a).

5.5.2 CBCT correction at the projection level

An approach to overcome these limitations of DIR-based vCT generation was originally proposed in the scope of photon therapy by Niu et al (2010, 2012).

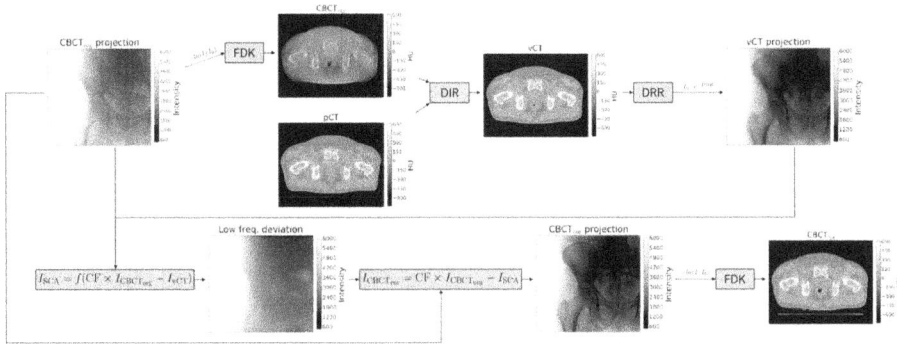

Figure 5.3. Illustration of the projection-level CBCT intensity correction algorithm. First a vCT is generated by DIR of the planning CT (pCT) to the reconstructed (using, e.g., the Feldkamp-Davis-Kress (FDK) algorithm) raw $CBCT_{org}$. The vCT is then forward projected (DRR) according to the considered CBCT geometry. The obtained vCT projections in intensity space are then subtracted from the raw measured CBCT projections weighted by a scan-protocol specific calibration factor (CF). A generous smoothing filter f is applied on the difference to estimate low frequency deviations in the measured projections. These deviations (I_{SCA}) are then subtracted from the raw projections and a set of corrected projections is obtained that can be reconstructed with FDK following translation to log-space, yielding a corrected $CBCT_{cor}$. Reproduced with permission from Landry *et al* (2019). © 2019 Institute of Physics and Engineering in Medicine. All rights reserved.

It employs the vCT as prior to perform a projection-based shading correction of low frequency deviations, such as scatter and beam hardening. In the scope of proton therapy, it could also be shown that this technique enables accurate CBCT-based dose calculation (Park *et al* 2015, Kurz *et al* 2016a, Hofmaier *et al* 2017, Andersen *et al* 2020). The main steps of the projection-level scatter correction algorithm are depicted in figure 5.3. Briefly, the algorithm starts by forward projecting the vCT according to the CBCT scanner geometry used for data acquisition. The obtained presumably scatter-free projections are then subtracted from the raw measured CBCT projections (weighted by a scan-protocol specific calibration factor (CF) accounting for the settings of x-ray source exposure time and tube current). Since the method aims at correcting only low spatial frequency deviations, the calculated differences of measured and vCT forward projections are blurred by a generous smoothing filter to estimate these deviations. By eventually subtracting the obtained estimated low frequency components from the raw measured projections, a set of corrected projections is retrieved and can be used to reconstruct an intensity-corrected CBCT image.

As was shown in several studies (Park *et al* 2015, Kurz *et al* 2016a), dose calculation accuracies similar to the vCT approach can be achieved for body regions with moderate anatomical changes and high DIR performance, e.g., in the head and neck (see figure 5.4). However, in cases where DIR is less accurate, e.g., in the pelvis, it could be demonstrated that by using the vCT only as prior, these geometric inaccuracies can be overcome by correction at projection level due to the generous smoothing operation applied when estimating the low frequency deviations (Kurz *et al* 2016a).

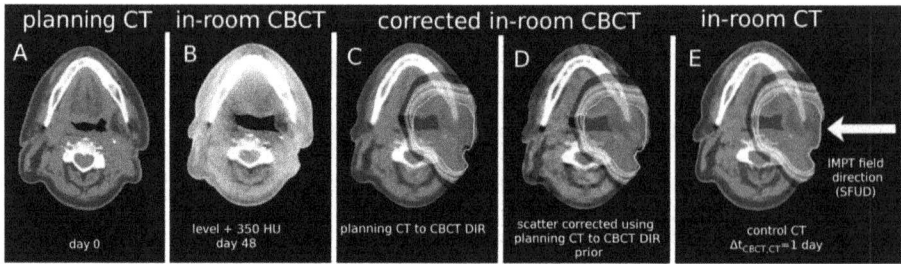

Figure 5.4. Example of in-room volumetric imaging data for dose calculation. All images acquired in the context of photon IMRT and used for illustration purposes. (A) Planning CT scan. (B) Late treatment in-room CBCT scan showing weight loss. (C,D,E) Dose distributions for a single field uniform dose (SFUD) adapted plan using IMPT. (C,D) The doses were recomputed on CBCT images corrected using (C) deformable image registration (DIR) of the planning CT to the daily CBCT image (Landry *et al* 2015) and (D) using the result of the deformation as prior information to estimate a scatter correction at projection level (Park *et al* 2015). In (E) an in-room equivalent control CT acquired 1 day after the CBCT was used to calculate the adapted plan and serves as reference. Figure adapted with permission from Kurz *et al* (2016a). John Wiley & Sons. © 2016 American Association of Physicists in Medicine.

5.5.3 4DCBCT

Another active field of research is the extension of these CBCT intensity correction methods to 4D. More specifically, it is aimed at reconstructing and correcting respiratory-correlated CBCT images in a phase-by-phase fashion. This is of particular interest for treatment sites that are affected by respiratory motion, e.g., in the thorax. It is well known that respiratory motion can vary from fraction to fraction, due to baseline shifts, variable breathing amplitude or other inter-fractional anatomical changes (Dhont *et al* 2018). Thus, inferring the motion of the treatment day is important for reconstructing the applied time-resolved dose under consideration of the daily motion or, in the future, for daily online treatment plan adaptation.

Typically, it is aimed at reconstructing 6–10 equally spaced (phase-based sorting) breathing phases. To this aim, the acquired CBCT projection data need to be binned into single breathing phases. In most cases, no external motion surrogate is available, such that binning relies on extracting the breathing phase from the acquired projection data themselves. The method at hand is the so-called Amsterdam-Shroud algorithm, which aims at extracting the motion signal in superior-inferior (SI) direction from a 1D signal generated by compressing the 2D projection data onto a single dimension (SI). According to the extracted breathing signal, projection data are then attributed to the single respiratory phases. For a typical CBCT scan protocol, this will leave only about 60–70 projections per phase for reconstruction. In consequence, CBCT quality is substantially degraded when performing analytical reconstruction using, e.g., the Feldkamp-Davis-Kress (FDK) algorithm. Considerably improved reconstruction quality can be achieved by iterative reconstruction algorithms, such as those based on conjugate gradient, in combination with total variation in either space or even space and time, as, e.g., in the Motion-Aware RecOnstructiOn method using Spatial and TEmporal Regularization (MA-ROOSTER) algorithm (Christoffersen *et al* 2013, Mory *et al* 2016, den Otter *et al* 2020).

Once a reasonable CBCT reconstruction quality is achieved, the same methods used for 3D CBCT correction can be employed. A vCT can be obtained either by performing DIR of a given 4DCT phase to the individual 4DCBCT phases (Niepel *et al* 2019), or by first generating Mid Position CT and CBCT images (Wolthaus *et al* 2008), which are then deformably registered to each other yielding a Mid Position vCT. The latter can then be animated according to the deformations applied during Mid Position CBCT generation to obtain a 4D vCT (Bondesson *et al* 2022). Based on the 4D vCT, also phase-by-phase projection-based intensity correction is feasible and was shown to yield similar 4D proton dose calculation accuracy as the 4D vCT approach (Schmitz *et al* 2021, Schmitz *et al* 2023a). The workflow of the projection-level CBCT correction in 4D is illustrated in figure 5.5.

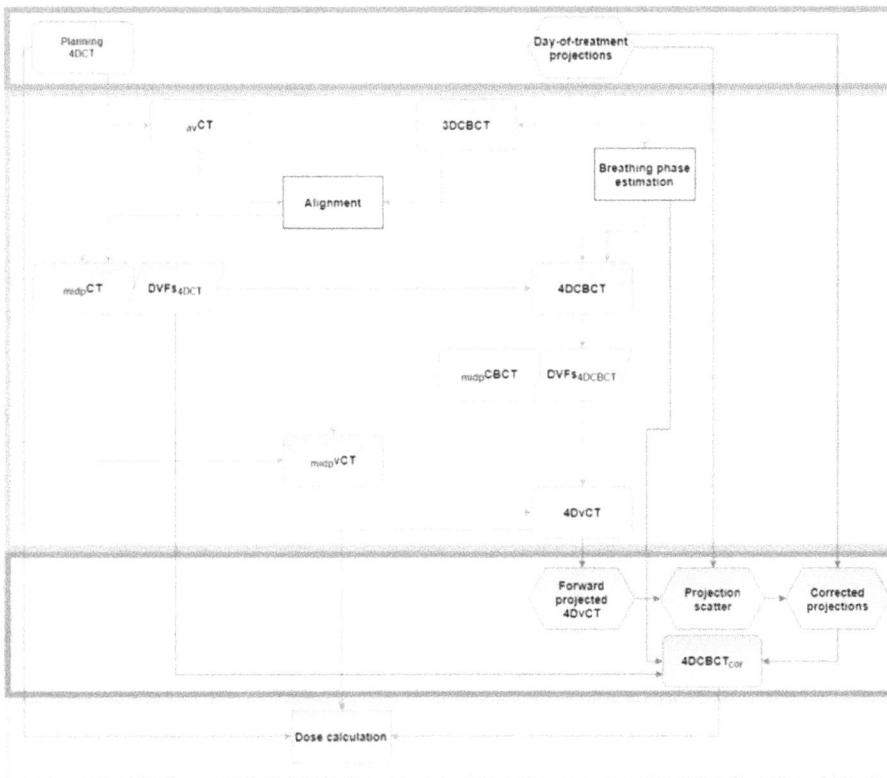

Figure 5.5. Illustration of a 4D projection-level CBCT correction approach. A planning 4DCT and the measured daily CBCT projections serve as input (blue). Rigid alignment of CT and CBCT space is performed using the respective average 3D images. Next CBCT projection data are split into the single motion phases. A mid-position (midp) CT is generated, and the obtained deformation vector fields (DVFs) are used as prior information in a motion aware 4DCBCT reconstruction. A mid-position CBCT is generated and used for mid-position CT to CBCT DIR, yielding a mid-position vCT which is then animated to 4D using the CBCT mid-position DVFs (orange). For projection-based correction (shown in red), each phase of the 4DvCT is forward projected according to the CBCT geometry and used to estimate low frequency deviations in the measured projections phase-by-phase (see figure 5.3). The corrected phase-specific projections can then be reconstructed by the same algorithm as the 4DCBCT, yielding the final 4DCBCT$_{cor}$ (red). Reproduced from Schmitz *et al* (2021). © 2021 The Author(s). Published on behalf of Institute of Physics and Engineering in Medicine by IOP Publishing Ltd. CC BY 4.0.

Recently alternative approaches making use of deep learning have also been used for 4DCBCT (Dong *et al* 2022, Thummerer *et al* 2022, Schmitz *et al* 2023b).

5.6 Outlook

In terms of x-ray in-room imaging, PT was lagging behind conventional photon therapy for many years. However, within the last decade, planar in-room x-ray imaging has been gradually replaced by volumetric in-room CT imaging, using either in-room diagnostic CT scanners mounted on rails or dedicated CBCT systems. Currently, the acquired 3D in-room images are still mainly used for accurate patient alignment even though particle therapy could greatly benefit from in-room imaging-based online treatment adaptation. In the case of CBCT, a first crucial step in this direction is to render the acquired in-room images suitable for accurate dose calculation. As outlined in this chapter, many approaches for CBCT intensity correction exist. An important drawback of the presented methods, rather than their accuracy, is their correction speed, typically in the order of several minutes, which is not acceptable in an online adaptive workflow. Thus, current efforts focus on the implementation of deep learning techniques for accurate and fast (seconds) CBCT correction, as described in detail in chapter 8 (Hansen *et al* 2018, Kida *et al* 2018, Landry *et al* 2019, Kurz *et al* 2019).

For enabling online adaptive workflows, further hurdles, such as fast (semi-) automatic target and organ-at-risk delineation and online quality assurance, will have to be overcome. Again, photon therapy has already taken a step ahead, by the clinical implementation of online adaptive workflows based either on in-room MRI (Corradini *et al* 2019, Kurz *et al* 2020, Keall *et al* 2022) or CBCT images (Sibolt *et al* 2021, de Jong *et al* 2021). Nevertheless, in the context of PT, many research efforts are currently taken to pave the way towards clinical CBCT- or MRI-guided (see chapter 7) online adaptive approaches.

References

Albrecht J *et al* 2022 Cone-beam CT from complete data using saddle trajectories on a mobile robotic CBCT scanner *Med. Phys.* **49** E123

Andersen A G, Park Y K, Elstrom U V, Petersen J B B, Sharp G C, Winey B, Dong L and Muren L P 2020 Evaluation of an *a priori* scatter correction algorithm for cone-beam computed tomography based range and dose calculations in proton therapy *Phys. Imaging Radiat. Oncol.* **16** 89–94

Antonuk L E 2002 Electronic portal imaging devices: a review and historical perspective of contemporary technologies and research *Phys. Med. Biol.* **47** R31–65

Arai K *et al* 2017 Feasibility of CBCT-based proton dose calculation using a histogram-matching algorithm in proton beam therapy *Phys. Med.* **33** 68–76

Balter J M and Kessler M L 2007 Imaging and alignment for image-guided radiation therapy *J. Clin. Oncol.* **25** 931–7

Bernier J, Hall E J and Giaccia A 2004 Radiation oncology: a century of achievements *Nat. Rev. Cancer* **4** 737–47

Biggs P J, Goitein M and Russell M D 1985 A diagnostic x ray field verification device for a 10 MV linear accelerator *Int. J. Radiat. Oncol. Biol. Phys.* **11** 635–43

Bondesson D *et al* 2022 Anthropomorphic lung phantom based validation of in-room proton therapy 4D-CBCT image correction for dose calculation *Z. Med. Phys.* **32** 74–84

Booth J T and Zavgorodni S F 2001 Modelling the dosimetric consequences of organ motion at CT imaging on radiotherapy treatment planning *Phys. Med. Biol.* **46** 1369–77

Bortfeld T R and Loeffler J S 2017 Three ways to make proton therapy affordable *Nature* **549** 451–3

Chow V U Y, Cheung M L M, Kan M W K and Chan A T C 2022 Shift detection discrepancy between ExacTrac Dynamic system and cone-beam computed tomography *J. Appl. Clin. Med. Phys.* **23** e13567

Christoffersen C P, Hansen D, Poulsen P and Sorensen T S 2013 Registration-based reconstruction of four-dimensional cone beam computed tomography *IEEE Trans. Med. Imaging* **32** 2064–77

Corradini S *et al* 2019 MR-guidance in clinical reality: current treatment challenges and future perspectives *Radiat. Oncol.* **14** 92

Dawson L A and Jaffray D A 2007 Advances in image-guided radiation therapy *J. Clin. Oncol.* **25** 938–46

de Jong R, Visser J, van Wieringen N, Wiersma J, Geijsen D and Bel A 2021 Feasibility of conebeam CT-based online adaptive radiotherapy for neoadjuvant treatment of rectal cancer *Radiat. Oncol.* **16** 136

den Otter L A, Chen K, Janssens G, Meijers A, Both S, Langendijk J A, Rosen L R, Wu H T and Knopf A C 2020 Technical note: 4D cone-beam CT reconstruction from sparse-view CBCT data for daily motion assessment in pencil beam scanned proton therapy (PBS-PT) *Med. Phys.* **47** 6381–7

Dhont J *et al* 2018 The long- and short-term variability of breathing induced tumor motion in lung and liver over the course of a radiotherapy treatment *Radiother. Oncol.* **126** 339–46

Dong G, Zhang C, Deng L, Zhu Y, Dai J, Song L, Meng R, Niu T, Liang X and Xie Y 2022 A deep unsupervised learning framework for the 4D CBCT artifact correction *Phys. Med. Biol.* **67** 055012

Engelsman M, Schwarz M and Dong L 2013 Physics controversies in proton therapy *Semin. Radiat. Oncol.* **23** 88–96

Fattori G *et al* 2015 Image guided particle therapy in CNAO room 2: implementation and clinical validation *Phys. Med.* **31** 9–15

Fotina I, Hopfgartner J, Stock M, Steininger T, Lutgendorf-Caucig C and Georg D 2012 Feasibility of CBCT-based dose calculation: comparative analysis of HU adjustment techniques *Radiother. Oncol.* **104** 249–56

Giacometti V, Hounsell A R and McGarry C K 2020 A review of dose calculation approaches with cone beam CT in photon and proton therapy *Phys. Med.* **76** 243–76

Gragoudas E S, Goitein M, Koehler A, Wagner M S, Verhey L, Tepper J, Suit H D, Schneider R J and Johnson K N 1979 Proton irradiation of malignant melanoma of the ciliary body *Br. J. Ophthalmol.* **63** 135–9

Habermehl D, Henkner K, Ecker S, Jakel O, Debus J and Combs S E 2013 Evaluation of different fiducial markers for image-guided radiotherapy and particle therapy *J. Radiat. Res.* **54** i61–8

Hansen D C, Landry G, Kamp F, Li M, Belka C, Parodi K and Kurz C 2018 ScatterNet: a convolutional neural network for cone-beam CT intensity correction *Med. Phys.* **45** 4916–26

Herman G T 1979 Correction for beam hardening in computed tomography *Phys. Med. Biol.* **24** 81–106

Hofmaier J *et al* 2017 Multi-criterial patient positioning based on dose recalculation on scatter-corrected CBCT images *Radiother. Oncol.* **125** 464–9

Hua C, Yao W, Kidani T, Tomida K, Ozawa S, Nishimura T, Fujisawa T, Shinagawa R and Merchant T E 2017 A robotic C-arm cone beam CT system for image-guided proton therapy: design and performance *Br. J. Radiol.* **90** 20170266

Jaffray D A, Siewerdsen J H, Wong J W and Martinez A A 2002 Flat-panel cone-beam computed tomography for image-guided radiation therapy *Int. J. Radiat. Oncol. Biol. Phys.* **53** 1337–49

Kamada T, Tsujii H, Mizoe J E, Matsuoka Y, Tsuji H, Osaka Y, Minohara S, Miyahara N, Endo M and Kanai T 1999 A horizontal CT system dedicated to heavy-ion beam treatment *Radiother. Oncol.* **50** 235–7

Kamino Y, Takayama K, Kokubo M, Narita Y, Hirai E, Kawawda N, Mizowaki T, Nagata Y, Nishidai T and Hiraoka M 2006 Development of a four-dimensional image-guided radiotherapy system with a gimbaled x-ray head *Int. J. Radiat. Oncol. Biol. Phys.* **66** 271–8

Keall P J *et al* 2022 Integrated MRI-guided radiotherapy—opportunities and challenges *Nat. Rev. Clin. Oncol.* **19** 458–70

Kida S, Nakamoto T, Nakano M, Nawa K, Haga A, Kotoku J, Yamashita H and Nakagawa K 2018 Cone beam computed tomography image quality improvement using a deep convolutional neural network *Cureus* **10** e2548

Kress J, Minohara S, Endo M, Debus J and Kanai T 1999 Patient position verification using CT images *Med. Phys.* **26** 941–8

Kurz C, Buizza G, Landry G, Kamp F, Rabe M, Paganelli C, Baroni G, Reiner M, Keall P J and van den Berg C A 2020 Medical physics challenges in clinical MR-guided radiotherapy *Radiat. Oncol.* **15** 16

Kurz C, Dedes G, Resch A, Reiner M, Ganswindt U, Nijhuis R, Thieke C, Belka C, Parodi K and Landry G 2015 Comparing cone-beam CT intensity correction methods for dose recalculation in adaptive intensity-modulated photon and proton therapy for head and neck cancer *Acta Oncol.* **54** 1651–7

Kurz C *et al* 2016a Investigating deformable image registration and scatter correction for CBCT-based dose calculation in adaptive IMPT *Med. Phys.* **43** 5635–46

Kurz C, Maspero M, Savenije M H F, Landry G, Kamp F, Pinto M, Li M, Parodi K, Belka C and van den Berg C A T 2019 CBCT correction using a cycle-consistent generative adversarial network and unpaired training to enable photon and proton dose calculation *Phys. Med. Biol.* **64** 225004

Kurz C, Nijhuis R, Reiner M, Ganswindt U, Thieke C, Belka C, Parodi K and Landry G 2016b Feasibility of automated proton therapy plan adaptation for head and neck tumors using cone beam CT images *Radiat. Oncol.* **11** 64

Landry G, Hansen D, Kamp F, Li M, Hoyle B, Weller J, Parodi K, Belka C and Kurz C 2019 Comparing Unet training with three different datasets to correct CBCT images for prostate radiotherapy dose calculations *Phys. Med. Biol.* **64** 035011

Landry G and Hua C H 2018 Current state and future applications of radiological image guidance for particle therapy *Med. Phys.* **45** e1086–e95

Landry G *et al* 2015 Investigating CT to CBCT image registration for head and neck proton therapy as a tool for daily dose recalculation *Med. Phys.* **42** 1354–66

Leong J 1986 Use of digital fluoroscopy as an on-line verification device in radiation therapy *Phys. Med. Biol.* **31** 985–92

Li H *et al* 2016 SU-F-J-188: clinical implementation of in room mobile CT for image guided Proton therapy *Med. Phys.* **43** 3451

Ling c c, Yorke E and Fuks Z 2006 From IMRT to IGRT: frontierland or neverland? *Radiother. Oncol.* **78** 119–22

MacKay R I 2018 Image guidance for proton therapy *Clin. Oncol. (R. Coll. Radiol.)* **30** 293–8

Mackie T R, Holmes T, Swerdloff S, Reckwerdt P, Deasy J O, Yang J, Paliwal B and Kinsella T 1993 Tomotherapy: a new concept for the delivery of dynamic conformal radiotherapy *Med. Phys.* **20** 1709–19

Mackie T R *et al* 2003 Image guidance for precise conformal radiotherapy *Int. J. Radiat. Oncol. Biol. Phys.* **56** 89–105

McCarter S D and Beckham W A 2000 Evaluation of the validity of a convolution method for incorporating tumour movement and set-up variations into the radiotherapy treatment planning system *Phys. Med. Biol.* **45** 923–31

Mori S, Sakata Y, Hirai R, Furuichi W, Shimabukuro K, Kohno R, Koom W S, Kasai S, Okaya K and Iseki Y 2019 Commissioning of a fluoroscopic-based real-time markerless tumor tracking system in a superconducting rotating gantry for carbon-ion pencil beam scanning treatment *Med. Phys.* **46** 1561–74

Mory C, Janssens G and Rit S 2016 Motion-aware temporal regularization for improved 4D cone-beam computed tomography *Phys. Med. Biol.* **61** 6856–77

Niepel K *et al* 2019 Feasibility of 4DCBCT-based proton dose calculation: an *ex vivo* porcine lung phantom study *Z. Med. Phys.* **29** 249–61

Niu T, Al-Basheer A and Zhu L 2012 Quantitative cone-beam CT imaging in radiation therapy using planning CT as a prior: first patient studies *Med. Phys.* **39** 1991–2000

Niu T, Sun M, Star-Lack J, Gao H, Fan Q and Zhu L 2010 Shading correction for on-board cone-beam CT in radiation therapy using planning MDCT images *Med. Phys.* **37** 5395–406

Ohnesorge B, Flohr T, Schwarz K, Heiken J P and Bae K T 2000 Efficient correction for CT image artifacts caused by objects extending outside the scan field of view *Med. Phys.* **27** 39–46

Oliver J A, Zeidan O A, Meeks S L, Shah A P, Pukala J, Kelly P, Ramakrishna N R and Willoughby T R 2017 The mobius AIRO mobile CT for image-guided proton therapy: characterization & commissioning *J. Appl. Clin. Med. Phys.* **18** 130–6

Park Y K, Sharp G C, Phillips J and Winey B A 2015 Proton dose calculation on scatter-corrected CBCT image: feasibility study for adaptive proton therapy *Med. Phys.* **42** 4449–59

Peroni M, Ciardo D, Spadea M F, Riboldi M, Comi S, Alterio D, Baroni G and Orecchia R 2012 Automatic segmentation and online virtualCT in head-and-neck adaptive radiation therapy *Int. J. Radiat. Oncol. Biol. Phys.* **84** e427–33

Poludniowski G, Evans P M, Kavanagh A and Webb S 2011 Removal and effects of scatter-glare in cone-beam CT with an amorphous-silicon flat-panel detector *Phys. Med. Biol.* **56** 1837–51

Rit S, Clackdoyle R, Keuschnigg P and Steininger P 2016 Filtered-backprojection reconstruction for a cone-beam computed tomography scanner with independent source and detector rotations *Med. Phys.* **43** 2344

Safai S, Bula C, Meer D and Pedroni E 2012 Improving the precision and performance of proton pencil beam scanning *Transl. Cancer Res.* **1** 196–206

Schmitz H *et al* 2021 Validation of proton dose calculation on scatter corrected 4D cone beam computed tomography using a porcine lung phantom *Phys. Med. Biol.* **66** 175022

Schmitz H, Rabe M, Janssens G, Rit S, Parodi K, Belka C, Kamp F, Landry G and Kurz C 2023a Scatter correction of 4D cone beam computed tomography to detect dosimetric effects due to anatomical changes in proton therapy for lung cancer *Med. Phys.* **50** 4981–92

Schmitz H, Thummerer A, Kawula M, Lombardo E, Parodi K, Belka C, Kamp F, Kurz C and Landry G 2023b ScatterNet for projection-based 4D cone-beam computed tomography intensity correction of lung cancer patients *Phys. Imaging Radiat. Oncol.* **27** 100482

Schulte R W and Li T 2006 Innovative strategies for image-guided proton treatment of prostate cancer *Technol. Cancer Res. Treat.* **5** 91–100

Shimizu S, Miyamoto N, Matsuura T, Fujii Y, Umezawa M, Umegaki K, Hiramoto K and Shirato H 2014 A proton beam therapy system dedicated to spot-scanning increases accuracy with moving tumors by real-time imaging and gating and reduces equipment size *PLoS One* **9** e94971

Shirato H *et al* 2000 Physical aspects of a real-time tumor-tracking system for gated radiotherapy *Int. J. Radiat. Oncol. Biol. Phys.* **48** 1187–95

Sibolt P, Andersson L M, Calmels L, Sjostrom D, Bjelkengren U, Geertsen P and Behrens C F 2021 Clinical implementation of artificial intelligence-driven cone-beam computed tomography-guided online adaptive radiotherapy in the pelvic region *Phys. Imaging Radia.t Oncol.* **17** 1–7

Siewerdsen J H and Jaffray D A 1999 Cone-beam computed tomography with a flat-panel imager: effects of image lag *Med. Phys.* **26** 2635–47

Siewerdsen J H and Jaffray D A 2001 Cone-beam computed tomography with a flat-panel imager: magnitude and effects of x-ray scatter *Med. Phys.* **28** 220–31

Slater J M, Archambeau J O, Miller D W, Notarus M I, Preston W and Slater J D 1992 The proton treatment center at Loma Linda University Medical Center: rationale for and description of its development *Int. J. Radiat. Oncol. Biol. Phys.* **22** 383–9

Thing R S, Bernchou U, Mainegra-Hing E, Hansen O and Brink C 2016 Hounsfield unit recovery in clinical cone beam CT images of the thorax acquired for image guided radiation therapy *Phys. Med. Biol.* **61** 5781–802

Thummerer A *et al* 2022 Deep learning-based 4D-synthetic CTs from sparse-view CBCTs for dose calculations in adaptive proton therapy *Med. Phys.* **49** 6824–39

van Herk M, Remeijer P and Lebesque J V 2002 Inclusion of geometric uncertainties in treatment plan evaluation *Int. J. Radiat. Oncol. Biol. Phys.* **52** 1407–22

Veiga C *et al* 2016 First clinical investigation of cone beam computed tomography and Deformable registration for adaptive proton therapy for lung cancer *Int. J. Radiat. Oncol. Biol. Phys.* **95** 549–59

Veiga C, McClelland J, Moinuddin S, Lourenco A, Ricketts K, Annkah J, Modat M, Ourselin S, D'Souza D and Royle G 2014 Toward adaptive radiotherapy for head and neck patients: Feasibility study on using CT-to-CBCT deformable registration for 'dose of the day' calculations *Med. Phys.* **41** 031703

Verellen D, De Ridder M and Storme G 2008 A (short) history of image-guided radiotherapy *Radiother. Oncol.* **86** 4–13

Verhey L J, Goitein M, McNulty P, Munzenrider J E and Suit H D 1982 Precise positioning of patients for radiation therapy *Int. J. Radiat. Oncol. Biol. Phys.* **8** 289–94

Wolthaus J W, Sonke J J, van Herk M and Damen E M 2008 Reconstruction of a time-averaged midposition CT scan for radiotherapy planning of lung cancer patients using deformable registration *Med. Phys.* **35** 3998–4011

Xing L, Thorndyke B, Schreibmann E, Yang Y, Li T F, Kim G Y, Luxton G and Koong A 2006 Overview of image-guided radiation therapy *Med. Dosim.* **31** 91–112

Yoshimura T *et al* 2020 Analysis of treatment process time for real-time-image gated-spot-scanning proton-beam therapy (RGPT) system *J. Appl. Clin. Med. Phys.* **21** 38–49

Zechner A, Stock M, Kellner D, Ziegler I, Keuschnigg P, Huber P, Mayer U, Sedlmayer F, Deutschmann H and Steininger P 2016 Development and first use of a novel cylindrical ball bearing phantom for 9-DOF geometric calibrations of flat panel imaging devices used in image-guided ion beam therapy *Phys. Med. Biol.* **61** N592–605

IOP Publishing

Imaging in Particle Therapy
Current practice and future trends
Chiara Paganelli, Chiara Gianoli and Antje Knopf

Chapter 6

Ion imaging in particle therapy

C Gianoli, J Bortfeldt and R Schulte

6.1 Introduction

Direct range verification techniques are based on phenomena pertaining to the primary therapeutic radiation[1]. Ion imaging falls into this description, as based on the transmission of the primary beam. If ion beams have sufficient energy to traverse the object of interest, the tissue stopping properties can be retrieved by measuring the residual energy or the energy losses of energetic ions passing through the object of interest by means of dedicated detectors. Ion imaging can in principle enable direct assessment of the tissue stopping power and its variations due to inter-fractional anatomical changes. For this reason, ion imaging is not only an imaging technique for treatment verification, but its role is fundamentally relevant to treatment planning and adaptation in ion beam therapy. Ion imaging systems are approaching commercialization, and an increasing number of groups worldwide are currently investigating different ion imaging technologies and methodologies in perspective of clinical application (Meijers *et al* 2021).

6.2 Detector technologies in ion imaging

Ion imaging exploits the measured, spatially resolved energy loss of charged ions that traverse the object to be imaged. Particle path information is obtained by spatially resolving detectors, typically in front of and behind the object. Prototype imaging systems have been realized that only feature a rear tracking station (Bucciantonio *et al* 2013) or that use averaged pencil beam position information from the beam delivery system (Rinaldi *et al* 2014). These systems, however, offer a considerably worse spatial resolution, as the resulting particle scattering in the object cannot be experimentally assessed. The energy loss inside the object is usually determined by subtracting the measured residual energy or range of the transmitted

---

[1] *Ionoacoustic and electromagnetometry, based on the measurement of the acoustic and electromagnetic fields respectively, are emerging techniques that can also be referred to as direct range verification techniques.

doi:10.1088/978-0-7503-5117-1ch6

particles from the known initial particle energy. Subject to the availability of large-area high-temporal resolution detectors, the residual energy can also be determined by measuring the time of flight (TOF) and thus the velocity of transmitted particles (Krah *et al* 2022, Ulrich-Pur *et al* 2022). Complementary image information to the relative stopping power can be obtained with multiple high-spatial-resolution tracking stages upstream and downstream of the imaged object, by assessing the scattering angle, referred to as scattering power, of transmitted ions (Taylor *et al* 2016).

6.2.1 Particle detector physics: interaction mechanisms and observables

In line with the two major energy loss processes (i.e., excitation and ionization), two principal particle detector classes can be distinguished: (1) detectors exploiting the production of light from the subsequent de-excitation and recombination, and (2) detectors exploiting the production of charge.

6.2.1.1 Charged-based detectors

In charge-based detectors the charge carriers, produced by ionization processes inside the detector's active volume with thickness d, are separated by an electric field. The resulting currents (for an in-depth discussion see e.g., Riegler 2016) can be measured on electrodes, adjacent to the active volume, typically by a charge integrating readout electronics. The total energy loss of the particle $\Delta E = dE/dx.d$ is proportional to the measured charge $Q = (dE/dx.d)/W_I$, where W_I is the average energy lost per created electron–ion pair. W_I only has a very weak particle energy dependence. The electrodes are typically segmented in pixels or strips, but non-segmented electrodes are also possible.

Ionization chambers (ICs) are the simplest representative of this detector class. Two electrodes sandwich a volume, filled with gas, typically a noble gas-based mixture or air. A high voltage applied to one of the electrodes creates an electric field of typically 1 kV cm^{-1}. Upon passage of an ionizing particle, the created electrons and positive ions drift within approximately 200 ns and 200 µs, respectively, towards the electrodes, where they are neutralized. A single 200 MeV proton, e.g., would produce in a typically 6 mm wide ionization gap, filled with air, order of 85 electron–ion pairs (Berger *et al* 2005). This small amount of charge is very challenging to measure, such that ICs are typically used for integrating particle beam detection, rather than for individual particles.

As the energy loss per unit path of charged particles is proportional to the density of the detection material, the ionization charge produced in solid state detectors is by approximately three orders of magnitude larger than in gaseous detectors and thus directly measurable. Silicon-based semiconductor detectors combine the additional advantage of small $W_I = 3.65$ eV (Workman *et al* 2022) with the possibility to create finely segmented electrode structures and integrated amplification elements by doping and photo-lithographical structuring. A 200 MeV proton produces accordingly in a typically 300 µm thick active layer of a silicon strip detector a directly measurable charge of 6.9×10^4 electron–hole pairs (Berger *et al* 2005). Gaseous detectors with single particle sensitivity contain narrow high electric field regions, in which the ionization electrons are sufficiently accelerated, to create further electron–ion pairs in collisions with gas atoms/molecules. In these electron avalanches a so-called gas gain of order 10^4 is reachable.

6.2.1.2 Light-based detectors

Scintillation detectors exploit the production of visible or ultra-violet (UV) light from de-excitation and charge recombination after the passage of a charged particle. Similar to charge-based detectors, the deposited energy inside the scintillator with thickness d is related to the produced number of photons $N_\gamma = (dE/dx.d)/W_\gamma$, where W_γ describes the necessary energy for the production of one photon and is typically of order 100 eV. Especially in regions with high energy loss dE/dx, e.g., towards the end of the particle range, W_γ can increase considerably, as non-radiative de-excitation becomes more dominant. Two different classes with characteristic behavior exist: organic scintillators with lower density and inorganic scintillators with high density, larger atomic number and accordingly larger stopping power.

The most widespread organic scintillators are solid plastic and liquid scintillators, consisting of molecules with aromatic structure. As scintillators are not transparent for their own scintillation light, at least two fluorophores are added, that successively absorb the primary scintillation light in the UV range and re-emit it at longer wavelengths in the visible range. As the energy loss is converted to light within individual molecules, the rise and decay times are typically in the order of nano-seconds, thus enabling a considerable rate capability. Plastic scintillators can be cast, machined or extruded to almost arbitrary shape. A moderate segmentation in e.g., millimeter diameter fibers, allows, depending on the arrangement of several fiber layers, for constructing also position sensitive tracking detectors.

Inorganic scintillators are crystals that either scintillate by themselves, such as Barium Fluoride (BaF_2), or a doped with an additional element for enhanced light yield e.g., cesium iodide, doped with thallium (CsI:Tl). Due to their production method, inorganic scintillators are limited in size, often hygroscopic and fairly expensive. Traditional materials such as CsI:Tl or bismuth germanate (BGO) have relatively long signal decay times of 1.2 μs and 300 ns, respectively, and thus limited rate capability. In recent years other materials with high light yield and considerably shorter decay time have been developed, e.g., cerium doped lanthanum bromide ($LaBr_3$:Ce) with 20 ns decay time (for an overview of inorganic scintillators and their properties see e.g., table 35.4 in Workman *et al* 2022).

Inherent for all scintillators is that they need to be interfaced by a light detector, that converts a fraction of the produced visible light to a voltage signal, proportional to the number of collected photons. Vacuum photomultiplier tubes (PMTs) contain a photocathode of a material with high atomic number and low work function. Visible photons produce electrons by photo-effect on the cathode. These are repeatedly accelerated by an electric field onto so-called dynodes, where each impacting electron liberates two to six additional electrons. In vacuum tubes with 8–12 dynodes, high-voltage dependent amplification factors between 10^5 and 10^7 are reached. The multiplied electrons are collected by an anode. Multi-anode photomultipliers feature separated anode pads and an at least partially separated dynode structure in the same tube, thus enabling an individual readout of a larger number of scintillators. Avalanche photodiodes (APDs) are solid state detectors, combining n- and p-type semiconducting regions. They are reversed biased via the p-n-junction. Electrons, liberated inside the charge-depleted silicon by impinging optical photons, are accelerated inside the thus created electric field and can create order of 100 additional electrons. APDs thus have a moderate photon sensitivity and are typically cooled during operation. Low gain avalanche detectors (LGADs) are variants of APDs and are operated at moderate gains of order 10. When traversed by an ionizing particle, the ionization electrons are amplified in avalanches, resulting in an excellent timing resolution of order 25 ps. Current challenges are the available size, segmentation and radiation hardness (Cartiglia *et al* 2017, Carulla *et al* 2019). Order of 1000 APDs operated in Geiger-mode, i.e., at a reverse bias voltage few volts above the breakdown voltage of the p-n-junction, can be combined to mm^2-sized silicon photomultipliers (SiPMs). A single optical photon that produces a photoelectron in one of the APD cells, creates an electron avalanche and leads to a breakdown of the field in that cell. The avalanche is interrupted, when the cell voltage over an internal quenching resistor falls below the breakdown threshold. The mV signal amplitude is independent of the number of primary photoelectrons produced in the specific cell. By internally summing the quasi-digital output of all APD cells in the SiPM, the overall amplitude is proportional to the number of impinging photons, provided that a considerable fraction is absorbed in a sufficiently small number of different cells. Production of SiPMs is very cost effective and recent improvements have considerably decreased the spontaneously created single-electron noise rate from originally order of 100 kHz.

6.2.2 Detector technologies for ion imaging

6.2.2.1 *Tracking detector technology*

Two-dimensional position information in a single module can be obtained in double-sided silicon strip detectors with perpendicular readout strips on both sides. Alternatively, single-sided silicon strip detectors can be arranged perpendicularly or in triplet configurations with 60° mutual rotation. Also pixelized semiconductor detectors are possible, at the cost of quadratically increased readout channel count. Depending on the strip/pixel pitch, a spatial resolution as low as 10 μm is realistic.

Micro-pattern gaseous detectors combine the high segmentation of semiconductor detectors with an inherently low material budget and the possibility to construct large area detectors. This reduces the internal multiple scattering and avoids dead regions or layer overlaps, necessary in semiconductor detectors, which feature a typical module size of 10×10 cm^2. Thus, distortions of the measured particle trajectory and artifacts in the reconstructed image are mitigated. The small ionization charge in mm-wide gas layers needs to be internally amplified in narrow regions with high electric fields of order 50 kV cm^{-1} by gas electron avalanches. Suitable Gas Electron Multiplier (GEM) foils consist of few micrometers thick copper structures, separated by an insulating Polyimide foil of typically 50 μm thickness (Sauli 1997), into which O(80 μm) holes with a periodicity O(150 μm) have been etched. Applying a voltage of several 100 V between the two conductive sides of a GEM foil leads to considerable gas electron amplification inside the GEM holes and an efficient collection of equally produced positive ions renders GEM foils high-rate capable. Typically, three to four GEM foils are stacked above the segmented readout structure, the GEM copper electrodes are supplied individually with high-voltage via a resistor chain or an active voltage divider. Overall gas gains above 10^4 are stably possible, constant even at fluences of $10^6 \, \mathrm{mm}^{-1} \, \mathrm{s}^{-1}$ (Benlloch *et al* 1998). Other amplification structures such as Micromegas [Micromesh Gaseous Structure, (Giomataris *et al* 1996)] are under investigation for ion imaging applications (e.g., Bortfeldt *et al* 2017, Meyer *et al* 2020). Electron amplification can also be realized in the radially increasing field around stretched metallic wires with diameters O (20 μm). Spatial resolution can be obtained in multi-wire proportional chambers (MWPCs) by individually reading out signals from two perpendicular layers of wires with O(2 mm) spacing.

Combining hundreds of scintillating plastic fibers (SciFis) with O(1 mm^2) cross section each, closely spaced into layers, allows to use fast scintillation detectors as tracking stages in front of and behind the imaged object. Typically, at least two shifted layers of SciFis are used for each measurement dimension, to improve the quite coarse segmentation and mitigate the challenging light collection at the end of the fibers. This layer stacking is however limited by the considerable material budget of SciFis, which can significantly distort the particle trajectories, especially for the low energy, downstream particles. Fibers can be smartly grouped and read-out from both sides to considerably reduce the number of multi-anode PMT channels or SiPMs, used to convert the visible light into electronic signals.

6.2.2.2 Energy detector technology

Contrast information in ion imaging stems from a determination of the integral energy loss of individual or a collection of particles inside the imaged object. For transmitted ions with known initial energy, it is obtained by measuring either the residual energy calorimetrically or the residual range in a multi-layer range telescope. Alternatively, the residual momentum or energy of the transmitted particles can be determined in thin detectors with good energy loss measurement capabilities, by tracking the bent particle trajectory in a magnetic field (Takada *et al* 1988) or by measuring their velocity in detector pairs with good temporal resolution (Ulrich-Pur *et al* 2022).

Monolithic inorganic scintillators with high light yield enable a reliable calorimetric determination of the residual energy. Due to their high density and thus high stopping power, a moderate calorimeter thickness of order 15 cm is sufficient for e.g., 230 MeV protons, that can be read out with one or several light detectors. Limited transverse size however restricts the active area of the calorimeter, if transverse stitching and corresponding image artifacts are to be avoided.

This issue can be avoided in plastic or liquid organic scintillators. Due to their lower stopping power, thicknesses of order 35 cm are necessary. If additional position information is desired in the calorimeter, thick bundles of scintillator fibers can be used.

Calorimeters need to be calibrated to residual energy or to water equivalent path length (WEPL) of the transmitted particles. This calibration can either rely on scanning the particle energy with the clinical accelerator, thus injecting particles with well defined energy into the calorimeter, or on degrading the monoenergetic particle beam with materials of known water equivalent thickness (WET). It needs to be regularly repeated, due to non-stable environmental conditions, that impact the amount of produced and detected visible light. If the calorimeter has a lateral dependence of the light output, calibration is necessary for different lateral positions, which can render the procedure tedious (e.g., Bashkirov *et al* 2016b, Scaringella *et al* 2023).

Calibration issues can be largely mitigated in multi-layer range detectors. The WEPL resolution is not limited by the thickness of the range detector layers, if the WET of individual layers is lower than the range straggling of delivered ions, which corresponds to 1.1% of total range in water (Bashkirov *et al* 2016b). For clinical beams of highest available energy, this corresponds to approximately 3 mm. Fully active range detectors can consist of e.g., order of 100 optically insulated, 3 mm thick plastic scintillator plates. Wavelength shifting (WLS) fibers, optically coupled to the edges of the plates, help guiding the optical photons to light detectors. Sampling range detectors instead contain passive absorbers of approximately 3 mm WET, alternating with active layers, in which the particle passage is registered. These active layers can be simple detectors such as ICs, which are then however not able to detect individual particles or, e.g., highly-segmented silicon detectors, providing good multi-hit capability. If the layer thickness is well controlled, the calibration of range detectors is long-term stable. If the sensitive layers only register the presence of particles however, without a measure of their respective energy loss, the range determination for those particles, that lose a considerable fraction of their energy in less frequent nuclear interactions, or that laterally scatter out of the range detector, is error prone. Their range is systematically misestimated as too short. Also, hybrid range calorimeters with only few layers are used, that combine a range measurement with a registration of the deposited energy in each or only in the last hit layer.

6.2.3 Detector systems for ion imaging

In the following section, actually realized prototypes and concept studies of ion radiography and tomography scanners will be listed (figure 6.1 and tables 6.1–6.3). Further information needs to be found in the respective publications.

6.2.3.1 Full tracking detector systems
The development of full tracking systems, also referred to as list-mode detector configuration, has been pioneered by the Paul Scherrer Institute in Villigen and later

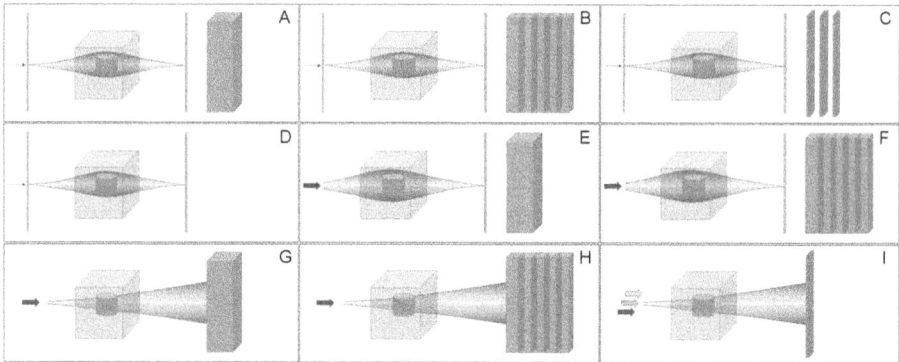

Figure 6.1. Schematic of the list-mode prototypes: double tracking (A, B, C, D) and single tracking (rear, E, F) and integration-mode prototypes (G, H, I). In red the object of interest, blue the beam (broad beam or pencil beams), green the energy detector and yellow the tracking detector.

the Ludwig-Maximilians-Universität in Munich. Two hodoscopes, consisting of four layers of perpendicular 2×2 mm^2 SciFis each, measured particle position upstream and downstream of the imaged object. Two SciFi layers inside each hodoscope were directly adjacent and shifted by half pitch to increase the effective segmentation per dimension to 1 mm. The residual range detector consisted of 3 mm thick plastic scintillator tiles, coupled to wavelength shifting fibers (WLS). The WLS and the smartly grouped SciFis were read out by ten 16 channel PMTs. The system was able to register 10^6 protons/s (Pemler *et al* 1999, Schneider *et al* 2004). Conceptual studies had been performed on an earlier prototype system, combining a particle position measurement each in a MWPC up- and down- stream of the object with the calorimetric residual energy detection in an inorganic sodium iodide (NaI) scintillator. The system had limited rate capability of 1 kHz and limited energy acceptance, necessitating energy scanning of the imaging beam (Schneider and Pedroni 1995).

The currently most capable imaging system, measuring particle track position and direction upstream and downstream the object, is the so-called Phase-II scanner, developed by the US pCT collaboration[2]. Each tracking module consists of four layers of single-sided silicon strip detectors, and each layer contains four individual and closely spaced sensors with 9×9 cm^2 active area. Two layers, with strips oriented vertically and horizontally, respectively, are mounted back-to-back, forming a double-layer with 2D resolution. The two double layers inside each tracking module are spaced by 50 mm. In the Phase-II scanner, a hybrid five-layer calorimetric range detectors consisting of five plastic scintillators and read out by a PMT each substitutes a cesium iodide (CsI) calorimeter (Sadrozinski *et al* 2004). The system allows for a particle rate of order 1 MHz (Johnson *et al* 2015, Bashkirov *et al* 2016a).

---

[2] http://scipp.ucsc.edu/pCT/

Table 6.1. Overview of list-mode prototypes (double tracking).

Schematic	Project/prototype	Tracking detector technology		Energy detector technology		Imaging
		Entrance position	Exit position	Absorption detectors	Light to charge/ voltage converter	
Figure 6.1(A)	Paul Scherrer Institute	Multi-wire proportional chambers	Multi-wire proportional chambers	Plastic scintillating counter (trigger) and NaI crystal scintillating calorimeter	Photomultiplier tubes	Back-projection (Schneider and Pedroni 1995)
Figure 6.1(B)	Paul Scherrer Institute	Plastic scintillating fibre	Plastic scintillating fibre	Range telescope (stack of plastic scintillator tiles)	Photomultiplier tubes	Radiography (Pemler et al 1999)
Figure 6.1(A)	Loma Linda University (LLU), University of California Santa Cruz (UCSC) and Northern Illinois University (NIU)	Silicon strip detectors	Silicon strip detectors	CsI crystal calorimeter	Photomultiplier tubes	Analytical and numerical tomographic image reconstruction (Schulte et al 2004)
Figure 6.1(B)	Loma Linda University (LLU), University of California Santa Cruz (UCSC) and Northern Illinois University (NIU)			Hybrid range detector/ calorimeter stack of plastic scintillator blocks	Photomultiplier tubes	Analytical and numerical tomographic image reconstruction (Bashkirov et al 2016a)
Figure 6.1(C)	INFN and INAF (Cagliari and Catania), PREDATE	Scintillating fibres	Scintillating fibres	Scintillating fibres	Silicon photomultiplier array	Hardware prototype (Lo Presti et al 2014)

Figure	Institution	Tracker	Tracker	Range/Calorimeter	Readout	Type
Figure 6.1(B)	NICADD/NIU, FNAL, Dehli	Scintillating fibres	Scintillating fibres	Range telescope (stack of plastic scintillatortiles)	Silicon photomultipliers (tracker), photomultiplier tubes (range)	Hardware prototype (Naimuddin et al 2016)
Figure 6.1(A)	INFN (Firenze and Catania), PRIMA	Silicon strip trackers	Silicon strip trackers	YAG;Ce crystal calorimeter	Silicon photodiodes	Hardware prototype (Scaringella et al 2013)
						Analytical image reconstruction (Scaringella et al 2023)
Figure 6.1(A)	Niigata University, Japan	Silicon strip trackers	Silicon strip trackers	Crystal calorimeter	Photomultiplier tube	Hardware prototype (Saraya et al 2014)
Figure 6.1(C)	University of Liverpool, Universities of Birmingham, Lincoln and Surrey, University Hospitals in Birmingham and Coventry, and iThemba Laboratories in Cape Town, South Africa (PraVDA consortium)	Silicon strip detectors	Silicon strip detectors	Silicon strip detectors + PMMA absorbers	—	Hardware prototype (Esposito et al 2018)
Figure 6.1(A)		Silicon strip detectors	Silicon strip detectors	Segmented scintillators (foreseen)	—	Hardware prototype (Winter et al 2023)

(Continued)

Table 6.1. (*Continued*)

Schematic	Project/prototype	Tracking detector technology		Energy detector technology		Imaging
		Entrance position	Exit position	Absorption detectors	Light to charge/voltage converter	
Figure 6.1(B)	Universities of Birmingham, Institut de Fisica d'Altes Energies (IFAE), Barcelona, University of Geneva	Position sensitive detectors (CMOS/DMAPS)	Position sensitive detectors (CMOS/DMAPS)	Range telescope as stack of plastic scintillator bars	Silicon photomultiplier array	Hardware prototype (Granado-González et al 2022)
Figure 6.1(B)	University of Padova, in collaboration with INFN (Padova and Trento) and CERN	Position sensitive detectors (CMOS/MAPS)	Position sensitive detectors (CMOS/MAPS)	Range telescope as stack of plastic scintillator bars	Silicon photomultipliers	Hardware prototype (Baruffaldi et al 2018)
Figure 6.1(D)	Austrian Academy of Sciences, TU Wien	LGAD timing/tracking station	LGAD timing/tracking station	Time-of-flight (TOF) measurement between 4D-tracking stations	—	Analytical tomographic image reconstruction (Ulrich-Pur et al 2022)

Table 6.2. Overview of list-mode prototypes (single tracking or rear tracking).

Schematic	Project/prototype	Tracking detector technology		Energy detector technology		Imaging
		Entrance position	Exit position	Absorption detectors	Light to charge/voltage converter	
Figure 6.1(A)	Lawrence Berkeley Laboratory, California	Multi-wire proportional chambers	—	Range telescope as a stack of scintillating counters	Photomultiplier tubes	Analytical and numerical tomographic image reconstruction (helium ions) (Crowe *et al* 1975)
Figure 6.1(E) (earlier experiments), figure 6.1(F) (later experiments)	University of California, Los Alamos Scientific Laboratory	—	Multi-wire proportional chambers	Crystal scintillating calorimeter (earlier experiments), range telescope as stack of plastic scintillators (later experiments)	Photomultiplier tubes	Analytical tomographic image reconstruction (protons) (Hanson 1979)
Figure 6.1(F)	Bergen pCT collaboration	—	Multiple layers of pixelated silicon detectors (CMOS/APS)	Multiple layers of pixelated silicon detectors (CMOS/APS)	—	Radiography (Pettersen *et al* 2017)
		—	Multiple layers of pixelated silicon detectors (ALPIDE)	Multiple layers of pixelated silicon detectors (ALPIDE) + aluminium absorbers	—	Radiography (Alme *et al* 2020)

(*Continued*)

Table 6.2. (*Continued*)

Schematic	Project/prototype	Tracking detector technology		Energy detector technology		Imaging
		Entrance position	Exit position	Absorption detectors	Light to charge/ voltage converter	
Figure 6.1(F)	INFN and INAF (Cagliari and Catania)	—	Scintillating fibres	Scintillating fibres	Silicon photomultiplier array	Hardware prototype (Lo Presti *et al* 2016)
Figure 6.1(F)	CERN and Tera foundation	—	Gas electron multipliers (GEMs)	Range telescope as stack of plastic scintillator tiles	Silicon photomultipliers	Hardware prototype (Amaldi *et al* 2011)

Table 6.3. Overview of integration-mode prototypes.

Schematic	Project/prototype	Energy detector technology		Imaging
		Absorption detectors	Light to charge/voltage converter	
Figure 6.1(G)	Harvard University	Photographic film	—	First radiography (broad beam) (Koehler Science 1968)
Figure 6.1(G)	Harvard University, Tufts University	Crystal scintillating counter	Photomultiplier tubes	First tomography, analytical image reconstruction (broad beam) (Cormack and Koehler Phys. Med. Biol. 1976)
Figure 6.1(H)	Heidelberg University Hospital, Heidelberg Ion Therapy Center, GSI Helmholtz Center for Heavy Ion Research	Range telescope as a stack of plastic absorption tiles	Ionization chambers	Numerical tomographic image reconstruction based on numerical decomposition of the integrated signal of each pencil beams (Magallanes et al 2019)
Figure 6.1(I)	Heidelberg University Hospital, Heidelberg Ion Therapy Center, German Cancer Research Center	Pixelated (commercial) silicon detector	—	Analytical tomographic image reconstruction based on passive and active energy variations of the pencil beams (Telsemeyer et al 2012)
Figure 6.1(I)	Massachusetts General Hospital, Harvard University Medical School	Pixelated (commercial) silicon detector	—	Numerical tomographic image reconstruction based on passive energy variations of broad beam (Testa et al 2013)
Figure 6.1(I)	Ludwig-Maximilians-Universität München	Pixelated (commercial) silicon detector	—	Radiography (Würl et al 2022)
Figure 6.1(I)	Ludwig-Maximilians-Universität München	Pixelated silicon detectors (CMOS)	—	Radiography (Schnürle et al 2023)
Figure 6.1(G)	The University of Texas MD Anderson Cancer CenterF	Monolithic plastic scintillator	Optical cameras	Radiography (Darne et al 2022)

ProtonVDA LLC[3] has developed the only non-academic scanner. It is a compact device, using two tracking modules with four directly adjacent layers of 1 mm^2 scintillating fibers each, two oriented vertically and two horizontally, to determine proton position upstream and downstream of the imaged object. Always two layers are displaced by half pitch; the SciFis are read out by SiPMs. Residual energy is determined in a 40×40 cm^2 plastic scintillator block with sensitive thickness of only 10 cm, coupled to 16 PMTs. Due to aggressive SciFi grouping and the reduced calorimeter thickness, the device relies on imaging radiation delivered by a pencil beam treatment plan, featuring several energy layers (DeJongh *et al* 2021). A direct comparison of Phase-II and ProtonVDA scanner can be found in Dedes *et al* (2022).

The PRaVDA collaboration[4] has developed a high rate-capable, all-silicon prototype system with upstream and downstream tracking stations featuring six single-layer silicon strip detectors each. The sampling range detector uses the same silicon strip detectors, interleaved with 2 mm PMMA plates and has a limited energy range of 30–80 MeV (Esposito *et al* 2018). The efforts are continued by the OPTIma project[5], aiming for a tracker with a total of 12 single-sided silicon strip detectors, based on the ATLAS Inner Tracker (ITk) sensors (ATLAS Collaboration 2017), followed by a calorimeter of segmented scintillators (Winter *et al* 2023).

The Istituto Nazionale di Fisica Nucleare (INFN) scanner features a four-layer tracker. Each 20×5 cm^2 layer consists of eight 5×5 cm^2 single-sided silicon strip modules, glued back-to-back to provide 2D position information. Residual energy is measured in a 10 cm deep calorimeter, consisting of 2×7 YAG:Ce scintillators of 3×3 cm^2 cross section, interfaced by SiPMs. Due to the relatively long signal and shaping time of the calorimeter, the readout rate is below 100 kHz (Scaringella *et al* 2023).

A collaboration of Northern Illinois University (USA), Fermi National Accelerator Laboratory (USA) and University of Delhi (India) developed a 2 MHz rate capable scanner, foreseen to be gantry-mountable. The tracker consists of 0.5 mm diameter SciFis. Four layers are arranged into a tracking module with 2D position information, and two tracking modules upstream and downstream of the object provide position and direction information. 96 layers of 3.2 mm thick plastic scintillator, as the trackers interfaced by SiPMs, provide the residual range information (Naimuddin *et al* 2016). The collaboration funding ended before remaining issues with defective SiPMs and the self-triggered DAQ system could be resolved (Johnson 2017).

The iMPACT project[6] aims at developing a scanner, capable of handling 10^9 particles per second. The tracker should consist of monolithic active pixel sensors. For prototyping the ALPIDE sensor, originally developed for the inner tracker of ALICE, CERN, has been selected. The segmented calorimeter is envisaged to employ rectangular fingers of plastic scintillator, individually coupled to SiPMs

---

[3] https://protonvda.com/
[4] https://www.liverpool.ac.uk/particle-physics/experiments/pravda/
[5] https://gow.epsrc.ukri.org/NGBOViewGrant.aspx?GrantRef=EP/R023220/1
[6] https://cordis.europa.eu/project/id/6490311

(Baruffaldi *et al* 2018). In a concept study, only able to image small animal sizes, Timepix semiconductor detectors have been used as readout structure for gaseous Time Projection Chambers. The calorimeter is a BaF_2 crystal, coupled to a PMT (Biegun *et al* 2015).

6.2.3.2 Rear tracking detector systems

Several prototype scanners with only a downstream tracking and range station have been developed. The main advantage is the reduced complexity, thus potentially facilitating clinical integration, at the cost of reduced image quality.

The TERA foundation developed in the AQUA project an imaging device with[7], an imaging device with a 30×30 cm^2 active area and 1 MHz rate capable DAQ system. Position and direction of transmitted particles are determined in two triple-GEM detectors with 2D-readout. The residual range is measured in 48 layers of 3.2 mm thick plastic scintillators, each coupled via a WLS fiber to a single SiPM (Bucciantonio *et al* 2013).

An all-silicon imaging device has been proposed by the Bergen pCT collaboration[8]. The two downstream tracking layers and the 41 layers in the sampling range detector are formed by 108 ALPIDE sensors each, developed for the inner tracker of the ALICE experiment, CERN. The only difference between tracking and range detector layers is the sensor backing material: 0.2 mm thick carbon-epoxy sandwich structures and 3.5 mm aluminum, respectively (Alme *et al* 2020).

On a much smaller scale, suited only for small animal imaging, a system based on Timepix3 sensors has been developed. The position of transmitted particles is measured in several pixelized sensors, and the residual energy is determined from the measured particle energy loss inside each pixel (Würl *et al* 2020).

Equally suitable for small animal imaging, both with respect to active area and possible particle energy, is a full-SciFi imaging system. Four layers of 0.5×0.5 mm^2 SciFis, two oriented in the same direction, measure the position of transmitted particles. Smart grouping reduces the necessary number of SiPMs for fiber readout. The range detector consists of 60 layers of the same SciFis, coupled layer-wise with two WLS fibers to a SiPM (Lo Presti *et al* 2016).

6.2.3.3 Particle integrating detector systems

Systems with further reduced complexity are built to register the mean residual range or energy of an ensemble of particles referred to as integration-mode detector configuration. While these systems can be cost effective and relatively straightforward in analysis, the imaging dose is considerably higher than in single particle tracking systems.

An ion imaging system, completely omitting spatially resolving detectors has been realized based on a 30×30 cm^2 sampling multi-layer ion chamber. The spatial information is instead provided by the clinical beam delivery and monitoring system. 61 3 mm thick PMMA absorbers, alternating with 6 mm wide planar, air-filled ICs,

---

[7] https://project-aqua.web.cern.ch/home.html
[8] https://www.uib.no/en/ift/1423566/medical-physics-bergen-pct-project

determine the average range of typically 100 or more particles per spot. While the system has the major advantage to use clinically available beam parameters, the resolution, especially at interfaces between different materials, is only moderate (Rinaldi *et al* 2014). More recent results have been reported from a similar system, using a commercial multi-layer-IC (Krah *et al* 2018).

A spatially resolving particle integrating system has been realized by combining liquid organic scintillator, contained in an acrylic cube (20 cm side length), with a cooled charge-coupled-device (CCD) camera. The camera registers the scintillation light production in beam direction via a 45° mirror. The amount of scintillation light in each pixel can be calibrated to average energy loss (Darne *et al* 2019). The concept can be extended to a plastic scintillator system with multiple camera view directions (Darne *et al* 2022).

The above-mentioned integrating systems operate with monoenergetic scanned pencil beams. If, alternatively, the particle energy is scanned, integrating particle imaging systems can be realized with a single layer of pixelized, energy-loss sensitive detectors. Each pixel measures an increasing energy loss, i.e., signal amplitude, as the beam energy is decreased. When the particle range is smaller than the WET of the object upstream of the respective pixel, the measured amplitude drops to zero. These amplitude-energy relations can be calibrated to WET.

A commercial diode-array detector, consisting of 249 semiconductor diodes at 7 mm pitch, has been used to record the temporal variation of dose per pixel, created by a quickly spinning moderator wheel. Although limited in spatial resolution, the system is very fast and in principle able to image moving structures (Testa *et al* 2013).

A similar concept, using energy modulation by active beam delivery, has been realized with a commercial CMOS pixel detector. Its size of 11.4×6.5 cm 2 is sufficient for small animal imaging. Due to the small pixel pitch of 49.5 μm, the achievable spatial resolution is competitive (Schnürle *et al* 2023).

6.3 Methodological fundamentals and detector configurations for ion imaging

Although the current clinical workflow in ion beam therapy is based on x-ray imaging, the native imaging technique for ion beam therapy is ion imaging (Parodi 2014, Johnson 2017). The most promising prototypes for ion imaging are conceived as 'list-mode' detectors (Schneider and Pedroni 1995, Pemler *et al* 1999, Sadrozinski *et al* 2004, Schulte *et al* 2004, Bashkirov *et al* 2016a). This detector configuration is typically based on the synchronization of a residual energy detector with a tracking system. Individual ions are therefore tracked and fully or partially absorbed. The energy detector can be designed either as a thick absorber measuring the residual energy or the energy loss and thus, the range of the ion traversing the object of interest (section 6.2). The tracking system typically consists of thin trackers upstream and downstream of the object of interest (ref. Detector technologies in ion imaging). With pencil beam scanning systems, the upstream tracking can be also removed. Fast tracking systems can in principle retrieve directly the residual energy by the TOF measurement between different tracking positions, placed downstream of the object of interest (Ulrich-Pur *et al* 2022). The residual energy or range is then calibrated to WET relying on proper detector characterization. List-mode data are defined by assigning the WET to the trajectory of each ion.

Simplified imaging prototypes composed of only the energy detector without an additional tracking system are proposed for pencil beam scanning, typically referred to as 'integration-mode' detectors. This detector configuration infers the mixed residual energy or range components of the pencil beam (due to lateral and traversal inhomogeneities) through either the total energy loss in multiple absorption and detection layers (Rinaldi *et al* 2013, Magallanes *et al* 2019) or the time resolved energy loss of multiple initial beam energies in a single thin absorption and detection layer (Telsemeyer *et al* 2012, Testa *et al* 2013, Schnürle *et al* 2023). These mixed components for each pencil beam can be resolved by means of linear decomposition of the laterally segmented spatial signal (total energy loss in multiple absorption and detection layers) or the temporal signal (multiple energy losses in a single thin absorption and detection layer). This way, information about range variations due to lateral inhomogeneities can be retrieved (Krah *et al* 2015, Meyer *et al* 2017). The retrieval of traversal inhomogeneities requires instead also the traversal spatial segmentation of the signal relevant to the pencil beam (Chen *et al* 2022). With respect to that, semiconductor detectors working as thin absorption and detection layers (and as downstream tracking systems) can offer fine pixelation of this signal.

Relying on the calibration of the resolved components to WET, a WET histogram expressing the relative occurrence of each WET component is therefore obtained for each pencil beam. Integration-mode data are defined by the WET histogram assigned to the straight pencil beam direction, as provided by the synchronization of the absorption detector with the pencil beam scanning system. The WET histogram enables the computation of a weighted mean WET (WET components weighted by the relative occurrences and averaged) and a mode WET (WET component with the most frequent relative occurrence), thus referring to integration-mode mean and mode, respectively (Gianoli *et al* 2019). It is worth noticing that in literature, integration-mode mode is also referred to as integration-mode max to avoid the 'mode' word repetition.

List-mode or integration-mode data covering the object of interest at a certain projection angle are referred to as an ion radiography (iRad). By mounting the detector on the rotating gantry (or by rotating the object of interest via patient couch or chair), several iRads can be acquired. Since the WET is modeled as the integral RSP along an estimated ion trajectory, the iRads correspond to a forward-projection of the unknown ion computed tomography (iCT). In particular, the estimate of ion trajectory is based on the tracking for list-mode data and assumed to coincide with the straight line along the pencil beam direction for integration-mode data. The iCT can be therefore obtained by means of tomographic image reconstruction of the iRads acquired at different projection angles.

6.3.1 Tomographic ion imaging

The accuracy and spatial resolution of iCT greatly depend on the estimate of ion trajectory and therefore, on the detector configuration. To estimate the tracked ion trajectory inside the object of interest for list-mode data, multiple Coulomb scattering (MCS) models of ion trajectories are adopted. The scattering model for list-mode detector configuration can be described as a bi-variate Gaussian distribution with increasing standard deviation along the initial ion direction (i.e., the direction in air prior to scattering in the object of interest) and with decreasing standard deviation along the final ion direction (i.e., the direction in air after scattering in the object of interest), according to a 'scattering spindle' (figure 6.1). The most probable ion trajectory inside the object of interest is typically derived relying on the Bayes formalism of the maximum likely path (MLP; Schulte et al 2008) or its approximations (Collins-Fekete et al 2015). The scattering spindle is the statistical description of the uncertainties of the MLP relevant to each ion. Different from the MLP, the scattering spindle does not provide the most probable ion trajectory but rather the statistical description of the ion trajectories constrained by the ion tracking upstream and downstream of the object of interest. The MLP can be embedded in the forward-projection model of numerical algorithms for tomographic image reconstruction. This methodology, eventually provided with superiorization (Penfold and Censor 2015), is the current state-of-the-art for list-mode data and potentially enables eliminating (or reducing to less than 1%) the intrinsic inaccuracies of the treatment planning x-ray CT (Meyer et al 2019). Computationally faster analytical algorithms based on modified filtered back-projection along the scattering curves can be also considered when list-mode data satisfy the required mathematical hypotheses about continuity (Rit et al 2013). The MLP as the most probable ion trajectory turns into a straight line along the pencil beam direction for integration-mode detector configuration. This direction corresponds to the pencil beam direction deduced from the treatment planning system or the beam monitoring system. The statistical description of the uncertainties of the straight line along the pencil beam direction is referred to as 'scattering cone' (figure 6.1). For this reason, tomographic image reconstruction for integration-mode data is traditionally limited to the use of the straight lines in either analytical or numerical algorithms. However, the straight line describes only the most probable range component (mode WET) of the pencil beam. The use of scattering models for integration-mode data is reported in literature (Rescigno et al 2015, Seller Oria et al 2018). Analytical algorithms based on filtered back-projection along the scattering cones are proposed for the unresolved range component of the pencil beam (Rescigno et al 2015). The scattering cone for each range component of the pencil beam is also directly embedded in the forward-projection model of numerical algorithms, guaranteeing reduced noise break-up and better convergence of the tomographic image reconstruction (Seller Oria et al 2018).

The scattering models behind the scattering curve are typically given in homogeneous water. Lateral and traversal inhomogeneities of the object of interest makes the scattering model inconsistent to both list-mode and integration-mode data.

The inconsistency of the scattering curves is demonstrated to affect the accuracy of tomographic image reconstruction of list-mode data, nevertheless remaining superior to integration-mode data (Gianoli *et al* 2019). To cope with the inconsistency of the scattering model due to inhomogeneities, different adjustments of the scattering curve for list-mode data are implemented relying on prior anatomical information. The elemental composition and mass density of the water are replaced by those of the biological tissue as given in the stoichiometric calibration (Collins-Fekete *et al* 2017). Alternatively, maintaining the elemental composition of water but scaling the mass density according to the RSP along an estimate of ion trajectory, as implemented in analytical dose calculation algorithms, the scattering model is extended to water equivalent inhomogeneity (Gianoli *et al* 2019).

6.3.1.1 *Clinical considerations for tomographic ion imaging*
Tomographic ion imaging can be obtained when the beam line and the detector are embedded in a rotating gantry for patients positioned on beds or by rotating the treatment seat for ocular and cranial patients, thus probing the object of interest from different angles with a series of ion radiographies for tomographic image reconstruction. Research towards the development of cost-effective rotational beam lines are currently ongoing (Meer and Psoroulas 2015). However, in addition to geometrical limitations, the need to minimize the (extra) imaging dose to the patient puts constraints on the possibilities to obtain a full iCT image on a daily basis (Murphy *et al* 2007, Hansen *et al* 2014a). Hence, dedicated reconstruction methodologies are currently under investigation with the purpose of optimizing image quality in presence of geometrical limitations and dosimetric constraints, based on priors coming from other imaging acquisitions such as the pCT image, under the assumption of CT-iCT registration (Hansen *et al* 2014b).

The flexibility of pencil beam scanning offers unique opportunities to reduce imaging dose, similar to what is performed in x-ray imaging with tube current intensity modulation (Dickmann *et al* 2021) by optimizing the theoretical noise of the region of interest (Rädler *et al* 2018). A non-uniform sampling of the iRads can be obtained by varying the beam fluence or intensity per pencil beam, thus maintaining the image quality in the region of interest and to penalize only less interesting regions without a loss of relevant information. In particular, an optimal fluence/intensity modulation pattern, minimizing dose exposure and maximizing information in regions of interest can be defined based on priors coming from treatment planning x-ray CT image.

6.3.2 Radiographic ion imaging
Alternatively to the replacement of the treatment planning x-ray CT based on tomographic image reconstruction of several iRads, the use of a limited number of iRads is proposed to potentially minimize the intrinsic inaccuracies of the semi-empirical calibration of the treatment planning x-ray CT (Schneider *et al* 2005) due to tissue-specific and patient-specific RSP variations. The stoichiometric calibration is optimized relying on the forward-projection of the treatment planning x-ray CT

along the estimated ion trajectory, yielding the water equivalent Digitally Reconstructed Radiography (weDRR). Relying on this forward-projection model, the optimization algorithm maximizes the matching between the iRad and the weDRR, expressed as a function of the unknown adjustments of the stoichiometric calibration. This optimization can be implemented as a linear minimization if prior segmentation of the treatment planning x-ray CT is applied. Alternatively, an optimization algorithm embedding forward-projection and segmentation of the iteratively adjusted treatment planning x-ray CT can be adopted. Despite the computational advantage of a linear minimization (Collins-Fekete *et al* 2017, Krah *et al* 2019, Zhang *et al* 2019), the adoption of a non-linear optimization algorithm enables overcoming the limitation of the prior segmentation and the forward-projection of the treatment planning x-ray CT (Schneider *et al* 2005, Doolan *et al* 2015, Gianoli *et al* 2020).

Depending on the detector configuration, the trajectory is either estimated for each ion (list-mode data; Collins-Fekete *et al* 2017, Gianoli *et al* 2020) or assumed to be a straight line for each pencil beam (integration-mode data; Doolan *et al* 2015, Zhang *et al* 2019, Krah *et al* 2019, Gianoli *et al* 2020). Exact registration between the treatment planning x-ray CT and the iRad is assumed. Therefore, clinical application of the optimization of the treatment planning x-ray CT based on iRads can only rely on compensation of anatomical changes based on 2D-3D deformable image registration (DIR) for treatment planning adaptation (Palaniappan *et al* 2021, Palaniappan *et al* 2022). The use of a limited number of iRads is therefore proposed also to compensate anatomical changes in adaptive proton therapy.

The optimization of the treatment planning x-ray CT based on iRads has been investigated by excluding non-straight proton trajectories from the optimization in a pioneering imaging prototype of a list-mode detector in a dog patient (Schneider *et al* 2005) or by excluding regions relevant to range mixing in real tissue samples in an integration-mode detector (Doolan *et al* 2015). However, in these two works the ground truth iCT was not available, thus making the optimization of the objective function hardly interpretable as a minimization of the intrinsic inaccuracies in the optimized calibration curve. Such optimization of the treatment planning x-ray CT based on iRads has been also numerically investigated in anthropomorphic phantoms for proton list-mode data at relatively high initial beam energy (Collins-Fekete *et al* 2017) and regularized based on information about the inaccurate calibration curve (Zhang *et al* 2019) or the (actually unknown) true one (Krah *et al* 2019). In these studies, realistic calibration curves have been adopted as inaccurate, without controlling the applied inaccuracies. The extensive application of controlled inaccuracies with respect to the ground truth iCT has been numerically investigated in realistic Monte Carlo simulations of clinical data, for proton, helium and carbon ion pencil beams (Gianoli *et al* 2020). List-mode and integration-mode data have been compared. The use of a scattering model consistent to the integration-mode data has also been introduced. The robustness against controlled inaccuracies applied to the realistic calibration curve has been proven in analytical simulations of an anthropomorphic phantom. However, in clinical data the optimization of the treatment planning x-ray CT based on iRads has been limited by the inconsistencies of the forward-projection model. These inconsistencies between the iRad and the weDRR of the ground truth iCT have been quantified to be in the same order of magnitude as the intrinsic inaccuracies of the treatment planning x-ray CT. In Monte Carlo simulations of clinical data, an accuracy of 2%–5% for integration-mode data and 1%–3% for list-mode data has been found, thus resulting insufficient to minimize the intrinsic inaccuracies in the calibration curve (Gianoli *et al* 2020).

6.4 Artificial intelligence in ion imaging

In the last few years, the use of artificial intelligence has been proposed in ion imaging. In particular, machine learning has been adopted to improve the forward-projection model and speed up its calculation for list-mode data (Lazos *et al* 2021), which is typically based on the MLP. Further, machine learning has been proposed to overcome the forward-projection model itself by means of a data-driven approach, as the inconsistencies of the model are comparable to the intrinsic inaccuracies of the treatment planning x-ray CT (Gianoli *et al* 2022). Machine learning has been used for the correction of the iCT (proton CT) along with the prediction of the uncertainties of the image in terms of noise and scattering (Collins-Fekete *et al* 2020, Nomura *et al* 2021) and for the estimation of treatment planning x-ray CT based on dual-energy x-ray CT (Wang *et al* 2020). Machine learning has been proposed also to identify possible sources of range mismatches on proton radiographies (Seller Oria *et al* 2020) and to estimate the scattering on proton radiographies when multi-energy proton imaging system is available (van der Heyden *et al* 2021).

References

Alme J, Barnaföldi G G, Barthel R, Borshchov V, Bodova T, Van den Brink A and Yokoyama H 2020 A high-granularity digital tracking calorimeter optimized for proton CT *Front. Phys.* **8** 568243

Amaldi U, Bianchi A, Chang Y H, Go A, Hajdas W, Malakhov N and Watts D 2011 Construction, test and operation of a proton range radiography system *Nucl. Instrum. Methods Phys. Res. Sect.* A **629** 337–44

ATLAS Collaboration 2017 *Technical Design Report for the ATLAS Inner Tracker Strip Detector* (No. PUBDB-2017-09975) (LHC/ATLAS Experiment)

Baruffaldi F, Iuppa R, Ricci E and Snoeys W 2018 iMPACT: an innovative tracker and calorimeter for proton computed tomography *IEEE Trans. Radiat. Plasma Med. Sci.* **2** 345–52

Bashkirov V A, Johnson R P, Sadrozinski H F W and Schulte R W 2016a Development of proton computed tomography detectors for applications in hadron therapy *Nucl. Instrum. Methods Phys. Res. Sect.* A **809** 120–9

Bashkirov V A, Schulte R W, Hurley R F, Johnson R P, Sadrozinski H W, Zatserklyaniy A and Giacometti V 2016b Novel scintillation detector design and performance for proton radiography and computed tomography *Med. Phys.* **43** 664–74

Benlloch J, Bressan A, Buttner C, Capeans M, Gruwe M, Hoch M and Veenhof R 1998 Development of the gas electron multiplier (GEM) *IEEE Trans. Nucl. Sci.* **45** 234–43

Berger M J, Coursey J S, Zucker M A and Chang J 2005 Calculated using online database: ESTAR, PSTAR, and ASTAR: computer programs for calculating stopping-power and range tables for electrons, protons, and helium ions (version 1.2. 3) *Physics. Nist. Gov/StarS* (Gaithersburg, MD: National Institute of Standards and Technology) https://www.nist.gov/pml/stopping-power-and-range-tables-electrons-protons-and-helium-ions-version-history

Biegun A K, Visser J, Klaver T, Ghazanfari N, van Goethem M J, Koffeman E and Brandenburg S 2015 Proton radiography with timepix based time projection chambers *IEEE Trans. Med. Imaging* **35** 1099–105

Bortfeldt J, Biebel O, Flierl B, Hertenberger R, Klitzner F, Lösel P and Zibell A 2017 Low material budget floating strip Micromegas for ion transmission radiography *Nucl. Instrum. Methods Phys. Res., Sect.* A **845** 210–4

Bucciantonio M, Amaldi U, Kieffer R, Sauli F and Watts D 2013 Development of a fast proton range radiography system for quality assurance in hadrontherapy *Nucl. Instrum. Methods Phys. Res. Sect. A: Accel. Spectrom. Detector. Assoc. Equip.* **732** 564–7

Cartiglia N, Staiano A, Sola V, Arcidiacono R, Cirio R, Cenna F and Zavrtanik M 2017 Beam test results of a 16 ps timing system based on ultra-fast silicon detectors *Nucl. Instrum. Methods Phys. Res., Sect.* A **850** 83–8

Carulla M, Doblas A, Flores D, Galloway Z, Hidalgo S, Kramberger G and Zhao Y 2019 50 μm thin low gain avalanche detectors (LGAD) for timing applications *Nucl. Instrum. Methods Phys. Res., Sect.* A **924** 373–9

Chen X, Medrano M, Sun B, Hao Y, Reynoso F J, Darafsheh A and Zhao T 2022 A reconstruction approach for proton computed tomography by modeling the integral depth dose of the scanning proton pencil beam *Med. Phys.* **49** 2602–20

Collins-Fekete C A, Bär E, Volz L, Bouchard H, Beaulieu L and Seco J 2017 Extension of the Fermi–Eyges most-likely path in heterogeneous medium with prior knowledge information *Phys. Med. Biol.* **62** 9207

Collins-Fekete C A, Brousmiche S, Hansen D C, Beaulieu L and Seco J 2017 Pre-treatment patient-specific stopping power by combining list-mode proton radiography and x-ray CT *Phys. Med. Biol.* **62** 6836

Collins-Fekete C A, Dikaios N, Royle G and Evans P M 2020 Statistical limitations in proton imaging *Phys. Med. Biol.* **65** 085011

Collins-Fekete C A, Doolan P, Dias M F, Beaulieu L and Seco J 2015 Developing a phenomenological model of the proton trajectory within a heterogeneous medium required for proton imaging *Phys. Med. Biol.* **60** 5071

Crowe K M, Budinger T F, Cahoon J L, Elischer V P, Huesman R H and Kanstein L L 1975 Axial scanning with 900 MeV alpha particles *IEEE Trans. Nucl. Sci.* **22** 1752–4

Darne C D, Alsanea F, Robertson D G, Guan F, Pan T, Grosshans D and Beddar S 2019 A proton imaging system using a volumetric liquid scintillator: a preliminary study *Biomed. Phys. Eng. Express* **5** 045032

Darne C D, Robertson D G, Alsanea F, Collins-Fekete C A and Beddar S 2022 A novel proton-integrating radiography system design using a monolithic scintillator detector: experimental studies *Nucl. Instrum. Methods Phys. Res., Sect.* A **1027** 166077

Dedes G, Drosten H, Götz S, Dickmann J, Sarosiek C, Pankuch M and Landry G 2022 Comparative accuracy and resolution assessment of two prototype proton computed tomography scanners *Med. Phys.* **49** 4671–81

DeJongh E A, DeJongh D F, Polnyi I, Rykalin V, Sarosiek C, Coutrakon G and Welsh J S 2021 A fast and monolithic prototype clinical proton radiography system optimized for pencil beam scanning *Med. Phys.* **48** 1356–64

Dickmann J, Kamp F, Hillbrand M, Corradini S, Belka C, Schulte R W and Landry G 2021 Fluence-modulated proton CT optimized with patient-specific dose and variance objectives for proton dose calculation *Phys. Med. Biol.* **66** 064001

Doolan P J, Testa M, Sharp G, Bentefour E H, Royle G and Lu H M 2015 Patient-specific stopping power calibration for proton therapy planning based on single-detector proton radiography *Phys. Med. Biol.* **60** 1901

Esposito M, Waltham C, Taylor J T, Manger S, Phoenix B, Price T and Allinson N M 2018 PRaVDA: the first solid-state system for proton computed tomography *Phys. Med.* **55** 149–54

Gianoli C, Göppel M, Meyer S, Palaniappan P, Rädler M, Kamp F, Belka C, Riboldi M and Parodi K 2020 Patient-specific CT calibration based on ion radiography for different detector configurations in 1H, 4He and 12C ion pencil beam scanning *Phys. Med. Biol.* **65** 245014

Gianoli C, Meyer S, Magallanes L, Paganelli C, Baroni G and Parodi K 2019 Analytical simulator of proton radiography and tomography for different detector configurations *Phys. Med.* **59** 92–9

Gianoli C, Zlatić M, Würl M, Schnürle K, Meyer S, Bortfeldt J, Englbrecht F S, Palaniappan P, Riboldi M and Parodi K 2022 Model-based and data-driven calibration of the x-ray CT Image based on proton radiographies *Nuclear Science Symposium and Medical Imaging Conference (NSS/MIC)* 2022 (Piscataway, NJ: IEEE) pp 1–3

Giomataris Y, Rebourgeard P, Robert J P and Charpak G 1996 MICROMEGAS: a high-granularity position-sensitive gaseous detector for high particle-flux environments *Nucl. Instrum. Methods Phys. Res., Sect. A* **376** 29–35

Granado-González M, Jesús-Valls C, Lux T, Price T and Sánchez F 2022 A novel range telescope concept for proton CT *Phys. Med. Biol.* **67** 035013

Hansen D C, Bassler N, Sørensen T S and Seco J 2014a The image quality of ion computed tomography at clinical imaging dose levels *Med. Phys.* **41** 111908

Hansen D C, Petersen J B B, Bassler N and Sørensen T S 2014b Improved proton computed tomography by dual modality image reconstruction *Med. Phys.* **41** 031904

Hanson K M 1979 Proton computed tomography *IEEE Trans. Nucl. Sci.* **26** 1635–40

van der Heyden B, Cohilis M, Souris K, de Freitas Nascimento L and Sterpin E 2021 Artificial intelligence supported single detector multi-energy proton radiography system *Phys. Med. Biol.* **66** 105001

Johnson R P 2017 Review of medical radiography and tomography with proton beams *Rep. Prog. Phys.* **81** 016701

Johnson R P, Bashkirov V, Giacometti V, Hurley R F, Piersimoni P, Plautz T E and Zatserklyaniy A 2015 A fast experimental scanner for proton CT: technical performance and first experience with phantom scans *IEEE Trans. Nucl. Sci.* **63** 52–60

Krah N, Dauvergne D, Létang J M, Rit S and Testa E 2022 Relative stopping power resolution in time-of-flight proton CT *Phys. Med. Biol.* **67** 165004

Krah N, De Marzi L, Patriarca A, Pittá G and Rinaldi I 2018 Proton radiography with a commercial range telescope detector using dedicated post processing methods *Phys. Med. Biol.* **63** 205016

Krah N, Patera V, Rit S, Schiavi A and Rinaldi I 2019 Regularised patient-specific stopping power calibration for proton therapy planning based on proton radiographic images *Phys. Med. Biol.* **64** 065008

Krah N, Testa M, Brons S, Jäkel O, Parodi K, Voss B and Rinaldi I 2015 An advanced image processing method to improve the spatial resolution of ion radiographies *Phys. Med. Biol.* **60** 8525

Lazos D, Collins-Fekete C A, Bober M, Evans P and Dikaios N 2021 Machine learning for proton path tracking in proton computed tomography *Phys. Med. Biol.* **66** 105013

Magallanes L, Meyer S, Gianoli C, Kopp B, Voss B, Jäkel O and Parodi K 2019 Upgrading an integrating carbon-ion transmission imaging system with active scanning beam delivery toward low dose ion imaging *IEEE Trans. Radiat. Plasma Med. Sci.* **4** 262–8

Meer D and Psoroulas S 2015 Gantries and dose delivery systems *Mod. Phys. Lett.* A **30** 1540021

Meijers A, Seller Oria C, Free J, Langendijk J A, Knopf A C and Both S 2021 First report on an *in vivo* range probing quality control procedure for scanned proton beam therapy in head and neck cancer patients *Med. Phys.* **48** 1372–80

Meyer S, Bortfeldt J, Lämmer P, Englbrecht F S, Pinto M, Schnürle K and Parodi K 2020 Optimization and performance study of a proton CT system for pre-clinical small animal imaging *Phys. Med. Biol.* **65** 155008

Meyer S, Gianoli C, Magallanes L, Kopp B, Tessonnier T, Landry G, Dedes G, Voss B and Parodi K 2017 Comparative Monte Carlo study on the performance of integration-and list-mode detector configurations for carbon ion computed tomography *Phys. Med. Biol.* **62** 1096

Meyer S, Kamp F, Tessonnier T, Mairani A, Belka C, Carlson D J, Gianoli C and Parodi K 2019 Dosimetric accuracy and radiobiological implications of ion computed tomography for proton therapy treatment planning *Phys. Med. Biol.* **64** 125008

Murphy M J *et al* 2007 The management of imaging dose during image-guided radiotherapy: report of the AAPM task group 75 *Med. Phys.* **34** 4041–63

Naimuddin M, Coutrakon G, Blazey G, Boi S, Dyshkant A, Erdelyi B and Wilson P 2016 Development of a proton computed tomography detector system *J. Instrum.* **11** C02012

Nomura Y, Tanaka S, Wang J, Shirato H, Shimizu S and Xing L 2021 Calibrated uncertainty estimation for interpretable proton computed tomography image correction using Bayesian deep learning *Phys. Med. Biol.* **66** 065029

Palaniappan P, Meyer S, Kamp F, Belka C, Riboldi M, Parodi K and Gianoli C 2021 Deformable image registration of the treatment planning CT with proton radiographies in perspective of adaptive proton therapy *Phys. Med. Biol.* **66** 045008

Palaniappan P, Meyer S, Rädler M, Kamp F, Belka C, Riboldi M, Parodi K and Gianoli C 2022 X-ray CT adaptation based on a 2D-3D deformable image registration framework using simulated in-room proton radiographies *Phys. Med. Biol.* **67** 045003

Parodi K 2014 Heavy ion radiography and tomography *Phys. Med.* **30** 539–43

Pemler P, Besserer J, de Boer J, Dellert M, Gahn C, Moosburger M *et al* 1999 A detector system for proton radiography on the gantry of the Paul-Scherrer-Institute *Nucl. Instrum. Methods Phys. Res., Sect.* A **432** 483–95

Penfold S and Censor Y 2015 Techniques in iterative proton CT image reconstruction *Sens. Imaging* **16** 1–21

Pettersen H E S, Alme J, Biegun A, Van Den Brink A, Chaar M, Fehlker D and Röhrich D 2017 Proton tracking in a high-granularity digital tracking calorimeter for proton CT purposes *Nucl. Instrum. Methods Phys. Res., Sect.* A **860** 51–61

Presti D L, Bonanno D, Longhitano F, Pugliatti C, Aiello S, Cirrone G A P and Ventura C 2014 A real-time, large area, high space resolution particle radiography system *J. Instrum.* **9** C06012

Presti D L, Bonanno D L, Longhitano F, Bongiovanni D G, Russo G V, Leonora E and Gallo G I U S E P P E 2016 Design and characterisation of a real time proton and carbon ion radiography system based on scintillating optical fibres *Phys. Med.* **32** 1124–34

Rädler M, Landry G, Rit S, Schulte R W, Parodi K and Dedes G 2018 Two-dimensional noise reconstruction in proton computed tomography using distance-driven filtered back-projection of simulated projections *Phys. Med. Biol.* **63** 215009

Rescigno R, Bopp C, Rousseau M and Brasse D 2015 A pencil beam approach to proton computed tomography *Med. Phys.* **42** 6610–24

Riegler W 2016 Electric fields, weighting fields, signals and charge diffusion in detectors including resistive materials *J. Instrum.* **11** P11002

Rinaldi I, Brons S, Gordon J, Panse R, Voss B, Jäkel O and Parodi K 2013 Experimental characterization of a prototype detector system for carbon ion radiography and tomography *Phys. Med. Biol.* **58** 413

Rinaldi I, Brons S, Jäkel O, Voss B and Parodi K 2014 Experimental investigations on carbon ion scanning radiography using a range telescope *Phys. Med. Biol.* **59** 3041

Rit S, Dedes G, Freud N, Sarrut D and Létang J M 2013 Filtered backprojection proton CT reconstruction along most likely paths *Med. Phys.* **40** 031103

Sadrozinski H F W, Bashkirov V, Keeney B, Johnson L R, Peggs S G, Ross G *et al* 2004 Toward proton computed tomography *IEEE Trans. Nucl. Sci.* **51** 3–9

Saraya Y, Izumikawa T, Goto J, Kawasaki T and Kimura T 2014 Study of spatial resolution of proton computed tomography using a silicon strip detector *Nucl. Instrum. Methods Phys. Res. Sect.* A **735** 485–9

Sauli F 1997 GEM: a new concept for electron amplification in gas detectors *Nucl. Instrum. Methods Phys. Res. Sect.* A **386** 531–4

Scaringella M, Brianzi M, Bruzzi M, Bucciolini M, Carpinelli M, Cirrone G A P and Zani M 2013 The PRIMA (PRoton IMAging) collaboration: development of a proton computed tomography apparatus *Nucl. Instrum. Methods Phys. Res. Sect.* A **730** 178–83

Scaringella M, Bruzzi M, Farace P, Fogazzi E, Righetto R, Rit S and Civinini C 2023 The INFN proton computed tomography system for relative stopping power measurements: calibration and verification *Phys. Med. Biol.* **68** 154001

Schneider U, Besserer J, Pemler P, Dellert M, Moosburger M, Pedroni E and Kaser-Hotz B 2004 First proton radiography of an animal patient *Med. Phys.* **31** 1046–51

Schneider U and Pedroni E 1995 Proton radiography as a tool for quality control in proton therapy *Med. Phys.* **22** 353–63

Schneider U, Pemler P, Besserer J, Pedroni E, Lomax A and Kaser-Hotz B 2005 Patient specific optimization of the relation between CT-hounsfield units and proton stopping power with proton radiography *Med. Phys.* **32** 195–9

Schnürle K, Bortfeldt J, Englbrecht F S, Gianoli C, Hartmann J, Hofverberg P and Würl M 2023 Development of integration mode proton imaging with a single CMOS detector for a small animal irradiation platform *Front. Phys.* **10** 1384

Schulte R, Bashkirov V, Li T, Liang Z, Mueller K, Heimann J and Williams D C 2004 Conceptual design of a proton computed tomography system for applications in proton radiation therapy *IEEE Trans. Nucl. Sci.* **51** 866–72

Schulte R W, Penfold S N, Tafas J T and Schubert K E 2008 A maximum likelihood proton path formalism for application in proton computed tomography *Med. Phys.* **35** 4849–56

Seller Oria C, Marmitt G G, Both S, Langendijk J A, Knopf A C and Meijers A 2020 Classification of various sources of error in range assessment using proton radiography and neural networks in head and neck cancer patients *Phys. Med. Biol.* **65** 235009

Seller Oria C, Meyer S, De Bernardi E, Parodi K and Gianoli C 2018 A dedicated tomographic image reconstruction algorithm for integration-mode detector configuration in ion imaging *2018 IEEE Nuclear Science Symposium and Medical Imaging Conference Proceedings (NSS/MIC)* (Piscataway, NJ: IEEE) pp 1–3

Takada Y, Kondo K, Marume T, Nagayoshi K, Okada I and Takikawa K 1988 Proton computed tomography with a 250 MeV pulsed beam *Nucl. Instrum. Methods Phys. Res. Sect.* A **273** 410–22

Taylor J T, Poludniowski G, Price T, Waltham C, Allport P P, Casse G L and Allinson N M 2016 An experimental demonstration of a new type of proton computed tomography using a novel silicon tracking detector *Med. Phys.* **43** 6129–36

Telsemeyer J, Jäkel O and Martišíková M 2012 Quantitative carbon ion beam radiography and tomography with a flat-panel detector *Phys. Med. Biol.* **57** 7957

Testa M, Verburg J M, Rose M, Min C H, Tang S, Bentefour E H and Lu H M 2013 Proton radiography and proton computed tomography based on time-resolved dose measurements *Phys. Med. Biol.* **58** 8215

Ulrich-Pur F, Bergauer T, Burker A, Hirtl A, Irmler C, Kaser S and Rit S 2022 Feasibility study of a proton CT system based on 4D-tracking and residual energy determination via time-of-flight *Phys. Med. Biol.* **67** 095005

Wang T, Lei Y, Harms J, Liu Y, Ghavidel B, Lin L and Yang X 2020 Stopping power map estimation from dual-energy CT using deep convolutional neural network *Medical Imaging 2020: Physics of Medical Imaging* **Vol 11312** (Bellingham, WA: International Society for Optics and Photonics) p 113124M

Winter A, Aitkenhead A, Allinson N, Allport P, Esposito M, Green S and Waltham C 2023 OPTIma: a tracking solution for proton computed tomography in high proton flux environments *J. Instrum.* **18** P04026

Workman R L, Burkert V D, Crede V, Klempt E, Thoma U and Quadt AParticle Data Group 2022 Review of particle physics *Prog. Theor. Exp. Phys.* **2022** 083C01

Würl M, Gianoli C, Englbrecht F S, Schreiber J and Parodi K 2022 A Monte Carlo feasibility study on quantitative laser-driven proton radiography *Z. Med. Phys.* **32** 109–19

Würl M, Schnürle K, Bortfeldt J, Oancea C, Granja C, Verroi E and Parodi K 2020 Proton radiography for a small-animal irradiation platform based on a miniaturized Timepix detector *2020 IEEE Nuclear Science Symposium and Medical Imaging Conference (NSS/MIC)* (Piscataway, NJ: IEEE) pp 1–6

Zhang R, Sharp G C, Jee K W, Cascio E, Harms J, Flanz J B and Lu H M 2019 Iterative optimization of relative stopping power by single detector based multi-projection proton radiography *Phys. Med. Biol.* **64** 065022

IOP Publishing

Imaging in Particle Therapy
Current practice and future trends
Chiara Paganelli, Chiara Gianoli and Antje Knopf

Chapter 7

Magnetic resonance imaging in particle therapy

C Paganelli, B Oborn, A Hoffmann and M Riboldi

7.1 Introduction

Up til now, computed tomography (CT) has been the clinical imaging standard for treatment planning, whereas image guidance during treatment commonly relies on 2D x-ray projections. More recently, volumetric imaging has become available (chapter 5), including gantry, nozzle, or couch-mounted cone beam computed tomography (CBCT), robotic C-arm CBCT, and CT-on-rails (Landry and Hua 2018). Although x-ray imaging is the current state-of-the-art modality, it presents several limitations such as the poor soft-tissue contrast, the inability to directly track moving tumours in real time and the need for extra non-therapeutic imaging dose. Due to the greater sensitivity of particles to anatomical and density changes along the beam path, advanced image guidance is therefore essential to make the most of particle therapy (PT) benefits.

In recent years magnetic resonance imaging (MRI) has gained importance in radiation therapy for different anatomical sites thanks to its intrinsic advantages: it is a radiation-free modality, with improved soft-tissue contrast compared to x-ray imaging, fast dynamic pulse sequences, and functional imaging (Hunt *et al* 2018, Paganelli *et al* 2018b, Corradini *et al* 2019, Kurz *et al* 2020). MRI in PT is expected to combine the ability of MRI to visualize anatomy and biological heterogeneity with the unique dose-deposition and biological properties of PT. This brings potential novel opportunities to improve cures by biological dose escalation in specific cancer types, including pancreatic, central lung, liver, oesophagus, brain and oligometastatic cancers (Keall *et al* 2022, Pham *et al* 2022), as well as in pediatric patients, where radiation levels must be carefully controlled.

Up-to-date MRI is adopted offline in the clinical routine of PT for precise tumour contouring and to support treatment planning and verification, with near-room systems installed in some of the facilities. However, the integration of MRI with linear accelerators (i.e. MRI-linac) is the most recent advancement in image-guided conventional radiotherapy, with different configurations being proposed, ranging

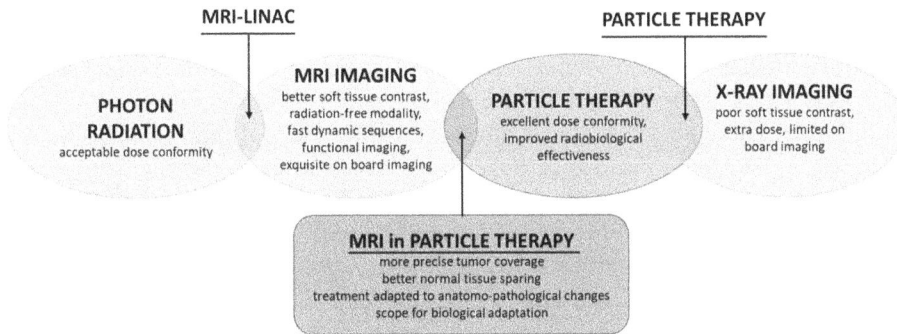

Figure 7.1. Potential of MRI in particle therapy with respect to x-ray imaging. Adapted from Pham *et al* (2022). Copyright (2022), with permission from Elsevier.

from in-room (Jaffray *et al* 2014) to in-beam modalities (Fallone 2014, Keall *et al* 2014, Lagendijk *et al* 2014, Mutic and Dempsey 2014). Among the latter, two commercial systems are currently available (ViewRay MRIdian and Elekta Unity; Olsen *et al* 2015, Raaymakers *et al* 2017, Klüter 2019), which have demonstrated significant improvement in clinical treatment outcomes, e.g., by enabling dose escalation for pancreatic cancer (Rudra *et al* 2019) or benefit from online plan adaptation (Intven *et al* 2021, Nierer *et al* 2022, Kishan *et al* 2023). Given the higher dosimetric sensitivity and biological effectiveness, PT would greatly benefit from MRI guidance, through online delivery monitoring and treatment adaptation (Pham *et al* 2022).

A true MRI-integrated proton therapy system could offer superior targeting accuracy compared with offline imaging options, especially for moving or hard to visualize tumours (figure 7.1). A recent study has shown that margin reduction enabled by a hypothetical MRI-integrated proton therapy could significantly decrease the normal tissue complication probability with respect to MRI-linac, offline MRI-guided proton therapy and online CBCT-guided proton therapy for liver tumours (Moteabbed *et al* 2021). Several challenges need to be accounted for in the integration of an MRI scanner with proton beam delivery, but a first pre-clinical prototype system is currently exploring the mutual interactions between the two systems (Gantz *et al* 2020) and the prospect of the first clinical MRI-integrated proton therapy prototype system is on the horizon (Oborn *et al* 2017, Hoffmann *et al* 2020). If MRI-integrated proton therapy seems to be the next engineering challenge, the integration of an MRI system with a carbon-ion beam seems more far from reality. In the meantime, however, a dedicated near-room MRI scanner in the PT suite to facilitate offline treatment adaptations and biological targeting could play an important role to improve treatment efficacy (Moteabbed *et al* 2021).

In this chapter, we will revise MR imaging modalities for static and moving organs (section 7.2), the perspectives for in-beam MRI proton therapy (section 7.3) and the features of an MRI-guided PT workflow (section 7.4). The book by Liney *et al* (Liney and Van der Heide 2019) can also complement this chapter.

7.2 MR imaging

MRI forms images via the detection of unpaired nuclear spins. Although a number of nuclei possess an unpaired nuclear spin and can in principle be detected using MRI, the hydrogen nucleus is by far the most commonly utilised due to its prevalence in the body and strong MRI signal. To enable detection of nuclear spins, the imaging object is placed in a static magnetic field. A combination of radio frequency pulses and magnetic field gradients is then applied to detect and localise the signal within the so-called k-space data, which is then transformed into the image domain via the application of an inverse Fourier transform. The flexibility of MRI in providing different contrasts and information makes this modality particularly suited to image the anatomo-pathological condition of the patient. In this section, we report an overview of the imaging modalities for static and moving organs that are currently available in off-line scanners or MRI-linac units and thus can be adopted in off-line workflows or potentially integrated in future in-room/in-beam MRI-PT systems. A deeper description of MRI basic physics is beyond the scope of this chapter, and can be found in McRobbie *et al* (2017).

7.2.1 Imaging of the static anatomy

MR imaging of the static anatomy is usually performed using 3D imaging protocols, relying on either stacked 2D slices or native 3D MR acquisition sequences. The former approach has been reported for low-field MRI-linacs using a bSSFP (balanced steady state free precession) sequence (Gao *et al* 2018), whereas the latter for 1.5 T MRI-linacs is relying on 3D SPGR (spoiled gradient recalled acquisition in steady state; Raaymakers *et al* 2017), 3D T1 weighted FFE (fast field echo; Werensteijn-Honingh *et al* 2019), or 3D T2-weighted scans (Intven *et al* 2021). These sequences can be also acquired off-line in conventional near-room diagnostic scanners and with contrast media to increase tumour visibility and subsequent delineation. Image resolution depends on the investigated anatomical site, ranging from 3 mm in the brain (Dirix *et al* 2014) to high resolution (e.g. 0.5 mm) for ocular treatments (Via *et al* 2021). Native 3D acquisitions are favorable as they can potentially minimize slice distortions that occur in 2D imaging due to B_0 inhomogeneity and facilitate the verification of the organ contours in the three anatomical planes (Kurz *et al* 2020). This is meant to facilitate inter-fractional treatment adaptation, by capturing daily images at minimal spatial distortion. Anatomical acquisitions can be also coupled with quantitative MRI data, such as MR perfusion and diffusion sequences (see chapter 11; Gurney-Champion *et al* 2020, Thorwarth *et al* 2020) which can support treatment planning for the definition of a biological target volume (BTV; Ling *et al* 2000) and thus, implement biological adaptation. An interesting application in this direction is the use of diffusion MRI for glioblastoma and sarcoma (Gao *et al* 2017), and central nervous system tumours (Lawrence *et al* 2021).

7.2.2 Imaging of the moving anatomy

At present, MRI approaches capable of resolving organ motion can be broadly classified as either time-resolved or respiratory-correlated (4D); the former delivers

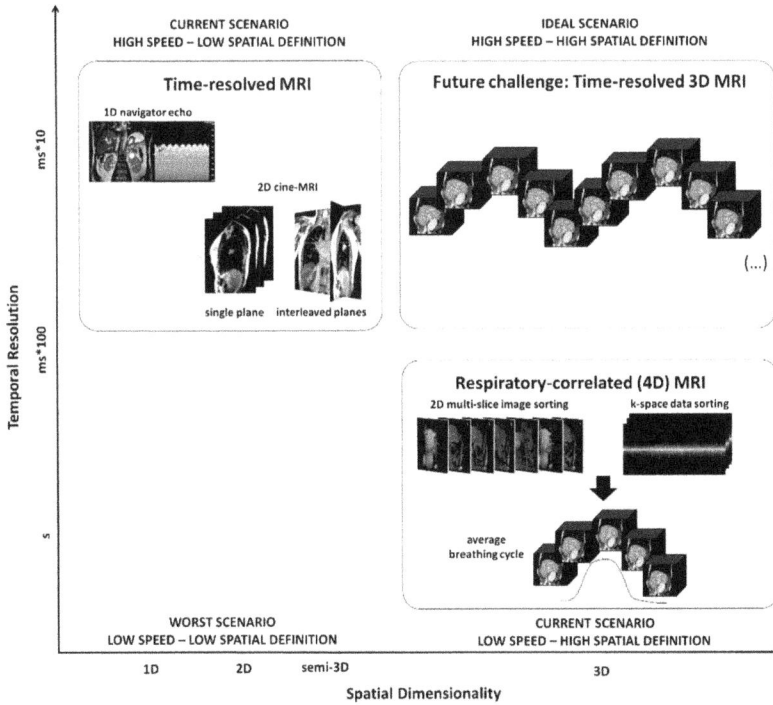

Figure 7.2. Image acquisition approaches for moving anatomy (adapted from Paganelli *et al* 2018b). © 2018 Institute of Physics and Engineering in Medicine. All rights reserved.

organ motion data in real-time at comparatively low spatial resolution, whilst the latter provides better spatial sampling, but relies on retrospective reconstruction (i.e., it is not real-time). Ideally, MRI for motion quantification would involve real-time 3D MRI (i.e., sub-second 3D imaging), but due to the intrinsic trade-off between spatial and temporal resolution, this is still a challenge (figure 7.2).

The limited frequency at which full 3D volumes can be acquired requires the patient to breathe slowly or limits image quality (Dinkel *et al* 2009); as such, images are created by retrospective sorting or prospective acquisition acquired over several breathing cycles to reconstruct one average representation, in a similar fashion to conventional 4DCT. Different techniques have been proposed in the literature for retrospective sorting, including navigator slices, image-based approaches or k-space data sorting (Stemkens *et al* 2018, Paganelli *et al* 2018b). Navigator slices are typically acquired interleaved with imaging data to be sorted and provide a robust internal surrogate (von Siebenthal *et al* 2007, Peteani *et al* 2023). Image-based approaches instead rely on extracting internal surrogates directly from MRI data and use such information for data labelling (Paganelli *et al* 2018a, Meschini *et al* 2019). Conversely, k-space techniques sort the raw data into respiratory bins prior to reconstructing into image space (Mickevicius and Paulson 2017a), by continuously sampling the center of the k-space in the form of the so-called self-gated or self-navigated acquisition. While image-based approaches can be easily implemented in conventional scanners by acquiring fast imaging sequences such as bSSFP, T2-weighted turbo spin echo and spoiled gradient echo, the navigator slice approach or k-space based sorting require proper implementation in the MR scanner. To improve spatial resolution while respecting a clinically feasible total acquisition time of a few minutes or less, parallel imaging and under-sampling schemes (Mickevicius and Paulson 2017b) can be utilized, as well as deep learning solutions to speed up reconstruction time (Terpstra *et al* 2020, Freedman *et al* 2021).

In time-resolved MRI instead, image acquisition is reduced to 2D information but continuously performed at sub-second frame rates (down to 125 ms; Kim *et al* 2021) with the so-called 2D cine MRI sequences, such as bSSFP or spoiled gradient echo, to capture cycle-to-cycle variations. 2D cine MRI, representing the state of the art for MRI-linacs, can be acquired either on a single plane or multiple planes (commonly in the sagittal direction), or in an orthogonal sagittal/coronal interleaved fashion centered in the tumour to achieve pseudo 3D information (Paganelli *et al* 2018b, Kurz *et al* 2020, Keall *et al* 2022).

7.3 In-beam MRI-guided proton therapy

As previously mentioned, MRI is currently adopted offline in PT, but the implementation of real-time MRI guidance with an integrated MRI scanner at the treatment isocenter is under investigation for proton therapy (Oborn *et al* 2017, Schellhammer *et al* 2018, Hoffmann *et al* 2020, Pham *et al* 2022). The availability of such a system would enable in-room time-resolved imaging able to directly monitor the internal anatomy just before and during treatment (i.e., to perform online adaptation and gating at first instance) coupled with better dose conformality provided by the proton beam. This configuration by nature means that the MRI scanner is expected to be operational while the proton beams are being delivered. This immediately introduces various complexities or additional requirements to the proton therapy. The most important requirements are listed in table 7.1 with a brief summary and discussed below in the following paragraphs.

7.3.1 Beam delivery, MR design and magnetic compatibility

One of the most important considerations for in-beam MRI-guided proton therapy is that the proton beam delivery must be pencil beam scanning (PBS; Oborn *et al* 2015). A passively scattered beam will lose its volumetric dose conformity after traversing through a magnetic field. This is due to the polyenergetic nature of the beams containing protons with energies that range over many MeV, i.e., the difference between the deepest and the most shallow Bragg peak for a given treatment field. Each of these protons will undergo a different magnetic deflection before coming to rest inside the patient. Therefore, the integrated MRI proton therapy system will need to be PBS based instead, and so dose planning, which needs to account for the magnetic field induced beam deflection, can be performed on a monoenergetic spot-by-spot basis.

As discussed in Hoffmann *et al* (2020) and Pham *et al* (2022), the magnet design either needs to be open or split-bore style, such that the proton beam has direct

Table 7.1. A summary of the unique requirements of a real-time MRI-guided proton therapy system.

Feature/requirement	Description
Beam delivery method	Pencil beam scanning is required. Passive scattering methods break down due to spatial degradation of polyenergetic beams during transport through the complex 3D spatially varying MRI magnetic fringe field (Oborn *et al* 2015).
Proton path to MRI isocenter	A clear path for the proton beam to reach the patient located inside an MRI scanner is required. This is possible with open or split-bore style MRI scanners (Burigo and Oborn 2022, Burigo and Oborn 2019).
Magnetic compatibility	There must be no detrimental impact on the MRI scanner operation by the proton beam and vice versa (Gantz *et al* 2020). This could be achieved via magnetic decoupling using magnetic shielding between the two systems.
Treatment planning	The Treatment Planning System (TPS) must be able to account for the transport of the proton beam through the MRI fringe field, as well as the calculation of proton beam dose in the presence of the main MRI field (Padilla-Cabal *et al* 2018, Padilla-Cabal *et al* 2020).
Dosimetry	Dosimetry should be conducted in the presence of the magnetic field of the MRI. Thus, the detectors and their performance must be evaluated and possibly modified to operate successfully in this environment. Magnetic field effects on their dose response can be accounted for via correction factors (Causer *et al* 2020, Fuchs *et al* 2021a).

access to the patient. For best practice, at least a partial gantry (e.g., 220° rotation) is required for beam access from any gantry angle (when coupled with a reversible patient couch). In a system with an almost complete split-gap the beam direction would be perpendicular to the main magnetic field (Oborn *et al* 2015). Alternatively, an open magnet design with a C-shaped or U-shaped rotating magnet could be integrated in the proton gantry, which requires the beam to pass through one of the magnet poles.

At least two research groups have already created prototype systems that have brought together a portable, open MRI scanner with a C-shaped permanent magnet design and a PBS assembly. At OncoRay in Dresden, Germany, three configurations using a compact MRI scanner for extremity imaging have been investigated (figure 7.3). These include (i) a 0.22 T MRI located at the end of a horizontal fixed proton beam line (Schellhammer *et al* 2018); (ii) the same 0.22 T MRI positioned at the end of a horizontal clinical-quality PBS assembly (non-gantry PBS; Gantz *et al* 2020); (iii) and a 0.32 T MRI scanner at the end of the same PBS assembly (Gebauer *et al* 2023). At the DKFZ in Heidelberg, Germany, a 0.25 T MRI has been integrated at the end of a PBS assembly with the potential for multiple ion species (Debus 2021). Finally, a dedicated 0.5 T bi-directional, whole-body MRI scanner using a cryogen-free superconducting magnet technology has been installed in late

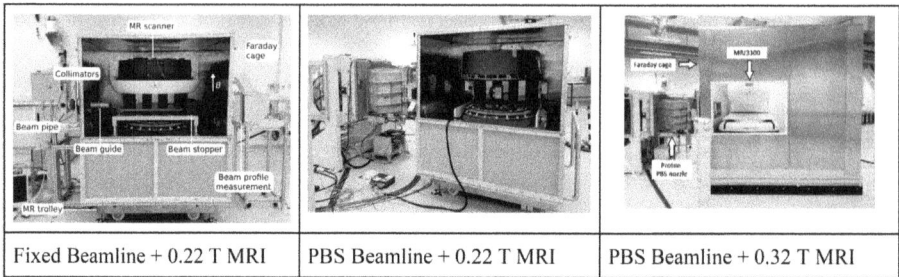

| Fixed Beamline + 0.22 T MRI | PBS Beamline + 0.22 T MRI | PBS Beamline + 0.32 T MRI |

Figure 7.3. The preclinical MRI-integrated proton therapy systems at OncoRay, Dresden, Germany.

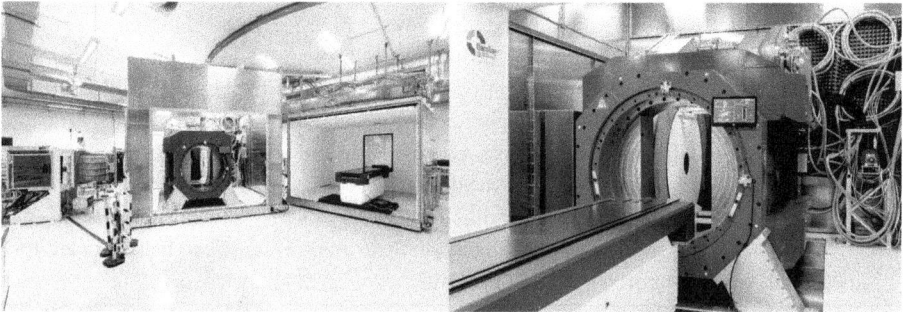

Figure 7.4. The 0.5 T bi-directional, whole-body in-beam MRI scanner installed at the horizontal proton PBS research beam line at OncoRay, Dresden, Germany.

2023 to serve as the next prototype at OncoRay. This system will allow for proton beam access either through a portal hole in the magnet yoke of the scanner or through the gap between the MRI cryostat halves. Figure 7.4 presents an impression of the proposed system with the proton beam incident from the perpendicular orientation. This system was installed at the end of 2023 and is currently being commissioned for first experimental use.

When integrating an MRI with a proton beam, electromagnetic interference effects between the PBS process and the MRI system are present. This primarily manifests itself as a strong ghosting image artefact present in the MR images during concurrent irradiation (Gantz *et al* 2020). The mechanism is linked to the magnetic fringe field of the PBS assembly slightly altering the B_0 field strength of the MRI scanner, all occurring with a frequency corresponding to the PBS dose delivery process. This ghosting is clearly a threat to the whole purpose of using the MRI to guide the treatment process in real-time. The most obvious approach for eliminating this concern is to magnetically decouple the PBS from the MRI scanner. Passive magnetic shielding of the PBS assembly would appear the simplest option. It is also worth considering software-based solutions to filter distorted images from the correct images, remembering that a combined system would allow for shared timestamps across the image construction and PBS spot settings. For example, reconstructing images from k-space information obtained between the delivery of PBS energy layers (i.e., when the MRI field is not impacted) would inherently produce accurate images.

7.3.2 Proton therapy dose calculation and dosimetry in a magnetic field

Considerable work has been conducted in the area of dose calculation of proton beams in the presence of magnetic fields, which is a necessary requirement for in-beam MRI-PT systems. In 2008, the deflection of a PBS broad proton beam incident on a phantom with uniform magnetic fields was calculated with Monte Carlo methods (Raaymakers *et al* 2008). In 2012, an analytical method was derived to calculate the expected proton beam deflections in uniform, transverse magnetic fields (Wolf and Bortfeld 2012). In 2014 and 2015, the dosimetric effects induced by uniform, transverse magnetic fields were assessed in patient treatment planning studies, showing that clinical grade treatment plans can be calculated in the presence of 0.5 and 1.5 T magnetic fields (Moteabbed *et al* 2014, Hartman *et al* 2015). Also in 2015, the transport of a proton beam towards a realistic MRI scanner was modelled (Oborn *et al* 2015), showing that the full 3D magnetic fringe field needs to be taken into account for treatment planning. In 2017, a fast and accurate numerical model was presented to predict and compensate for magnetic field induced beam deflections (Schellhammer and Hoffmann 2017). Fuchs *et al* (2017) next studied the changes to proton and carbon pencil beams incident on water phantoms using Monte Carlo methods: magnetic fields of up to 3 T were studied, and the concept of a beam retraction (or shallower Bragg peak depth) was first introduced. Padilla-Cabal and colleagues (Padilla-Cabal *et al* 2018) next investigated a pencil beam algorithm for prediction of the changes to a proton pencil beam in magnetic fields. In 2019, a small (up to 8% local dose increase) electron return effect produced by proton beams at 0.95 T was investigated experimentally and with Monte Carlo simulations (Lühr *et al* 2019). Also in 2019, pencil beam dose planning that accounts for inline magnetic fields was explored (Burigo and Oborn 2019). In 2020, a Monte Carlo-based dose calculation algorithm was investigated for use in proton beams in magnetic fields (Padilla-Cabal *et al* 2020). In 2021, the response and performance of various radiation detectors exposed to proton beams in the presence of magnetic fields was studied (Fuchs *et al* 2021b). Dose planning in the presence of perpendicular magnetic fields that accounts for the MRI fringe field has also been shown with success (Burigo and Oborn 2022). In 2023, the OncoRay group measured the effect of the MRI magnetic field (both fringe field and imaging field) on the proton beam path, dose spot pattern, dose spot form for their 0.32 T in-beam MRI scanner at the PBS beam line and quantified the lateral beam deflection, radiation field shape deformation and dose spot distortion as a function of beam energy and distance to the beam and MRI isocenter (Gebauer *et al* 2023). This data is valuable for the commissioning and evaluation of future treatment planning systems taking into account the full 3D magnetic field map of the in-beam MRI scanner.

As such, a wide range of both experimental and modelling based studies have been conducted in the field of dose calculation and dosimetry for the unique conditions that will be present in real-time MRI-guided proton beam therapy. So far, there have been no concerning findings; proton beam radiotherapy dose planning optimization and dosimetry that accounts for the presence of MR magnetic fields appears completely feasible.

7.4 MRI-guided PT workflow

Currently in PT, MRI can be adopted as an off-line modality to acquire ionizing dose-free repeated imaging to support treatment planning and, eventually, adaptation, and to perform follow-up examinations; but with future integrated systems, online adaptation is envisioned. Figure 7.5 shows the potential use of MRI in a current PT workflow and the optional treatment style of using integrated real-time MRI-guidance.

7.4.1 Treatment planning

One step towards maximal tumour control with minimal toxicity in PT is when high-resolution imaging is used for tumour and OARs contouring in treatment planning. CT remains the clinical standard in PT treatment planning as it provides high spatial resolution and does not suffer from geometric distortion, providing electron density information for different tissues. However, low soft-tissue contrast and large interobserver and intra-observer variations have been reported in the delineation of most solid tumours, potentially leading to marginal misses or suboptimal organ sparing or both (Dirix *et al* 2014). To overcome this, MR images can be fused on the planning CT images for accurate target and organs at risk delineation, providing more consistent and more accurate information than CT images alone, when

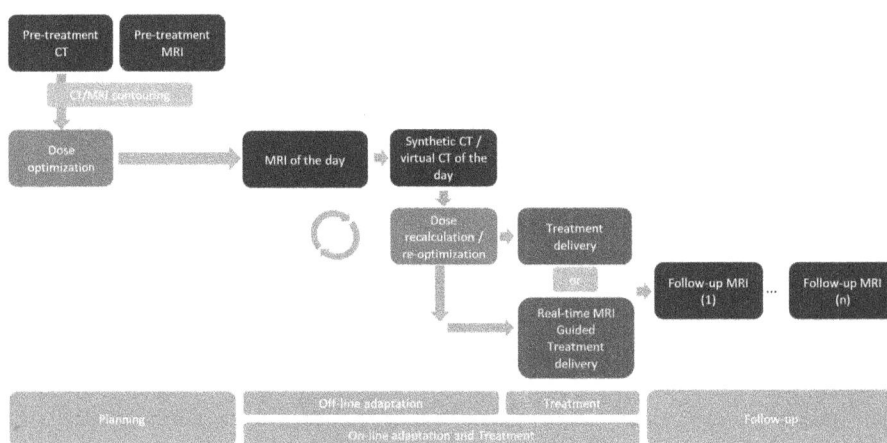

Figure 7.5. Potential use of MRI in an off-line and online workflow. The off-line workflow is intended for a current PT scenario with near room MR scanners, whereas the online workflow (highlighted in yellow) for in-beam integrated MRI-PT system.

compared with pathology (Dirix *et al* 2014). Nevertheless, although consensus guidelines and online available CT/MRI atlases have been created to support tumours and OARs delineation on CT/MRI data on head-and-neck, prostate and abdominal tumours (Heerkens *et al* 2017, Salembier *et al* 2018, Lukovic *et al* 2020, Eekers *et al* 2021) and show that MRI contributes to improved contouring, challenges in target volume definition with MRI are still present for some peculiar tumours such as ocular melanoma, where increased resolution or fusion with complementary ophthalmological imaging are required (Via *et al* 2021, Fleury *et al* 2021).

Apart from contouring, MRI can be useful to support treatment planning optimization. Several studies demonstrated the feasibility in deriving synthetic CT from MRI data with bulk density override, atlas-based analysis and more recently novel deep learning strategies (Johnstone *et al* 2018, Boulanger *et al* 2021), with promising results in terms of dose metrics for proton therapy applications ($<1\%$ of the prescribed dose in brain pediatric patients and $<3\%$ of the prescribed dose in abdominal pediatric patients; see Florkow *et al* 2020, Maspero *et al* 2020). This would allow optimizing the treatment plan directly on the MRI, thus (i) avoiding non-therapeutic dose to the patients for CT acquisitions and (ii) pushing towards MRI-only workflows, which perfectly match with the future availability of MRI-integrated proton therapy systems. Initial investigations on synthetic CT generation from MRI for PT have started. Although different methods have shown promising results in treatment planning studies (see table 10.1 in Hoffmann *et al* 2020), no validation studies have been performed so far. A comprehensive review on artificial intelligence strategies to derive synthetic CT is reported in chapter 8.

In the context of uveal melanoma, the feasibility and suitability of a 3D MRI-based treatment planning approach have been successfully tested, by implementing a full 3D MRI-based treatment planning approach with a gaze-angle proton dose optimization from 7 Tesla high-resolution MRI data (Fleury *et al* 2021).

MRI has also shown the potential to enhance the quantification of tissue parameters that are relevant for PT planning, such as the stopping power ratio (SPR; Scholey *et al* 2021). This brings the prospect of reducing systematic uncertainties in estimating the particle range, when compared to conventional stoichiometric calibration based on CT (Paganetti 2012).

The relevance of MRI in treatment planning has also been demonstrated in the literature for moving organs, where the plan, which currently relies on a single 4DCT before treatment ignoring respiratory variability, must be robust enough to account for inter- and intra-fraction variations. Specifically, respiratory-correlated 4DMRI was exploited to implement the so-called virtual 4DCT (v4DCT), which was first introduced by Boye *et al* (2013) and subsequently extended by Meschini *et al* (2020), and consisted of warping a planning static CT on respiratory phases depicted in a respiratory-correlated 4DMRI, thus producing additional respiratory phases with respect to those depicted in a planning 4DCT, which can be included in plan optimization or used to evaluate the plan robustness against unseen conditions (Bernatowicz *et al* 2016). Relying on this methodology, Krieger *et al* (2020) optimized 4D proton treatment plans on internal target volumes (ITVs) based on different v4DCTs. Different probabilistic ITVs were created by incorporating the voxels covered by the clinical target volume in at least 25%, 50%, or 75% (ITV25, ITV50, ITV75) of the cycles, and compared with the conservative ITV encompassing all possible target positions; results showed that probabilistic ITV50 provided an adequate compromise between target coverage and lung dose for most scenarios, with irregular respiration significantly affecting target coverage when ITVs were only defined by single 4DCTs. In pancreatic cancer, the v4DCT methodology was exploited to investigate the effectiveness of the gating procedure both in proton and carbon ions treatments (Dolde *et al* 2019a, Meschini *et al* 2022b) and to evaluate the interplay effect for pencil beam scanning proton therapy (Dolde *et al* 2019b). The method was also validated relying on physical phantoms and tested for its application in proton and carbon ions treatment of lung cancer (Annunziata *et al* 2023).

Cine-MRI data were also investigated to quantify off-line organ motion and evaluate margins in carbon ion therapy of abdominal lesions against cycle-to-cycle variations, showing that the gating procedure adopted in a clinical institution (i.e. National Center for Oncological Hadrontherapy, Pavia, Italy) was effective (Kalantzopoulos *et al* 2020, Meschini *et al* 2022a). Specifically, in Meschini *et al* (2022a), time-resolved virtual 3DCTs were generated for each cine-MRI frame (figure 7.6) allowing for dose recalculation, potential testing of RBE-weighted 4D

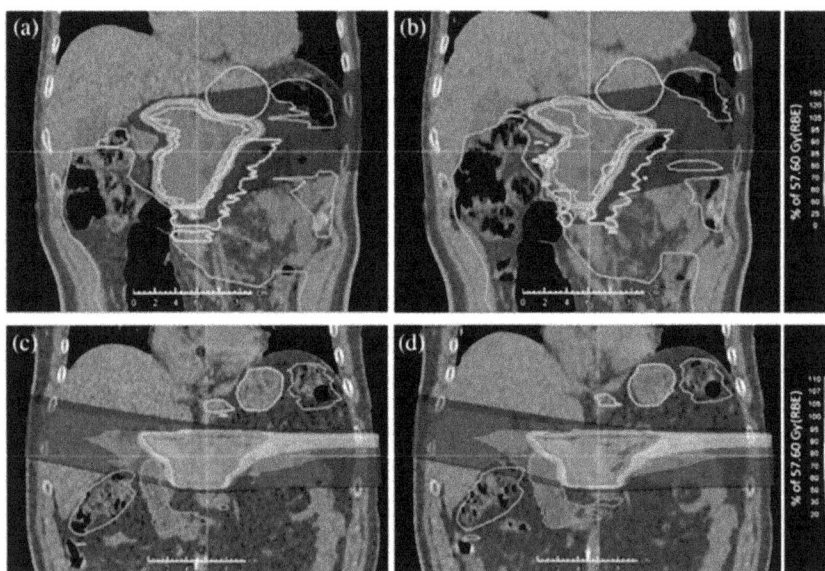

Figure 7.6. Treatment plan robustness evaluation. Planned dose on end-exhale CT (a and c) and recalculated dose on the virtual CT (vCT) (b and d) for two representative patients with high and limited anatomical variations, respectively. The contoured structures represent gross target volume (GTV; red), clinical target volume (CTV; pink), duodenum (light blue), stomach (green), and colon (orange). Picture taken from Meschini *et al* (2022a). John Wiley & Sons. © 2022 The Authors. Medical Physics published by Wiley Periodicals LLC on behalf of American Association of Physicists in Medicine.

particle dose calculation for non-periodic motion (Steinsberger *et al* 2021) and eventual dose accumulation.

7.4.2 Off-line adaptation

In current PT practice where no in-room/in-beam MRI systems are available, near-room MRI can be then adopted offline to adapt the original treatment plan on the basis of the daily patient-specific anatomo-pathological condition. This is most often encountered when changes in patient contour are seen, as on the current workflow based on CBCT, because of weight change or treatment response during conventionally fractioned courses. These changes trigger the creation of a new plan in an attempt to improve dosimetry and achieve the planned prescription for the remaining fractions (Hunt *et al* 2018). The current clinical approach adopted in MRI-linacs mainly consists of registering via DIR the planning CT scan on the in-room MRI acquisition, thus obtaining a virtual CT scan on which the plan can be recalculated and adapted on the anatomy of the day (Kurz *et al* 2020). This can be potentially translated in an offline scenario, where virtual CT (or virtual 4DCT in case of moving organs) can be exploited through repeated radiation-free MRI acquisitions and combined with automated contour propagation and plan re-optimization engines for more frequent plan adjustments (Landry *et al* 2015, Meschini *et al* 2022b). As previously mentioned, synthetic CT based on deep learning could also play a role in treatment adaptation, by directly generating a CT scan on the basis of the acquired MRI scan of the day, thus overcoming DIR limitations when markedly different anatomy is present between the planning CT and the MRI scan. In this context, any adaptation, even if implemented at a single time point during a conventionally fractionated treatment course, delivers dosimetric improvement above a single planning scan.

Recently, the potential value of MRI-based adaptation during PT has been investigated relying on MRI data acquired offline in the treatment position to detect anatomo-pathological changes. Patients demonstrating changes on MRI showed improved plan quality when reoptimized offline (Acharya *et al* 2021; figure 7.7).

The feasibility for an offline adaptive protocol with near-room MRI was implemented relying on a shuttle-based MRI workflow in pelvic tumours in conventional radiotherapy, but limitations, also transferrable to a PT scenario, are still present in terms of (i) long treatment workflow, (ii) prolonged patient immobilization and (iii) persistence of inter- and intra-fraction variations, especially in case of organs affected by respiratory motion (Bostel *et al* 2018).

7.4.3 Online adaptation

In in-beam MRI proton therapy systems, the generation of accurate volumetric and time-resolved or 4D MR images of the patient in the treatment position will immediately raise important questions regarding the impending fraction of radiation to be delivered pushing towards online adaptation (Hoffmann *et al* 2020). The obvious question is whether or not the patient's daily anatomy and positioning matches that of the planning stage. A dose recalculation on the new MRI scan of the

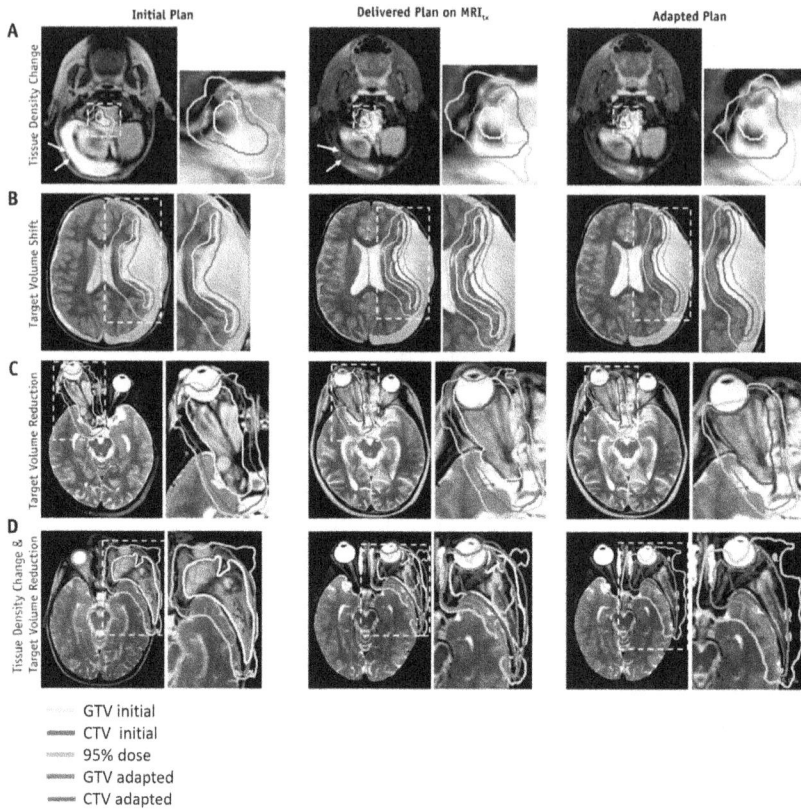

Figure 7.7. Gross tumour volume initial (yellow), clinical target volume initial (red), gross tumour volume adapted (blue), clinical target volume adapted (brown), and 95% isodose line (green) of the initial plan, the delivered plan on MRI$_{tx}$ (i.e. MRI acquired during treatment), and the adapted plan for (A) patient 1, demonstrating tissue density change; (B) patient 3, demonstrating target volume shift as the medial border of the resection cavity shifts laterally; (C) patient 8, demonstrating target volume reduction; and (D) patient 5, demonstrating tissue density change and target volume reduction. Reprinted from Acharya *et al* (2021). Copyright (2021), with permission from Elsevier.

day acquired online of the patient anatomy will need to be performed and the dose coverage and constraints be reassessed. All this needs to be completed in a timely fashion as well, since the patient will be waiting on the treatment couch. Also, in this case as for off-line adaptation, the generation of virtual/synthetic CT from MRI data would support the online workflow.

Further to this, delivering a proton beam fraction with real-time MRI images (i.e. cine-MRI) will open up the option to (i) treat with beam gating or even tumour tracking while directly imaging the tumour, and (ii) accumulate the delivered dose information for offline treatment replanning or re-optimization. Gated treatments could be expected as the default treatment style, where real-time MRI information provided by cine-MRI is used to confirm that the patient position has not changed significantly and that beam-on can continue as normal. For tumours that move, real-time motion mitigation could be achieved through synchronizing the dynamic MR images with the beam control system; simple lateral tumour motion (relative the beam direction) could be in principle tracked dynamically by globally shifting the PBS delivery pattern, but beam energy adaptation depending on the changes of the traversed anatomy, and in the more realistic case of true 3D tumour motion, could be challenging due to the degradation of the dose coverage (Mori *et al* 2018, Hoffmann *et al* 2020). Alternatively, multiphase 4D dose delivery schemes could be applied, as they require only lateral adaptation with online selection of a library of plans corresponding to different breathing phases (Steinsberger *et al* 2022).

The unique offerings of in-beam integrated MRI-guided proton therapy will give rise to an almost mandatory change in workflow. A similar workflow is observed in MRI-linac radiotherapy systems where daily replanning is required if the anatomy of the day is not consistent with the planning stages. It can be appreciated that proton therapy planning is more sensitive to anatomy changes than x-ray radiotherapy, dose calculation accuracy requirements are more demanding in proton therapy than in x-ray therapy, and so the integrated MRI-guided proton therapy workflow will need to be very robust to unlock the true potential of such hybrid systems.

7.4.4 Follow-up examinations

Finally, the treatment response is usually evaluated by acquiring follow-up MR images and measuring the change in size of the tumour either in one dimension (RECIST and RECIST 1.1—Response Evaluation Criteria in Solid Tumours) or in two dimensions (WHO criteria—World Health Organization; Suzuki *et al* 2008). The advantage of MRI to obtain functional imaging can be also exploited to evaluate with quantitative parameters (e.g. from diffusion and perfusion MRI) the structural characteristics of the tumour in response to therapy, along with potential toxicities in nearby healthy organs (Gurney-Champion *et al* 2020, Kurz *et al* 2020, Thorwarth *et al* 2020, Keall *et al* 2022). Refer to chapter 11 for more details on quantitative MRI.

7.5 Conclusion and future perspectives

MRI offers exquisite soft-tissue contrast, unparalleled fast image acquisition flexibility, ionizing dose-free imaging and functional imaging capabilities. Due to these advantages, commercial MRI-linac systems have been recently introduced in the clinic of conventional x-ray radiotherapy with potential improvements on treatment outcome. The potential of MRI guidance can be also exploited in PT to exploit the full benefit of its intrinsic geometrical selectivity and radiobiological effectiveness.

Currently, the utility of MRI has been already demonstrated in the literature relying on acquisitions with near-room MRI scanners. MRI can be used to support treatment planning, including contouring, treatment evaluation and robust optimization. For this latter application, the availability of time-resolved and respiratory-correlated 4DMRI in anatomical site that move as a function of respiration could provide more accurate information on respiratory motion variability than that depicted in conventional 4DCT. Also, the radiation-free nature of MRI allows for repeated acquisitions for treatment verification and adaptation; this is particularly important for PT, where anatomo-pathological changes need to be properly accounted for during treatment to avoid underdosage of the target and overdosage to surrounding healthy tissues. Further investigations are nevertheless required on the accuracy of virtual/synthetic CT, and novel MRI pulse sequences should be implemented to account for specific tissue properties (e.g., electron density or stopping power) for direct dose calculation (Scholey *et al* 2021).

The future availability of integrated MRI-guided proton therapy will further allow one to adapt the treatment online and directly image the internal anatomy of the patient in real-time while performing treatment delivery. Although integrated MRI-guided proton therapy is still in its infancy, several research groups have started addressing the major technical challenges and developments required for bringing this concept into clinical reality. Nevertheless, novel hardware solutions are required to properly decouple the MR magnetic field with the PBS and fast and accurate software is needed for online dose calculation. Also, technological and methodological solutions will be required towards the derivation of real-time volumetric MRI acquisitions (currently limited to 2D) to produce the required 3D information to perform lateral beam adjustments and energy adaptation for tumour tracking. The clinical benefit of such systems will also have to be assessed by implementing dedicated clinical trials in comparison with non-integrated MRI-guided PT workflows.

Finally, the potential adoption of MRI as modality for beam visualisation is under investigation by evaluating the contribution of the x-ray or proton beam on MR signal changes (Wancura *et al* 2022, Gantz *et al* 2023, Schieferecke *et al* 2023), or by exploiting proton beam's electromagnetic signal detectable through sensitive instrumentation, such as optical magnetometry (Rädler *et al* 2021, Rädler *et al* 2022). Although these studies are still at their infancy, promising perspectives are present to complement current solutions for in-vivo proton range verification (described in chapter 10) and push towards fully MRI-guided only workflows.

References

Acharya S, Wang C, Quesada S, Gargone M A, Ates O, Uh J, Krasin M J, Merchant T E and Hua C-h 2021 Adaptive proton therapy for pediatric patients: improving the quality of the delivered plan with on-treatment MRI *Int. J. Radiat. Oncol. Biol. Phys.* **109** 242–51

Annunziata S, Rabe M, Vai A, Molinelli S, Nakas A, Meschini G, Pella A, Vitolo V, Barcellini A and Imparato S 2023 Virtual 4DCT generated from 4DMRI in gated particle therapy: phantom validation and application to lung cancer patients *Phys. Med. Biol.* **68** 145004

Bernatowicz K, Peroni M, Perrin R, Weber D C and Lomax A 2016 Four-dimensional dose reconstruction for scanned proton therapy using liver 4DCT-MRI *Int. J. Radiat. Oncol. Biol. Phys.* **95** 216–23

Bostel T, Pfaffenberger A, Delorme S, Dreher C, Echner G, Haering P, Lang C, Splinter M, Laun F and Müller M 2018 Prospective feasibility analysis of a novel off-line approach for MR-guided radiotherapy *Strahlenther. Onkol.* **194** 425–34

Boulanger M, Nunes J-C, Chourak H, Largent A, Tahri S, Acosta O, De Crevoisier R, Lafond C and Barateau A 2021 Deep learning methods to generate synthetic CT from MRI in radiotherapy: a literature review *Phys. Med.* **89** 265–81

Boye D, Lomax T and Knopf A 2013 Mapping motion from 4D-MRI to 3D-CT for use in 4D dose calculations: a technical feasibility study *Med. Phys.* **40** 061702

Burigo L N and Oborn B M 2019 MRI-guided proton therapy planning: accounting for an inline MRI fringe field *Phys. Med. Biol.* **64** 215015

Burigo L N and Oborn B M 2022 Integrated MRI-guided proton therapy planning: accounting for the full MRI field in a perpendicular system *Med. Phys.* **49** 1853–73

Causer T J, Schellhammer S M, Gantz S, Lühr A, Hoffmann A L, Metcalfe P E, Rosenfeld A B, Guatelli S, Petasecca M and Oborn B M 2020 First application of a high-resolution silicon detector for proton beam Bragg peak detection in a 0.95 T magnetic field *Med. Phys.* **47** 181–9

Corradini S, Alongi F, Andratschke N, Belka C, Boldrini L, Cellini F, Debus J, Guckenberger M, Hörner-Rieber J and Lagerwaard F 2019 MR-guidance in clinical reality: current treatment challenges and future perspectives *Radiat. Oncol.* **14** 1–12

Debus J 2021 The ARTEMIS project Heidelberg *8th MR in RT Symp.* (Heidelberg, Germany: German Cancer Research Center)

Dinkel J, Hintze C, Tetzlaff R, Huber P E, Herfarth K, Debus J, Kauczor H U and Thieke C 2009 4D-MRI analysis of lung tumor motion in patients with hemidiaphragmatic paralysis *Radiother. Oncol.* **91** 449–54

Dirix P, Haustermans K and Vandecaveye V 2014 The value of magnetic resonance imaging for radiotherapy planning *Semin. Radiat. Oncol.* **24** 151–9

Dolde K, Naumann P, Dávid C, Kachelriess M, Lomax A J, Weber D C, Saito N, Burigo L N, Pfaffenberger A and Zhang Y 2019a Comparing the effectiveness and efficiency of various gating approaches for PBS proton therapy of pancreatic cancer using 4D-MRI datasets *Phys. Med. Biol.* **64** 085011

Dolde K, Zhang Y, Chaudhri N, Dávid C, Kachelrieß M, Lomax A J, Naumann P, Saito N, Weber D C and Pfaffenberger A 2019b 4DMRI-based investigation on the interplay effect for pencil beam scanning proton therapy of pancreatic cancer patients *Radiat. Oncol.* **14** 1–13

Eekers D B, Di Perri D, Roelofs E, Postma A, Dijkstra J, Ajithkumar T, Alapetite C, Blomstrand M, Burnet N G and Calugaru V 2021 Update of the EPTN atlas for CT-and MR-based contouring in neuro-oncology *Radiother. Oncol.* **160** 259–65

Fallone B G 2014 The rotating biplanar linac–magnetic resonance imaging system *Semin. Radiat. Oncol.* **24** 200–2

Fleury E, Trnková P, Erdal E, Hassan M, Stoel B, Jaarma-Coes M, Luyten G, Herault J, Webb A and Beenakker J W 2021 Three-dimensional MRI-based treatment planning approach for non-invasive ocular proton therapy *Med. Phys.* **48** 1315–26

Florkow M C, Guerreiro F, Zijlstra F, Seravalli E, Janssens G O, Maduro J H, Knopf A C, Castelein R M, van Stralen M and Raaymakers B W 2020 Deep learning-enabled MRI-only photon and proton therapy treatment planning for paediatric abdominal tumours *Radiother. Oncol.* **153** 220–7

Freedman J N, Gurney-Champion O J, Nill S, Shiarli A-M, Bainbridge H E, Mandeville H C, Koh D-M, McDonald F, Kachelrieß M and Oelfke U 2021 Rapid 4D-MRI reconstruction using a deep radial convolutional neural network: Dracula *Radiother. Oncol.* **159** 209–17

Fuchs H, Moser P, Gröschl M and Georg D 2017 Magnetic field effects on particle beams and their implications for dose calculation in MR-guided particle therapy *Med. Phys.* **44** 1149–56

Fuchs H, Padilla-Cabal F, Hummel A and Georg D 2021a Design and commissioning of a water phantom for proton dosimetry in magnetic fields *Med. Phys.* **48** 505–12

Fuchs H, Padilla-Cabal F, Zimmermann L, Palmans H and Georg D 2021b MR-guided proton therapy: impact of magnetic fields on the detector response *Med. Phys.* **48** 2572–9

Gantz S, Hietschold V and Hoffmann A L 2020 Characterization of magnetic interference and image artefacts during simultaneous in-beam MR imaging and proton pencil beam scanning *Phys. Med. Biol.* **65** 215014

Gantz S, Karsch L, Pawelke J, Schieferecke J, Schellhammer S, Smeets J, van der Kraaij E and Hoffmann A 2023 Direct visualization of proton beam irradiation effects in liquids by MRI *Proc. Natl Acad. Sci.* **120** e2301160120

Gao Y, Han F, Zhou Z, Cao M, Kaprealian T, Kamrava M, Wang C, Neylon J, Low D A and Yang Y 2017 Distortion-free diffusion MRI using an MRI-guided Tri-Cobalt 60 radiotherapy system: sequence verification and preliminary clinical experience *Med. Phys.* **44** 5357–66

Gao Y, Zhou Z, Han F, Cao M, Shaverdian N, Hegde J V, Bista B B, Steinberg M, Lee P and Raldow A 2018 Accelerated 3D bSSFP imaging for treatment planning on an MRI-guided radiotherapy system *Med. Phys.* **45** 2595–602

Gebauer B, Pawelke J, Hoffmann A and Lühr A 2023 Experimental dosimetric characterization of proton pencil beam distortion in a perpendicular magnetic field of an in-beam MR scanner *Med. Phys.* **50** 7294–303

Gurney-Champion O J, Mahmood F, van Schie M, Julian R, George B, Philippens M E, van der Heide U A, Thorwarth D and Redalen K R 2020 Quantitative imaging for radiotherapy purposes *Radiother. Oncol.* **146** 66–75

Hartman J, Kontaxis C, Bol G, Frank S, Lagendijk J, Van Vulpen M and Raaymakers B 2015 Dosimetric feasibility of intensity modulated proton therapy in a transverse magnetic field of 1.5 T *Phys. Med. Biol.* **60** 5955

Heerkens H D, Hall W, Li X, Knechtges P, Dalah E, Paulson E, van den Berg C, Meijer G, Koay E and Crane C 2017 Recommendations for MRI-based contouring of gross tumor volume and organs at risk for radiation therapy of pancreatic cancer *Pract. Radiat. Oncol.* **7** 126–36

Hoffmann A, Oborn B, Moteabbed M, Yan S, Bortfeld T, Knopf A, Fuchs H, Georg D, Seco J and Spadea M F 2020 MR-guided proton therapy: a review and a preview *Radiat. Oncol.* **15** 1–13

Hunt A, Hansen V, Oelfke U, Nill S and Hafeez S 2018 Adaptive radiotherapy enabled by MRI guidance *Clin. Oncol.* **30** 711–9

Intven M, van Otterloo S d M, Mook S, Doornaert P, de Groot-van Breugel E, Sikkes G, Willemsen-Bosman M, van Zijp H and Tijssen R 2021 Online adaptive MR-guided radiotherapy for rectal cancer; feasibility of the workflow on a 1.5 T MR-linac: clinical implementation and initial experience *Radiother. Oncol.* **154** 172–8

Jaffray D A, Carlone M C, Milosevic M F, Breen S L, Stanescu T, Rink A, Alasti H, Simeonov A, Sweitzer M C and Winter J D 2014 A facility for magnetic resonance–guided radiation therapy *Semin. Radiat. Oncol.* **24** 193–5

Johnstone E, Wyatt J J, Henry A M, Short S C, Sebag-Montefiore D, Murray L, Kelly C G, McCallum H M and Speight R 2018 Systematic review of synthetic computed tomography generation methodologies for use in magnetic resonance imaging–only radiation therapy *Int. J. Radiat. Oncol. Biol. Phys.* **100** 199–217

Kalantzopoulos C, Meschini G, Paganelli C, Fontana G, Vai A, Preda L, Vitolo V, Valvo F and Baroni G 2020 Organ motion quantification and margins evaluation in carbon ion therapy of abdominal lesions *Phys. Med.* **75** 33–9

Keall P J, Barton M and Crozier S 2014 The Australian magnetic resonance imaging–linac program *Semin. Radiat. Oncol.* **24** 203–6

Keall P J, Brighi C, Glide-Hurst C, Liney G, Liu P Z, Lydiard S, Paganelli C, Pham T, Shan S and Tree A C 2022 Integrated MRI-guided radiotherapy—opportunities and challenges *Nat. Rev. Clin. Oncol.* **19** 458–70

Kim T, Lewis B, Lotey R, Barberi E and Green O 2021 Clinical experience of MRI4D QUASAR motion phantom for latency measurements in 0.35 T MR-LINAC *J. Appl. Clin. Med. Phys.* **22** 128–36

Kishan A U, Ma T M, Lamb J M, Casado M, Wilhalme H, Low D A, Sheng K, Sharma S, Nickols N G and Pham J 2023 Magnetic resonance imaging–guided vs computed tomography–guided stereotactic body radiotherapy for prostate cancer: the MIRAGE randomized clinical trial *JAMA Oncol.* **9** 365–73

Klüter S 2019 Technical design and concept of a 0.35 T MR-Linac *Clin. Transl. Radiat. Oncol* **18** 98–101

Krieger M, Giger A, Salomir R, Bieri O, Celicanin Z, Cattin P C, Lomax A J, Weber D C and Zhang Y 2020 Impact of internal target volume definition for pencil beam scanned proton treatment planning in the presence of respiratory motion variability for lung cancer: a proof of concept *Radiother. Oncol.* **145** 154–61

Kurz C, Buizza G, Landry G, Kamp F, Rabe M, Paganelli C, Baroni G, Reiner M, Keall P J and van den Berg C A 2020 Medical physics challenges in clinical MR-guided radiotherapy *Radiat. Oncol.* **15** 1–16

Lagendijk J J, Raaymakers B W, Van den Berg C A, Moerland M A, Philippens M E and Van Vulpen M 2014 MR guidance in radiotherapy *Phys. Med. Biol.* **59** R349

Landry G and Hua C h 2018 Current state and future applications of radiological image guidance for particle therapy *Med. Phys.* **45** e1086–95

Landry G, Nijhuis R, Dedes G, Handrack J, Thieke C, Janssens G, Orban de Xivry J, Reiner M, Kamp F and Wilkens J J 2015 Investigating CT to CBCT image registration for head and neck proton therapy as a tool for daily dose recalculation *Med. Phys.* **42** 1354–66

Lawrence L S, Chan R W, Chen H, Keller B, Stewart J, Ruschin M, Chugh B, Campbell M, Theriault A and Stanisz G J 2021 Accuracy and precision of apparent diffusion coefficient measurements on a 1.5 T MR-Linac in central nervous system tumour patients *Radiother. Oncol.* **164** 155–62

Liney G and Van der Heide U 2019 *MRI for Radiotherapy: Planning, Delivery, and Response Assessment* (Berlin: Springer)

Ling C C, Humm J, Larson S, Amols H, Fuks Z, Leibel S and Koutcher J A 2000 Towards multidimensional radiotherapy (MD-CRT): biological imaging and biological conformality *Int. J. Radiat. Oncol. Biol. Phys.* **47** 551–60

Lühr A, Burigo L, Gantz S, Schellhammer S and Hoffmann A 2019 Proton beam electron return effect: Monte Carlo simulations and experimental verification *Phys. Med. Biol.* **64** 035012

Lukovic J, Henke L, Gani C, Kim T K, Stanescu T, Hosni A, Lindsay P, Erickson B, Khor R and Eccles C 2020 MRI-based upper abdominal organs-at-risk atlas for radiation oncology *Int. J. Radiat. Oncol. Biol. Phys.* **106** 743–53

Maspero M, Bentvelzen L G, Savenije M H, Guerreiro F, Seravalli E, Janssens G O, van den Berg C A and Philippens M E 2020 Deep learning-based synthetic CT generation for paediatric brain MR-only photon and proton radiotherapy *Radiother. Oncol.* **153** 197–204

McRobbie D W, Moore E A, Graves M J and Prince M R 2017 *MRI from Picture to Proton* (Cambridge: Cambridge University Press)

Meschini G, Paganelli C, Gianoli C, Summers P, Bellomi M, Baroni G and Riboldi M 2019 A clustering approach to 4D MRI retrospective sorting for the investigation of different surrogates *Phys. Med.* **58** 107–13

Meschini G, Vai A, Barcellini A, Fontana G, Molinelli S, Mastella E, Pella A, Vitolo V, Imparato S and Orlandi E 2022a Time-resolved MRI for off-line treatment robustness evaluation in carbon-ion radiotherapy of pancreatic cancer *Med. Phys.* **49** 2386–95

Meschini G, Vai A, Paganelli C, Molinelli S, Fontana G, Pella A, Preda L, Vitolo V, Valvo F and Ciocca M 2020 Virtual 4DCT from 4DMRI for the management of respiratory motion in carbon ion therapy of abdominal tumors *Med. Phys.* **47** 909–16

Meschini G, Vai A, Paganelli C, Molinelli S, Maestri D, Fontana G, Pella A, Vitolo V, Valvo F and Ciocca M 2022b Investigating the use of virtual 4DCT from 4DMRI in gated carbon ion radiation therapy of abdominal tumors *Z. Med. Phys.* **32** 98–108

Mickevicius N J and Paulson E S 2017a Investigation of undersampling and reconstruction algorithm dependence on respiratory correlated 4D-MRI for online MR-guided radiation therapy *Phys. Med. Biol.* **62** 2910

Mickevicius N J and Paulson E S 2017b Simultaneous orthogonal plane imaging *Magn. Reson. Med.* **78** 1700–10

Mori S, Knopf A C and Umegaki K 2018 Motion management in particle therapy *Med. Phys.* **45** e994–e1010

Moteabbed M, Schuemann J and Paganetti H 2014 Dosimetric feasibility of real-time MRI-guided proton therapy *Med. Phys.* **41** 111713

Moteabbed M, Smeets J, Hong T S, Janssens G, Labarbe R, Wolfgang J A and Bortfeld T R 2021 Toward MR-integrated proton therapy: modeling the potential benefits for liver tumors *Phys. Med. Biol.* **66** 195004

Mutic S and Dempsey J F 2014 The ViewRay system: magnetic resonance–guided and controlled radiotherapy *Semin. Radiat. Oncol.* **24** 196–9

Nierer L, Eze C, da Silva Mendes V, Braun J, Thum P, von Bestenbostel R, Kurz C, Landry G, Reiner M and Niyazi M 2022 Dosimetric benefit of MR-guided online adaptive radiotherapy in different tumor entities: liver, lung, abdominal lymph nodes, pancreas and prostate *Radiat. Oncol.* **17** 1–14

Oborn B, Dowdell S, Metcalfe P E, Crozier S, Mohan R and Keall P J 2015 Proton beam deflection in MRI fields: implications for MRI-guided proton therapy *Med. Phys.* **42** 2113–24

Oborn B M, Dowdell S, Metcalfe P E, Crozier S, Mohan R and Keall P J 2017 Future of medical physics: real-time MRI-guided proton therapy *Med. Phys.* **44** e77–90

Olsen J, Green O and Kashani R 2015 World's first applicaton of MR-guidance for radiotherapy *Mo. Med.* **112** 358

Padilla-Cabal F, Resch A F, Georg D and Fuchs H 2020 Implementation of a dose calculation algorithm based on Monte Carlo simulations for treatment planning towards MRI guided ion beam therapy *Phys. Med.* **74** 155–65

Padilla-Cabal F, Alejandro Fragoso J, Franz Resch A, Georg D and Fuchs H 2020 Benchmarking a GATE/Geant4 Monte Carlo model for proton beams in magnetic fields *Med. Phys.* **47** 223–33

Padilla-Cabal F, Georg D and Fuchs H 2018 A pencil beam algorithm for magnetic resonance image-guided proton therapy *Med. Phys.* **45** 2195–204

Paganelli C, Kipritidis J, Lee D, Baroni G, Keall P and Riboldi M 2018a Image-based retrospective 4D MRI in external beam radiotherapy: a comparative study with a digital phantom *Med. Phys.* **45** 3161–72

Paganelli C, Whelan B, Peroni M, Summers P, Fast M, Van de Lindt T, McClelland J, Eiben B, Keall P and Lomax T 2018b MRI-guidance for motion management in external beam radiotherapy: current status and future challenges *Phys. Med. Biol.* **63** 22TR03

Paganetti H 2012 Range uncertainties in proton therapy and the role of Monte Carlo simulations *Phys. Med. Biol.* **57** R99

Peteani G, Paganelli C, Giovannelli A C, Bachtiary B, Safai S, Rogers S, Pusterla O, Riesterer O, Weber D C and Lomax A J 2023 Retrospective reconstruction of four-dimensional magnetic resonance from interleaved cine imaging–a comparative study with four-dimensional computed tomography in the lung *Phys. Imaging Radiat. Oncol.* **29** 100529

Pham T T, Whelan B, Oborn B M, Delaney G P, Vinod S, Brighi C, Barton M and Keall P 2022 Magnetic resonance imaging (MRI) guided proton therapy: a review of the clinical challenges, potential benefits and pathway to implementation *Radiother. Oncol.* **170** 37–47

Raaymakers B W, Jürgenliemk-Schulz I, Bol G, Glitzner M, Kotte A, Van Asselen B, De Boer J, Bluemink J, Hackett S and Moerland M 2017 First patients treated with a 1.5 T MRI-Linac: clinical proof of concept of a high-precision, high-field MRI guided radiotherapy treatment *Phys. Med. Biol.* **62** L41

Raaymakers B W, Raaijmakers A J and Lagendijk J J 2008 Feasibility of MRI guided proton therapy: magnetic field dose effects *Phys. Med. Biol.* **53** 5615

Rädler M, Buizza G, Kawula M, Palaniappan P, Gianoli C, Baroni G, Paganelli C, Parodi K and Riboldi M 2022 Impact of secondary particles on the magnetic field generated by a proton pencil beam: a finite element analysis based on Geant4-DNA simulations *Med. Phys.* **50** 1000–18

Rädler M, Gianoli C, Palaniappan P, Parodi K and Riboldi M 2021 Electromagnetic signal of a proton beam in biological tissues for a potential range-verification approach in proton therapy *Phys. Rev. Appl.* **15** 024066

Rudra S, Jiang N, Rosenberg S A, Olsen J R, Roach M C, Wan L, Portelance L, Mellon E A, Bruynzeel A and Lagerwaard F 2019 Using adaptive magnetic resonance image-guided radiation therapy for treatment of inoperable pancreatic cancer *Cancer Med.* **8** 2123–32

Salembier C, Villeirs G, De Bari B, Hoskin P, Pieters B R, Van Vulpen M, Khoo V, Henry A, Bossi A and De Meerleer G 2018 ESTRO ACROP consensus guideline on CT-and MRI-based target volume delineation for primary radiation therapy of localized prostate cancer *Radiother. Oncol.* **127** 49–61

Schellhammer S M and Hoffmann A L 2017 Prediction and compensation of magnetic beam deflection in MR-integrated proton therapy: a method optimized regarding accuracy, versatility and speed *Phys. Med. Biol.* **62** 1548

Schellhammer S M, Hoffmann A L, Gantz S, Smeets J, Van Der Kraaij E, Quets S, Pieck S, Karsch L and Pawelke J 2018 Integrating a low-field open MR scanner with a static proton research beam line: proof of concept *Phys. Med. Biol.* **63** 23LT01

Schieferecke J, Gantz S, Hoffmann A and Pawelke J 2023 Investigation of contrast mechanisms for MRI phase signal-based proton beam visualization in water phantoms *Magn. Reson. Med.* **90** 1776–88

Scholey J E, Chandramohan D, Naren T, Liu W, Larson P E Z and Sudhyadhom A 2021 A methodology for improved accuracy in stopping power estimation using MRI and CT *Med. Phys.* **48** 342–53

Steinsberger T, Alliger C, Donetti M, Krämer M, Lis M, Paz A, Wolf M and Graeff C 2021 Extension of RBE-weighted 4D particle dose calculation for non-periodic motion *Phys. Med.* **91** 62–72

Steinsberger T, Donetti M, Lis M, Volz L, Wolf M, Durante M and Graeff C 2022 Experimental validation of an online adaptive 4D-optimized particle radiotherapy approach to treat irregularly moving tumors *Int. J. Radiat. Oncol. Biol. Phys.* **115** 1257–68

Stemkens B, Paulson E S and Tijssen R H 2018 Nuts and bolts of 4D-MRI for radiotherapy *Phys. Med. Biol.* **63** 21TR01

Suzuki C, Jacobsson H, Hatschek T, Torkzad M R, Bodén K, Eriksson-Alm Y, Berg E, Fujii H, Kubo A and Blomqvist L 2008 Radiologic measurements of tumor response to treatment: practical approaches and limitations *Radiographics* **28** 329–44

Terpstra *et al* 2020 Deep learning-based image reconstruction and motion estimation from undersampled radial k-space for real-time MRI-guided radiotherapy *Phys. Med. Biol.* **65** 155015

Thorwarth D, Ege M, Nachbar M, Mönnich D, Gani C, Zips D and Boeke S 2020 Quantitative magnetic resonance imaging on hybrid magnetic resonance linear accelerators: perspective on technical and clinical validation *Phys. Imaging Radiat. Oncol.* **16** 69–73

Via R, Hennings F, Pica A, Fattori G, Beer J, Peroni M, Baroni G, Lomax A, Weber D C and Hrbacek J 2021 Potential and pitfalls of 1.5 T MRI imaging for target volume definition in ocular proton therapy *Radiother. Oncol.* **154** 53–9

von Siebenthal M, Szekely G, Gamper U, Boesiger P, Lomax A and Cattin P 2007 4D MR imaging of respiratory organ motion and its variability *Phys. Med. Biol.* **52** 1547

Wancura J, Egan J, Sajo E and Sudhyadhom A 2022 MRI of radiation chemistry: first images and investigation of potential mechanisms *Med. Phys.* **50** 495–505

Werensteijn-Honingh A M, Kroon P S, Winkel D, Aalbers E M, van Asselen B, Bol G H, Brown K J, Eppinga W S, van Es C A and Glitzner M 2019 Feasibility of stereotactic radiotherapy using a 1.5 T MR-linac: multi-fraction treatment of pelvic lymph node oligometastases *Radiother. Oncol.* **134** 50–4

Wolf R and Bortfeld T 2012 An analytical solution to proton Bragg peak deflection in a magnetic field *Phys. Med. Biol.* **57** N329

IOP Publishing

Imaging in Particle Therapy
Current practice and future trends
Chiara Paganelli, Chiara Gianoli and Antje Knopf

Chapter 8

Artificial intelligence to generate synthetic CT for adaptive particle therapy

A Thummerer, P Zaffino, M F Spadea, A Knopf and M Maspero

8.1 Introduction

Artificial intelligence (AI) is a branch of computer science that deals with developing computer systems to perform tasks requiring human intelligence, such as visual perception, speech recognition, decision-making, and translation between languages (McCarthy 2007). The use of AI in healthcare is increasing (Rajpurkar *et al* 2022), and diagnostic medical imaging and radiotherapy are not immune to AI's impact (Meyer *et al* 2018, Oren *et al* 2020).

Specifically for radiotherapy (RT), one of the main pillars of cancer treatment (Delaney *et al* 2005), AI can play a role in all the steps of the radiotherapy workflow (Meyer *et al* 2018). AI promises to increase efficiency for the staff involved, improve the quality of treatments, and provide additional clinical information and treatment response predictions to assist and enhance clinical decision-making (Feng *et al* 2018, Huynh *et al* 2020).

This chapter focuses on AI for synthesizing computed tomography (CT) from magnetic resonance imaging (MRI) and cone-beam computed tomography (CBCT) for adaptive particle therapy (APT).

Traditionally, CT is considered the primary imaging modality in RT/PT, providing accurate and high-resolution patient geometry and enabling the estimation of electron density or charged particle stopping power ratio (SPR) needed for dose calculations (Chernak *et al* 1975, Schneider *et al* 1996).

CBCT-based image-guided radiotherapy (IGRT) is adopted in most clinics and crucial in accurate patient position verification. CBCT can facilitate online adaptive workflows by visualizing daily anatomical variations without recurring additional re-scanning on CT.

However, due to artifacts, CBCT image quality is inferior to CT in soft tissue contrast and CT number consistency (Schulze *et al* 2011). Therefore, CBCT is unsuitable for performing accurate dose calculations for photon therapy. Such issues become even more critical for PT, where CT inconsistencies have a larger impact (Paganetti and Bortfeld 2006). Thus, patients must be referred for a rescan CT when anatomical differences are noted between daily images and the planning CT (Ramella *et al* 2017).

Scheduling and acquiring a rescan CT adds logistic complexity and patient burden to the treatment, e.g., increased dose delivered to the patient and need for additional scheduling. On the contrary, with APT based on CBCT, many of these issues can be addressed.

A prerequisite for online APT based on CBCT is that the CT number accuracy is sufficient to enable dose calculation, which is crucial for dose calculations with particle beams. AI-based image synthesis can be adopted to improve CBCT image quality to CT level, generating the so-called synthetic CT (sCT).

AI-based corrections are meant to speed up CBCT correction, enabling daily adaptive scenarios. Other conventional methods that have been proposed to increase image intensity consistency include look-up table-based approaches (Dunlop *et al* 2015), deformable image registration of the planning CT to the daily anatomy on CBCT (Zhen *et al* 2012), i.e., virtual CT, and model- or Monte Carlo-based methods for scatter estimation and correction (Bootsma *et al* 2015, Zhao *et al* 2016). However, these techniques can be deployed on a time scale of minutes, which is unacceptable when aiming to use CBCT images for daily dose evaluation or online adaptation.

MRI-guided RT with novel MRI-linac units has been proposed (Raaymakers *et al* 2004) to increase daily target visibility and irradiation accuracy, which is beneficial for tumour control and the surrounding healthy tissues (Dawson and Sharpe 2006). Such motivations are even more relevant in PT due to the high sensitivity of beam range to daily geometrical inaccuracies or variations. MRI offers excellent and tunable soft-tissue contrast compared to x-ray-based imaging, making this imaging modality a preferable choice for organ delineation during the planning stage and for monitoring intra- and inter-anatomical changes. In addition, data acquisition in MRI can generate cine-MRI in the sagittal or coronal plane, as well as any other oblique orientation, thus allowing real-time tumour tracking during beam delivery. MRI can also provide functional and metabolic imaging, which can help monitor the treatment response and tailor or boost the dose in specific cases (Keall *et al* 2022). Finally, MRI avoids extra ionizing radiation to the patient, which could increase toxicity-associated risks and impact the patient's health and quality of life. The lack of radiation is relevant to pediatric patients, where radiation levels must be carefully controlled.

In-beam MRI guidance is not yet a clinical possibility for PT, but the first hardware design and experiments have been proposed (Oborn *et al* 2017, Hoffmann *et al* 2020).

As for the adaptive scenario based on CBCT, CT is still the standard planning imaging modality in MRI guidance, meaning that daily MRI needs to be registered to the planning CT, leading to a possible mismatch between planning images and daily anatomy. Recently, MR-only based RT has been proposed to investigate the generation of sCT from MRI to enable MR-based treatment planning. The main application is still photon therapy, but some particle therapies have begun to collect attention (Spadea *et al* 2021).

In the following, we will cover the most promising AI techniques. Afterward, sCT generation from CBCT and MRI will be reviewed, focusing on the steps required for clinical implementation in PT.

8.2 Neural network architectures, training, and evaluation

One of the most promising algorithms in the AI field is represented by convolutional neural networks (CNNs), given the significant impact demonstrated in image processing applications (Razzak *et al* 2018). CNNs are part of deep learning (DL), a subset of machine learning (ML) where the algorithm tries to perform a task by choosing its representation by learning a set of hierarchical features (figure 8.1).

To generate sCT from MRI or CBCT, the DL model should perform an image-to-image (I2I) translation task, mapping MRI or CBCT (initial domain) to CT (target domain; Zhu *et al* 2017). An I2I network uses a series of 2D or 3D convolutions to identify the non-linear association among input-target intensities. The weights of each kernel used to convolve the input image are found by an optimization process that minimizes the difference between translated and ground truth images. An extensive dataset must be used for training to let the network learn and generalize the task. Figure 8.2 shows a typical DL workflow where the to-be-

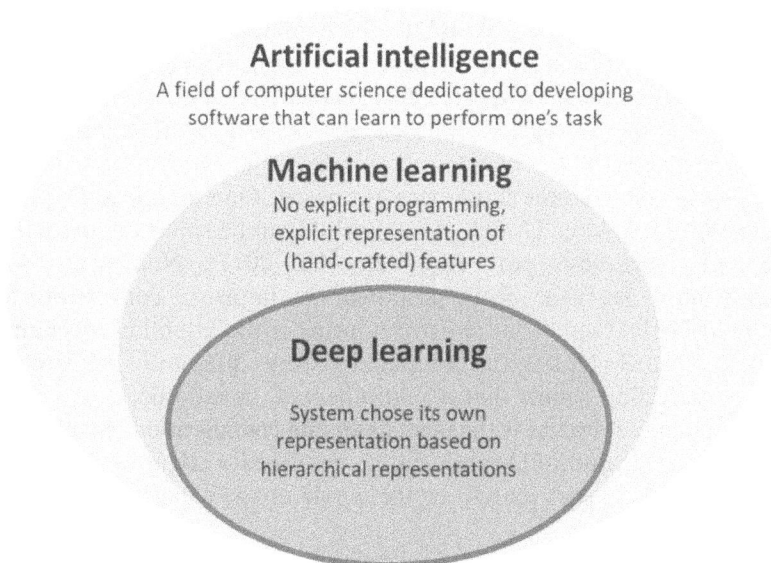

Artificial intelligence
A field of computer science dedicated to developing software that can learn to perform one's task

Machine learning
No explicit programming, explicit representation of (hand-crafted) features

Deep learning

System chose its own representation based on hierarchical representations

Figure 8.1. Sketch of the subfields of artificial intelligence (AI) comprising machine learning and deep learning (DL). The most promising architectures in this chapter are convolutional neural networks (CNNs), models subset of DL.

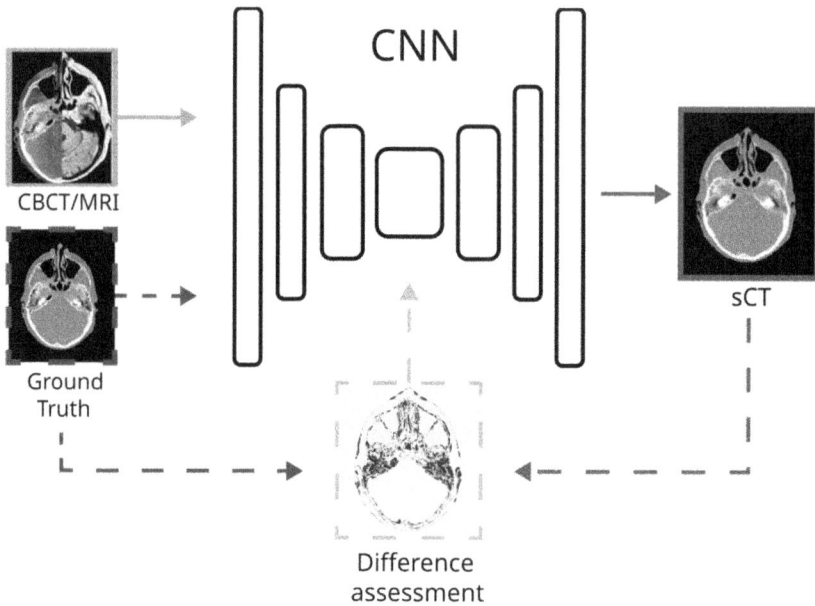

Figure 8.2. General DL workflow for sCT generation. Input is provided to the network, translating it into an sCT (red). Optimization minimizes the difference between sCT and ground truth image (light blue) during training. Dashed blocks are needed only during training.

converted image is provided to the model. The model, led by the similarity measure between remapped and ground truth images, iteratively learns to produce sCTs.

I2I translation is a complex task in DL where millions of parameters (e.g., kernel weights) must be tuned to achieve the best conversion. Due to the high modularity and customizability of the network, technical choices like model architecture, spatial configuration, training strategy, workflow structure, and loss function are critical to achieving good results.

Several **model architectures** have been proposed. One architecture that proved very effective in this field is 'U-Net'. This pipeline can be split into an analysis path (encoder) and a synthesis path (decoder; Han 2017). Numerous customized architectures have recently been proposed to improve conversion accuracy (Bahrami *et al* 2021). One of the most promising is the attention mechanism (Liu *et al* 2020), in which weighting the computed features differently helps the network focus on reconstructing details that would otherwise be ignored.

Another fundamental point is the **model's spatial configuration.** Available options are: 2D, 2D+, 2.5D, multi-2D, and 3D, as described in figure 8.3. For all these configurations, either a part (patch) or the whole image/volume can be considered (Spadea *et al* 2021).

The **training strategy** is another crucial point to maximizing conversion accuracy. Straightforward single architectures (CNN and U-Net) were the first proposed solutions (Han 2017). Later, multiple networks were used to accomplish the I2I translation. The most well-known example is the generative adversarial network

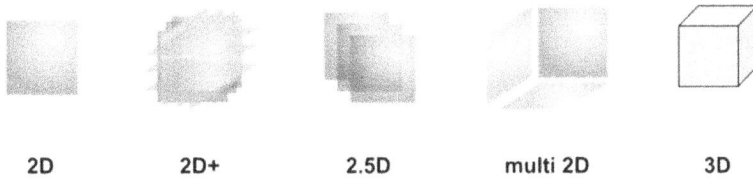

| 2D | 2D+ | 2.5D | multi 2D | 3D |

Figure 8.3. Sketch of the spatial configurations. From left to right, the conversion can be obtained by providing a single 2D slice per time, combining multiple 2D views in inference (2D+), providing neighboring slices along the same direction (2.5D), training a network showing all the possible views (multi 2D), or providing a volume (3D).

(GAN; Emami *et al* 2018), where the output of the I2I network is judged by another network trained to discriminate good sCT from bad sCT. This evaluation is considered during the training of the main network, leading to more reliable results. In the I2I field, the bleeding edge approach is represented by cycle GAN (Chartsias *et al* 2017). Two GANs convert an image back and forth, enabling non-paired and not-matching (unsupervised) training. In this case, the image (MRI or CBCT) is converted into an sCT (forward step), and this synthetic image is converted back to the original modality (reverse conversion). In a process like this, the main comparison is made between the input image and the one obtained from the reverse process (ideally, they should be identical).

The **loss function** to train the DL model is fundamental since it drives the algorithm toward the optimal parameters set (Li *et al* 2022). Optimizing the loss function during the training process can be made of a single metric or, as commonly happens, a combination of multiple metrics. Most of these metrics are also used offline to evaluate the conversion by providing an already-trained model. General quantification of the translation accuracy can be made by computing mean error (ME) or mean absolute error (MAE) (Han 2017), which quantifies the difference in intensity remapping but provides no information about spatial reconstruction. Complementary information can be obtained by computing structural similarity (SSIM) or dice similarity coefficient (DSC) between binary bone segmentation using intensity thresholding. Other common strategies are peak signal-to-noise ratio (PSNR) and dose evaluation, e.g., dose-volume histogram and gamma analysis, to assess the impact of the conversion process in hypothetical radiotherapy treatment.

Over the years, several studies have aimed to find the best setup. Still, the literature suggests that a straightforward absolute best design, irrespective of the anatomical site, has yet to be identified (Bahrami *et al* 2021, Spadea *et al* 2021).

8.3 CBCT-to-CT conversion

DL has proven to be a promising method to correct the shortcomings of daily CBCT, enabling accurate proton dose calculations based on CBCTs (Spadea *et al* 2021). The speed-up that deep learning brings compared to some conventional methods, such as DIR (Kurz *et al* 2016, Veiga *et al* 2017), prior-based scatter correction (Park *et al* 2015, Andersen *et al* 2020), or Monte Carlo simulations

(Thing *et al* 2013) is pivotal for online APT workflows. Conversion times ranging from a few seconds to a few minutes for a full image stack have been reported in the literature and facilitate the use in time-sensitive applications such as online APT (Li *et al* 2019, Barateau *et al* 2020, Maspero *et al* 2020). Another benefit of using deep learning for sCT generation is that once neural networks are trained, CBCT corrections are independent of previous images, such as planning CTs. In this sense, in contrast to some conventional approaches, trained deep learning models are insensitive to significant anatomical changes between CT and CBCT acquisitions. However, if acquisition parameters change, retraining with updated CT and CBCT pairs might be necessary to ensure accurate sCT generation.

CBCT correction using deep learning can be classified according to the domain the correction is applied: (a) the projection domain or (b) during image reconstruction, and thus going from projection to image domain or (c) the image domain (figure 8.4). In the projection domain, neural networks are trained using raw CBCT projections, affected by artifacts, as inputs and corrected CBCT projections as target images. Corrected CBCT projections can be generated using Monte Carlo simulations (Lalonde *et al* 2020) or prior-based corrections using CT images (Park *et al* 2015, Andersen *et al* 2020).

Deep learning techniques can be utilized for image reconstruction from projection data to either replace (Lu *et al* 2021) or assist conventional reconstruction algorithms (Chen *et al* 2018, Dilz *et al* 2019, Zhang *et al* 2019). Most deep learning-based image reconstruction work currently investigates conventional fan-beam CTs instead of CBCTs (Wang *et al* 2019, Arndt *et al* 2021).

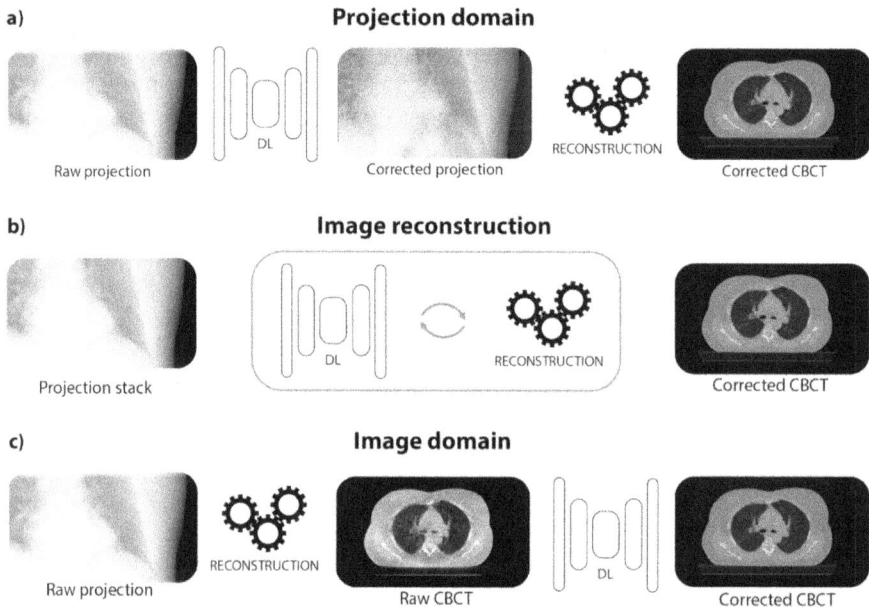

Figure 8.4. Sketch of CBCT correction approaches classified according to the imaging domain. CBCT corrections can be tackled by applying deep learning (DL) on the projections (a), integrating DL in a step of the reconstruction (b), or images (c).

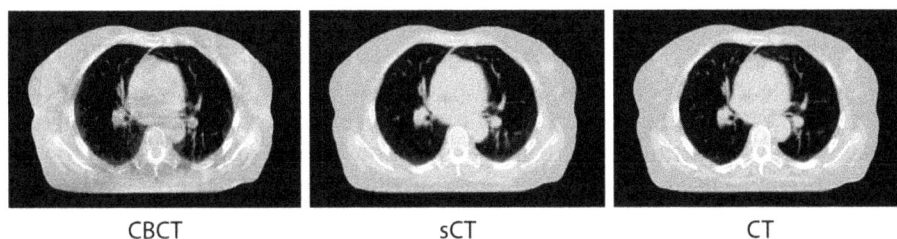

CBCT   sCT   CT

Figure 8.5. Example of CBCT-to-CT conversion for a lung cancer patient. It was generated using a deep convolutional neural network described by Thummerer *et al* (2021).

Finally, in the image domain, reconstructed CBCTs are used as input. The target images can be either conventional fan-beam CTs (Hansen *et al* 2018, Thummerer *et al* 2020) or artifact-corrected CBCTs (Landry *et al* 2019a).

Only one study by Landry *et al* compared projection and image-based approaches for prostate proton dose calculations, observing that reconstructed images outperformed projection-based training (Landry *et al* 2019a). Further investigation of projection-based techniques might be necessary to demonstrate the full potential of CBCT correction in the projection domain. Unfortunately, no studies have been conducted on deep learning CBCT reconstruction with direct application in photon or proton radiotherapy.

In the context of APT, CBCT-to-CT image synthesis has been investigated for a variety of anatomical locations, including head and neck (Thummerer *et al* 2020a, 2020, Zhang *et al* 2021), lung (Thummerer *et al* 2021, 2022) (figure 8.5), prostate (Kurz *et al* 2019, Landry *et al* 2019a) and pelvis (Zhang *et al* 2021). These studies showed the efficacy of deep learning-based sCT generation to correct CBCTs and enhance the proton dose calculation accuracy. Most studies on CBCT correction were performed in the image domain. Image similarity was commonly evaluated using MAE as a similarity metric. MAE values ranged from 24 ± 4 HU in head and neck patients (Zhang *et al* 2021) to 87 ± 5 HU in prostate patients (Kurz *et al* 2019). An average MAE of 34 ± 6 HU for lung patients was observed (Thummerer *et al* 2021). However, an inter-comparison of image similarity results between different studies is challenging since the results are affected by various factors such as training datasets, used registration (rigid vs. deformable), or varying field-of-view sizes.

Two different types of neural network architectures have been investigated for CBCT-to-CT synthesis. Landry *et al* and Thummerer *et al* used a U-Net-based architecture, while Kurz *et al* and Zhang *et al* used a GAN network architecture. There has yet to be clear evidence on which network architecture performs better for sCT generation in APT.

Proton beams are more sensitive to density variations along their beam path, generally requiring higher sCT HU accuracy than photon dose calculations. Several studies reported gamma pass ratios for proton dose calculations. The highest dose accuracy was found for head and neck patients, where an average 3%/3 mm gamma pass rate of 98.7% was reported (Thummerer *et al* 2020). Lower gamma pass rates were observed in the lung (average of 93.7%; Thummerer *et al* 2021) and prostate

(95.9% and >96.5%; Kurz *et al* 2019, Landry *et al* 2019b). Multiple studies also compared the accuracy of photon and proton dose calculations, with the conclusion that proton dose calculations show noticeably lower accuracy (Kurz *et al* 2019, Landry *et al* 2019b). The above studies have shown the fundamental suitability of deep learning to generate CBCT-based sCTs and to enable accurate proton dose calculations in head-and-neck, lung, and prostate cancer patients. However, no reports of clinical implementations within offline or online APT workflows exist. Existing challenges and the future direction of CBCT-based sCTs are addressed in section 8.5.

8.4 MR-to-CT conversion

While the potentialities of MRI in the PT workflow are evident (chapter 7), the investigation and the implementation in clinical practice are still slow compared to other imaging modalities. Slow implementation is due to several challenges that must be considered before fully integrating MRI scanners with PT systems. These include (1) the different patient positioning due to different scanning tables (flat for radiotherapy vs. curved for MRI scanner); (2) the compatibility of immobilization systems with the magnetic field and radio-frequency excitations; (3) the low MRI acquisition time, which can dramatically slow down the entire workflow; (4) the magnetic field distortion (Dumlu *et al* 2022), which causes geometric inaccuracies; (5) the integration of MRI scanners into the treatment room, where the interaction between the magnetic field and accelerated particles can degrade both image quality and beam delivery; (6) the missing information in MRI of electron density, which is necessary to estimate SPR. Numerous investigators have addressed this last issue by implementing methods to convert MRI into sCT. Deep-learning-based approaches are the most promising regarding image translation accuracy and conversion speed for real-time applications in adaptive treatments.

Most deep learning MRI-based methods for sCTs have been investigated for treatment planning due to the current unavailability of MRI during particle delivery irradiation.

The accuracy of PT dose calculation and range analysis on sCT obtained from brain MRI was considered by different authors (Neppl *et al* 2019, Shafai-Erfani *et al* 2019, Spadea *et al* 2019, Kazemifar *et al* 2019, Liu *et al* 2019a, 2019b, Maspero *et al* 2020, Florkow *et al* 2020, Thummerer *et al* 2020, Wang *et al* 2021, 2022, Knäusl *et al* 2022), with an example in figure 8.6. Indeed, the head represents an ideal site for these simulations, as there is no motion due to physiological activity (such as respiration and peristalsis). The analysis can focus on the accuracy of HU conversion. On the other hand, the main problem in the brain site is the presence of the skull bone, which gives a low signal in standard MRI contrasts, i.e., T1 and T2 weighted images, and can influence the beam range, as demonstrated by the first time in Neppl *et al* (2019). Here, the authors proposed both 2D and 3D U-Net MRI-to-CT conversion for proton planning, finding that overestimation of the bone in the upper part of the skull can lead to an extensive range shift. To address this issue, Shafai-Erfani *et al* (2019) implemented a 3D cycle GAN, and Spadea *et al* trained a

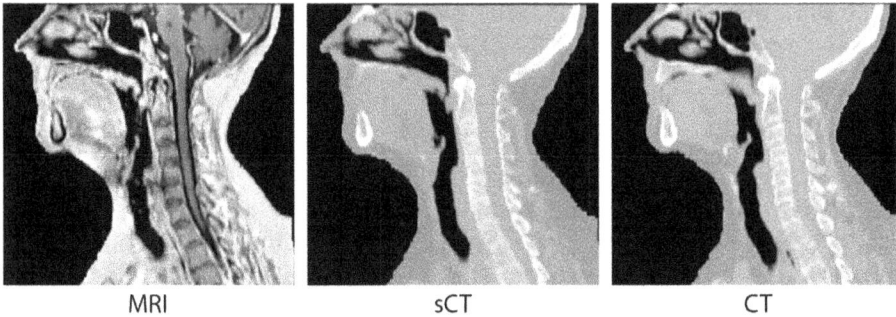

MRI   sCT   CT

Figure 8.6. Example of MRI-to-CT conversion for a head and neck cancer patient. It was generated with a previously trained network, described by Thummerer *et al* (2020a).

2D U-Net on multiple views (axial, sagittal, and coronal) (Spadea *et al* 2019). Both groups found improved bone and air cavity interface depiction, leading to range errors within the clinical acceptance threshold (gamma pass rate 2%/2 mm > 95% or beam-by-beam range shift of 3.5% + 1 mm and 2.5% + 1.5 mm). In the three above-cited works, the networks were trained on co-registered MRI-CT scan pairs. The registration quality profoundly influences the conversion accuracy. It can represent a limitation for implementing MRI-to-CT conversion into the clinical routine when well-matched pairs are unavailable for training. A step forward in this direction was made by Kazemifar *et al*. They implemented a conditional GAN where mutual information between MRI and CT was used as the metric for the generator's loss function to train non-aligned MRI-CT couples in the framework of intensity-modulated proton therapy (Kazemifar *et al* 2020). Recently, Knäusl *et al* (2022) tested a 3D U-Net-based MRI-to-CT conversion in a meningioma patient cohort treated with carbon ion beams. The study revealed the high sensitivity of heavy ions to wrong HU assignment in air cavities and to the lost generation of the thermo-plastic mask, which is transparent to the MR excitation. This poses a severe threat to this kind of treatment, where an additional challenge is the lower flexibility in-beam geometry configuration, due to the absence, in most cases, of a rotating gantry.

To date, sCT derivation from MRI in PT has been investigated in the extra-cranial districts only by two groups: Liu *et al* investigated using 3D cycle GAN for liver (Liu *et al* 2019a) and prostate (Liu *et al* 2019b) proton therapy, showing good performances of deep-learning-based conversion; Parella *et al* investigated using a conditional GAN to generate sCT in the abdomen for carbon ion therapy, showing acceptable dose accuracy (Parrella *et al* 2023).

Researchers also focused on the pediatric patient population, representing a challenging patient cohort due to considerable anatomical variation and tissue heterogeneity. At the same time, children are more radiation-sensitive than adults and could benefit more from MR-only PT, especially for adaptive treatment, where ionizing imaging is repeated. MR-to-CT conversion has been studied for PT planning of brain tumours (Maspero *et al* 2020), abdominal tumours (Florkow *et al* 2020), and pelvic sarcoma (Wang *et al* 2021). More recently, MRI-only APT for children was investigated by Wang *et al* where a cycle GAN with an attention gate was trained on

CT-MRI planning image pairs of 125 pediatric patients (Wang *et al* 2022). This first attempt showed the benefits of MRI-based replanning for offline APT.

8.5 Future direction

Translating AI-based technologies into clinical practice (Kelly *et al* 2019) is challenging, and such a challenge also applies to employing sCT in PT. Specifically, for sCT generation, the lack of ground truth data for commissioning commonly adopted quality assurance (QA) procedures (Vandewinckele *et al* 2020) and the difficulty of detecting outliers hinder implementation in clinical workflows. Recently, QA procedures based on proton range measurements (Seller Oria *et al* 2021) or uncertainty estimation (van Harten *et al* 2020, Tanno *et al* 2021) have been proposed to overcome some limitations. Digital phantoms may also be interesting for QA purposes. However, phantoms have been mainly proposed to evaluate the quality of inter-modality registrations and their use may not be trusted to verify the quality of sCT (Paganelli *et al* 2017, Bauer *et al* 2021). Further investigation is necessary here.

Additionally, most CBCT- and MR-based sCT studies investigate a single anatomical location with a consistent imaging system. The lack of multi-system or multi-center studies poses a crucial challenge to clinical implementation. It is unclear whether robust sCT generation can be achieved without retraining for each anatomy or whenever changes in the imaging system or settings occur. More in detail, MRI contrast is highly dependent on the particular sequence set, the strength of the magnetic field, and more in general, the scanner vendor. This makes it particularly difficult to build a proper dataset that can offer generalized capabilities of the network in converting MRI-to-CT. Future studies using more diverse datasets (e.g., multi-center, multi-anatomy, and multi-system) are required to investigate the robustness of deep learning-based sCTs. In this sense, it is worth mentioning that a Grand Challenge called SynthRAD023 (https://synthrad2023.grand-challenge.org/) has been launched making publicly available data from different centers for pelvis and brain for MRI-to-CT and CBCT-to-CT (Thummerer *et al* 2023). The results from such a challenge will be of interest to verify the robustness of different approaches on a common dataset.

For CBCT-based photon dose calculations, Maspero *et al* already showed that a single neural network could be trained for multiple anatomical sites (head-and-neck, lung, and breast) and varying imaging protocols with no reduction in dose calculation accuracy (Maspero *et al* 2020). This approach seems promising for more robust DL solutions suitable for clinical implementation.

Current studies focus primarily on the dose calculation accuracy of sCTs for a single fraction and less on how these sCTs compare to conventional CTs when it comes to adaptation decisions. sCTs can also potentially reduce or eliminate the need for repeated CT acquisitions during treatment, leading to an imaging dose reduction for the patient and a reduced workload for clinical staff.

Although sCTs can theoretically enable MRI-based (daily) APT, the above-mentioned technological challenges must be overcome to incorporate MRI into PT facilities. Currently, CBCT-based sCTs are suitable for implementation in daily APT workflows, while MR-based sCTs could enable MR-based treatment planning in PT. In conventional photon-based radiotherapy, MRI has recently been integrated into treatment systems (Cusumano *et al* 2020, Farjam *et al* 2021, Li *et al* 2022). Real-time MRI during treatment is required to close the loop and allow online MRI-based APT, and the first attempts to design and build such systems are being undertaken (Schellhammer *et al* 2018). Still, the clinical operation of such a system is far away.

The future availability of MRI-guided proton therapy combined with deep learning-based sCT generation (or SPR prediction) can potentially replace CBCT-based APT strategies. MRI-guided PT would combine the distinct advantages of higher soft-tissue contrast, no imaging dose, and the possibility of real-time imaging. However, this comes at the cost of technological complexity and affordability compared to CBCT-based APT.

The most critical factor contributing to range inaccuracies in PT is the uncertainty of estimating SPR from CT. Recently, dual-energy CT (DECT) has been proposed as an improved approach to SPR conversion (Yang *et al* 2012), and the first attempts to perform deep learning-based SPR prediction have recently led to promising results (Wang *et al* 2022).

To further move towards clinical implementation of sCTs as part of APT workflows, practical questions of reliability and QA in a clinical environment still must be addressed. The availability of commercial deep learning-based sCT generation could also accelerate the transition of sCTs into the clinic. For MR-to-CT conversion, commercial products already exist for the brain, head-and-neck, and pelvis region (Maspero *et al* 2017, Andersen *et al* 2020, Lerner *et al* 2021, Palmér *et al* 2021). Regarding network architectures, public datasets enable a fair comparison between different approaches and allow one to draw conclusions on which network architecture best suits sCT generation.

References

Andersen A G, Park Y K, Elstrøm U V, Petersen J B B, Sharp G C, Winey B, Dong L and Muren L P 2020 Evaluation of an *a priori* scatter correction algorithm for cone-beam computed tomography-based range and dose calculations in proton therapy *Phys. Imaging Radiat. Oncol.* **16** 89–94

Andres E A, Fidon L, Vakalopoulou M, Lerousseau M, Carré A, Sun R and Robert C 2020 Dosimetry-driven quality measure of brain pseudo computed tomography generated from deep learning for MRI-only radiation therapy treatment planning *Int. J. Radiat. Oncol. Biol. Phys.* **108** 813–23

Arndt C, Güttler F, Heinrich A, Bürckenmeyer F, Diamantis I and Teichgräber U 2021 Deep learning CT image reconstruction in clinical practice *RoFo: Fortschr. Geb. Rontgenstr. Nuklearmed.* **193** 252–61

Bahrami A, Karimian A and Arabi H 2021 Comparison of different deep learning architectures for synthetic CT generation from MR images *Phys. Med.* **90** 99–107

Barateau A *et al* 2020 Comparison of CBCT-based dose calculation methods in head and neck cancer radiotherapy: from Hounsfield unit to density calibration curve to deep learning *Med. Phys.* **47** 4683–93

Bauer D F, Russ T, Waldkirch B I *et al* 2021 Generation of annotated multimodal ground truth datasets for abdominal medical image registration *Int. J. CARS* **16** 1277–85

Bootsma G J, Verhaegen F and Jaffray D A 2015 Efficient scatter distribution estimation and correction in CBCT using concurrent Monte Carlo fitting *Med. Phys.* **42** 54–68

Chartsias A, Joyce T, Dharmakumar R and Tsaftaris S A 2017 Adversarial image synthesis for unpaired multi-modal cardiac data *International Workshop on Simulation and Synthesis in Medical Imaging* (Cham: Springer) pp 3–13

Chen B, Xiang K, Gong Z, Wang J and Tan S 2018 Statistical iterative CBCT reconstruction based on neural network *IEEE Trans. Med. Imaging* **37** 1511–21

Chernak E S, Rodriguez-Antunez A, Jelden G L, Dhaliwal R S and Lavik P S 1975 The use of computed tomography for radiation therapy treatment planning *Radiology* **117** 613–4

Cusumano D, Lenkowicz J, Votta C, Boldrini L, Placidi L, Catucci F and Valentini V 2020 A deep learning approach to generate synthetic CT in low field MR-guided adaptive radiotherapy for abdominal and pelvic cases *Radiother. Oncol.* **153** 205–12

Dawson L A and Sharpe M B 2006 Image-guided radiotherapy: rationale, benefits, and limitations *Lancet Oncol.* **7** 848–58

Delaney G, Jacob S, Featherstone C and Barton M 2005 The role of radiotherapy in cancer treatment: estimating optimal utilization from a review of evidence-based clinical guidelines *Cancer* **104** 1129–37

Dilz R J, Schröder L, Moriakov N, Sonke J J and Teuwen J 2019 Learned SIRT for cone beam computed tomography reconstruction *arXiv preprint* arXiv:1908.10715

Dumlu H S, Meschini G, Kurz C, Kamp F, Baroni G, Belka C and Riboldi M 2022 Dosimetric impact of geometric distortions in an MRI-only proton therapy workflow for lung, liver and pancreas *Z. Med. Phys.* **32** 85–97

Dunlop A, McQuaid D, Nill S, Murray J, Poludniowski G, Hansen V N and Oelfke U 2015 Comparison of CT number calibration techniques for CBCT-based dose calculation *Strahlenther. Onkol.* **191** 970–8

Emami H, Dong M, Nejad-Davarani S P and Glide-Hurst C K 2018 Generating synthetic CTs from magnetic resonance images using generative adversarial networks *Med. Phys.* **45** 3627–36

Farjam R, Nagar H, Kathy Zhou X, Ouellette D, Chiara Formenti S and DeWyngaert J K 2021 Deep learning-based synthetic CT generation for MR-only radiotherapy of prostate cancer patients with 0.35 T MRI linear accelerator *J. Appl. Clin. Med. Phys.* **22** 93–104

Feng M, Valdes G, Dixit N and Solberg T D 2018 Machine learning in radiation oncology: opportunities, requirements, and needs *Front. Oncol.* **8** 110

Florkow M C, Guerreiro F, Zijlstra F, Seravalli E, Janssens G O, Maduro J H and Seevinck P R 2020 Deep learning-enabled MRI-only photon and proton therapy treatment planning for paediatric abdominal tumours *Radiother. Oncol.* **153** 220–7

Han X 2017 MR-based synthetic CT generation using a deep convolutional neural network method *Med. Phys.* **44** 1408–19

Hansen L, Kamp L, C B, K P and C K 2018 ScatterNet: a convolutional neural network for cone-beam CT intensity correction David *Med. Phys.* **45** 4916–26

van Harten L D, Wolterink J M, Verhoeff J J and Išgum I 2020 Automatic online quality control of synthetic CTs *Medical Imaging 2020: Image Processing* vol **11313** (Bellingham, WA: SPIE) pp 399–405

Hoffmann A *et al* 2020 MR-guided proton therapy: a review and a preview *Radiat. Oncol.* **15** 1–3

Huynh E, Hosny A, Guthier C, Bitterman D S, Petit S F, Haas-Kogan D A and Mak R H 2020 Artificial intelligence in radiation oncology *Nat. Rev. Clin. Oncol.* **17** 771–81

Kazemifar S, Barragán Montero A M, Souris K, Rivas S T, Timmerman R, Park Y K and Owrangi A 2020 Dosimetric evaluation of synthetic CT generated with GANs for MRI-only proton therapy treatment planning of brain tumours *J. Appl. Clin. Med. Phys.* **21** 76–86

Keall P J, Brighi C, Glide-Hurst C *et al* 2022 Integrated MRI-guided radiotherapy—opportunities and challenges *Nat. Rev. Clin. Oncol.* **19** 458–70

Kelly C J, Karthikesalingam A, Suleyman M, Corrado G and King D 2019 Key challenges for delivering clinical impact with artificial intelligence *BMC Med.* **17** 195

Knäusl B, Kuess P, Stock M, Georg D, Fossati P, Georg P and Zimmermann L 2022 Possibilities and challenges when using synthetic computed tomography in an adaptive carbon-ion treatment workflow *Z. Med. Phys.* **33** 146–54

Kurz C, Kamp F, Park Y-K, Zöllner C, Rit S, Hansen D and Landry G 2016 Investigating deformable image registration and scatter correction for CBCT-based dose calculation in adaptive IMPT *Med. Phys.* **43** 5635–46

Kurz C, Maspero M, Savenije M H F, Landry G, Kamp F, Pinto M, Li M, Parodi K, Belka C and van den Berg C A T 2019 CBCT correction using a cycle-consistent generative adversarial network and unpaired training to enable photon and proton dose calculation *Phys. Med. Biol.* **64** 225004

Lalonde A, Winey B, Verburg J, Paganetti H and Sharp G C 2020 Evaluation of CBCT scatter correction using deep convolutional neural networks for head and neck adaptive proton therapy *Phys. Med. Biol.* **65** 245022

Landry G, Hansen D, Kamp F, Hoyle B, Weller J, Parodi K and Kurz C 2019a Comparing Unet training with three different datasets to correct CBCT images for prostate radiotherapy dose calculations *Phys. Med. Biol.* **64** 035011

Landry G, Hansen D, Kamp F, Li M, Hoyle B, Weller J, Parodi K, Belka C and Kurz C 2019b Comparing Unet training with three different datasets to correct CBCT images for prostate radiotherapy dose calculations *Phys. Med. Biol.* **64** 35011

Lerner M, Medin J, Jamtheim Gustafsson C *et al* 2021 Clinical validation of a commercially available deep learning software for synthetic CT generation for brain *Radiat. Oncol.* **16** 66

Li Y, Zhu J, Liu Z, Teng J, Xie Q, Zhang L, Liu X, Shi J and Chen L 2019 A preliminary study of using a deep convolution neural network to generate synthesized CT images based on CBCT for adaptive radiotherapy of nasopharyngeal carcinoma *Phys. Med. Biol.* **64** 145010

Li X, Yadav P and McMillan A B 2022 Synthetic computed tomography generation from 0.35 T magnetic resonance images for magnetic resonance–only radiation therapy planning using perceptual loss models *Pract. Radiat. Oncol.* **12** e40–8

Liu Y, Lei Y, Wang T, Fu Y, Tang X, Curran W J and Yang X 2020 CBCT-based synthetic CT generation using deep-attention cycleGAN for pancreatic adaptive radiotherapy *Med. Phys.* **47** 2472–83

Liu Y, Lei Y, Wang Y, Shafai-Erfani G, Wang T, Tian S and Yang X 2019a Evaluation of a deep learning-based pelvic synthetic CT generation technique for MRI-based prostate proton treatment planning *Phys. Med. Biol.* **64** 205022

Liu Y, Lei Y, Wang Y, Wang T, Ren L, Lin L and Yang X 2019b MRI-based treatment planning for proton radiotherapy: dosimetric validation of a deep learning-based liver synthetic CT generation method *Phys. Med. Biol.* **64** 145015

Lu K, Ren L and Yin F F 2021 A geometry-guided deep learning technique for CBCT reconstruction *Phys. Med. Biol.* **66** 15LT01

Maspero M, Bentvelzen L G, Savenije M H, Guerreiro F, Seravalli E, Janssens G O and Philippens M E 2020 Deep learning-based synthetic CT generation for paediatric brain MR-only photon and proton radiotherapy *Radiother. Oncol.* **153** 197–204

Maspero M, Houweling A C, Savenije M H F, van Heijst T C F, Verhoeff J J C, Kotte A N T J and van den Berg C A T 2020 A single neural network for cone-beam computed tomography-based radiotherapy of head-and-neck, lung, and breast cancer *Phys. Imaging Radiat. Oncol.* **14** 24–31

Maspero M, Van den Berg C A, Landry G, Belka C, Parodi K, Seevinck P R and Kurz C 2017 Feasibility of MR-only proton dose calculations for prostate cancer radiotherapy using a commercial pseudo-CT generation method *Phys. Med. Biol.* **62** 9159

McCarthy J 2007 What is artificial intelligence? http://www-formal.stanford.edu/jmc/whatisai.html

Meyer P, Noblet V, Mazzara C and Lallement A 2018 Survey on deep learning for radiotherapy *Comput. Biol. Med.* **98** 126–46

Neppl S, Landry G, Kurz C, Hansen D C, Hoyle B, Stöcklein S and Kamp F 2019 Evaluation of proton and photon dose distributions recalculated on 2D and 3D Unet-generated pseudo CTs from T1-weighted MR head scans *Acta Oncol.* **58** 1429–34

Oborn B M, Dowdell S, Metcalfe P E, Crozier S, Mohan R and Keall P J 2017 Future of medical physics: real-time MRI-guided proton therapy *Med. Phys.* **44** e77–90

Oren O, Gersh B J and Bhatt D L 2020 Artificial intelligence in medical imaging: switching from radiographic pathological data to clinically meaningful endpoints *Lancet Digit. Health* **2** e486–8

Paganetti H and Bortfeld T 2006 Proton therapy ed W Schlegel, T Bortfeld and A L Grosu *New Technologies in Radiation Oncology. Medical Radiology* (Berlin: Springer) pp 345–63

Paganelli C, Summers P, Gianoli C, Bellomi M, Baroni G and Riboldi M 2017 A tool for validating MRI-guided strategies: a digital breathing CT/MRI phantom of the abdominal site *Med. Biol. Eng. Comput.* **55** 2001–14

Palmér E, Karlsson A, Nordström F, Petruson K, Siversson C, Ljungberg M and Sohlin M 2021 Synthetic computed tomography data allows for accurate absorbed dose calculations in a magnetic resonance imaging only workflow for head and neck radiotherapy *Phys. Imaging Radiat. Oncol.* **17** 36–42

Parrella G *et al* 2023 Synthetic CT in carbon ion radiotherapy of the abdominal site *Bioengineering* **10** 250

Park Y K, Sharp G C, Phillips J and Winey B A 2015 Proton dose calculation on scatter-corrected CBCT image: feasibility study for adaptive proton therapy *Med. Phys.* **42** 4449–59

Raaymakers B W, Raaijmakers A J E, Kotte A N T J, Jette D and Lagendijk J J W 2004 Integrating a MRI scanner with a 6 MV radiotherapy accelerator: dose deposition in a transverse magnetic field *Phys. Med. Biol.* **49** 4109

Rajpurkar P, Chen E, Banerjee O and Topol E J 2022 AI in health and medicine *Nat. Med.* **8** 31–8

Razzak M I, Naz S and Zaib A 2018 Deep learning for medical image processing: overview, challenges and the future *Classification in BioApps* (Berlin: Springer) 323–50

Ramella S, Fiore M, Silipigni S, Zappa M C, Jaus M, Alberti A M and D'Angelillo R M 2017 Local control and toxicity of adaptive radiotherapy using weekly CT imaging: results from the LARTIA trial in stage III NSCLC *J. Thorac. Oncol.* **12** 1122–30

Thing R S, Bernchou U, Mainegra-Hing E and Brink C 2013 Patient-specific scatter correction in clinical cone beam computed tomography imaging made possible by the combination of Monte Carlo simulations and a ray tracing algorithm *Acta Oncol.* **52** 1477–83

Schellhammer S M, Hoffmann A L, Gantz S, Smeets J, Van Der Kraaij E, Quets S and Pawelke J 2018 Integrating a low-field open MR scanner with a static proton research beam line: proof of concept *Phys. Med. Biol.* **63** 23LT01

Schneider U, Pedroni E and Lomax A 1996 The calibration of CT hounsfield units for radiotherapy treatment planning *Phys. Med. Biol.* **41** 111

Schulze R, Heil U, Groβ D, Bruellmann D D, Dranischnikow E, Schwanecke U and Schoemer E 2011 Artefacts in CBCT: a review *Dentomaxillofac. Radiol.* **40** 265–73

Seller Oria C, Thummerer A, Free J, Langendijk J A, Both S, Knopf A C and Meijers A 2021 Range probing as a quality control tool for CBCT-based synthetic CTs: *in vivo* application for head and neck cancer patients *Med. Phys.* **48** 4498–505

Shafai-Erfani G, Lei Y, Liu Y, Wang Y, Wang T, Zhong J and Yang X 2019 MRI-based proton treatment planning for base of skull tumours *Int. J. Part. Ther.* **6** 12–25

Spadea M F, Maspero M, Zaffino P and Seco J 2021 Deep learning-based synthetic-CT generation in radiotherapy and PET: a review *Med. Phys.* **48** 6537–66

Spadea M F, Pileggi G, Zaffino P, Salome P, Catana C, Izquierdo-Garcia D and Seco J 2019 Deep convolution neural network (DCNN) multiplane approach to synthetic CT generation from MR images—application in brain proton therapy *Int. J. Radiat. Oncol. Biol. Phys.* **105** 495–503

Tanno R, Worrall D E, Kaden E, Ghosh A, Grussu F, Bizzi A, Sotiropoulos S N, Criminisi A and Alexander D C 2021 Uncertainty modelling in deep learning for safer neuroimage enhancement: demonstration in diffusion MRI *NeuroImage* **225** 117366

Thummerer A *et al* 2020 Comparison of the suitability of CBCT- and MR-based synthetic CTs for daily adaptive proton therapy in head and neck patients *Phys. Med. Biol.* **65** 235036

Thummerer A *et al* 2021 Clinical suitability of deep learning-based synthetic CTs for adaptive proton therapy of lung cancer *Med. Phys.* **48** 7673–84

Thummerer A, van der Bijl E, Galapon A, Verhoeff J J, Langendijk J A, Both S and Maspero M 2023 SynthRAD2023 grand challenge dataset: generating synthetic CT for radiotherapy *Med. Phys.* **50** 4664–74

Thummerer A, Zaffino P, Meijers A, Marmitt G G, Seco J, Steenbakkers R, Langendijk J A, Both S, Spadea M F and Knopf A C 2020a Comparison of CBCT-based synthetic CT methods suitable for proton dose calculations in adaptive proton therapy *Phys. Med. Biol.* **65** 95002

Thummerer A *et al* 2022 Deep learning-based 4D-synthetic CTs from sparse-view CBCTs for dose calculations in adaptive proton therapy *Med. Phys.* **49** 6824–39

Vandewinckele L, Claessens M, Dinkla A, Brouwer C, Crijns W, Verellen D and van Elmpt W 2020 Overview of artificial intelligence-based applications in radiotherapy: recommendations for implementation and quality assurance *Radiother. Oncol.* **153** 55–66

Veiga C, Janssens G and Baudier T 2017 A comprehensive evaluation of the accuracy of CBCT and deformable registration-based dose calculation in lung proton therapy *Biomed. Phys. Eng. Express* **3** 015003

Wang C, Uh J, He X, Hua C H and Sahaja A 2021 Transfer learning-based synthetic CT generation for MR-only proton therapy planning in children with Pelvic Sarcomas *Medical Imaging 2021: Physics of Medical Imaging* **vol 11595** (Bellingham, WA: International Society for Optics and Photonics) p 1159549

Wang C, Uh J, Merchant T E, Hua C H and Acharya S 2022 Facilitating MR-guided adaptive proton therapy in children using deep learning-based synthetic CT *Int. J. Part. Ther.* **8** 11–20

Wang C, Uh J, Patni T, Merchant T, Li Y, Hua C H and Acharya S 2022 Toward MR-only proton therapy planning for pediatric brain tumours: synthesis of relative proton stopping power images with multiple sequence MRI and development of an online quality assurance tool *Med. Phys.* **49** 1559–70

Wang G, Zhang Y, Ye X and Mou X 2019 *Machine Learning for Tomographic Imaging* (Bristol: IOP Publishing Ltd)

Zhen X, Gu X, Yan H, Zhou L, Jia X and Jiang S B 2012 CT to cone-beam CT deformable registration with simultaneous intensity correction *Phys. Med. Biol.* **57** 6807

Yang M, Zhu X R, Park P C, Titt U, Mohan R, Virshup G and Dong L 2012 Comprehensive analysis of proton range uncertainties related to patient stopping-power-ratio estimation using the stoichiometric calibration *Phys. Med. Biol.* **57** 4095

Zhang Y, Yue N, Su M, Liu B, Ding Y, Zhou Y, Wang H, Kuang Y and Nie K 2021 Improving CBCT quality to CT level using deep learning with generative adversarial network *Med. Phys.* **48** 2816–26

Zhang Y, Huang X and Wang J 2019 Advanced 4-dimensional cone-beam computed tomography reconstruction by combining motion estimation, motion-compensated reconstruction, bio-mechanical modeling, and deep learning *Vis. Comput. Ind. Biomed. Art.* **2** 23

Zhu J Y, Zhang R, Pathak D, Darrell T, Efros A A, Wang O and Shechtman E 2017 Toward multimodal image-to-image translation *31st Conf. on Neural Information Processing Systems (NIPS 2017)* (Red Hook, NY: Curran Associates) 30

Zhao W, Vernekohl D, Zhu J, Wang L and Xing L 2016 A model-based scatter artifacts correction for cone beam CT *Med. Phys.* **43** 1736–53

Chapter 9

Modelling strategies to enable time-resolved volumetric imaging

A Nakas, G Meschini, G Baroni and C Paganelli

9.1 Introduction

Particle therapy (PT) with protons or carbon ions has become an attractive option for the treatment of various tumor types, thanks to its increased radiobiological effectiveness and high geometrical selectivity, when compared with conventional photon radiotherapy (Durante *et al* 2017). To fully exploit the benefits of PT, optimal target coverage and sparing of surrounding healthy tissue must be ensured throughout the treatment course, which is a challenging task especially for tumors that are subject to respiratory motion, such as thoracic or abdominal tumors. Indeed, respiratory motion can introduce geometrical uncertainties into the process, leading to potential target underdosage and/or overdosage of normal tissues. In addition, density variations created along the beam path due to respiratory motion, cause changes of the radiological water equivalent path length (WEL) and, thus, undesired dose depositions (Keall *et al* 2006, Mori *et al* 2018, Pakela *et al* 2022). In this regard, it is mandatory to address inter- and intra-fraction variations due to organ motion, such as respiration, to improve treatment outcome (Keall *et al* 2006, Mori *et al* 2018, Pakela *et al* 2022).

Up to now, motion variabilities are accounted for during the treatment planning phase, by relying on respiratory-correlated 4D imaging, with 4D computed tomography (4DCT) being the current clinical standard, in combination with motion mitigation strategies such as compression masks, gating and/or rescanning during treatment delivery. However, 4DCT presents many limitations, including that: (i) the patients should breathe regularly to avoid artifacts in 4DCT reconstruction and this is not always guaranteed; (ii) the internal anatomy is assumed to be correlated with the external mono-dimensional respiratory surrogate used for retrospective sorting; and thus (iii) it provides an average description of the breathing cycle of the patient which is not always representative of the anatomy within a treatment fraction or between different fractions. Static in-room image modalities are currently adopted in PT to account for inter-fraction anatomical changes prior to treatment delivery (chapter 5), but time-resolved 3D information of the tumor location at all times would be required to account for range changes resulting from motion induced density variations to perform robust treatment planning and verification, and potentially to implement lateral beam adjustment and energy adaptation for tumor tracking (Riboldi *et al* 2012, Fassi *et al* 2014, Mori *et al* 2018).

Imaging techniques alternative to CT that are put forward to provide time-resolved information are currently under investigation. The most promising is magnetic resonance imaging (MRI), with commercial hybrid MRI-linac systems already available for conventional x-ray radiotherapy (RT; Olsen *et al* 2015, Raaymakers *et al* 2017, Paganelli *et al* 2018c) and feasibility studies investigating MRI-guided proton therapy (Hoffmann *et al* 2020). MRI indeed provides radiation-free acquisitions able to derive respiratory-correlated (4D) MRI and time-resolved MRI (i.e., fast 2D cine-MRI; Paganelli *et al* 2018c, Kurz *et al* 2020), along with multiple and extended examinations to address respiratory motion and its induced uncertainties. However, 4DMRI suffers from low temporal resolution and still represents an average description of the breathing cycle, whereas 2D cine-MRI provides time-resolved information but with low spatial dimensionality. Similarly, ultrasound imaging (US) can provide real-time radiation-free acquisitions; (Giger *et al* 2020, Krieger *et al* 2021) time-resolved 3D US technologies are under investigation (Al-Badri *et al* 2017, Ipsen *et al* 2019) and a few commercial systems available for x-ray RT (Grimwood *et al* 2018), but the limited field of view and the compatibility with a PT workflow are still a challenge.

Motion modelling techniques can be therefore exploited to overcome the limitations of current imaging modalities in providing time-resolved 3D information. Motion models were initially developed as an alternative to fluoroscopy at keV energies (Shirato *et al* 1999) for tumor tracking in x-ray RT as a relevant non-therapeutic dose was delivered to the patient (Shirato *et al* 2004) and implantation of radio-opaque fiducials were typically required to cope with the low tumor contrast in kV images (Hirai *et al* 2019). Specifically, indirect local motion modelling has been demonstrated with clinically used commercial tracking systems in conventional RT, such as Cyberknife and VERO (Kamino *et al* 2006, Kilby *et al* 2010) and with few feasibility studies for ion beam therapy (Seregni *et al* 2013). These models are built upon a correlation of a continuously acquired external surrogate (i.e., typically a respiratory belt or an optical system which measure the breathing activity of the patient) with the internal target anatomy sporadically acquired via x-ray projections. However, the robustness of this internal-external correlation has been a debated topic among many studies in literature (Riboldi *et al* 2012, Mylonas *et al* 2021) and the localized estimation at the target lack the quantification of surrounding tissues motion required for PT applications, which could be instead possible via global motion modelling (McClelland *et al* 2013).

The aim of this chapter is to present an overview of global motion models to derive time-resolved 3D information of the entire anatomy under investigation and discuss their application in PT. In general, motion models can be classified in two categories: (i) image-based motion models, where imaging data (CT, MRI or US) are needed to build the model via statistical (here referred to as conventional techniques) or artificial intelligence (AI) strategies and (ii) dose variation models, where predictions are made on the dose map.

9.2 Image-based motion modelling techniques

9.2.1 Conventional motion modelling techniques

Global respiratory motion modelling techniques (McClelland *et al* 2013) is a viable solution that was first investigated to derive 3D data not depicted in 4D imaging. The rationale behind global motion modelling is that a combination of 4D imaging and surrogate-based information can be used to predict and generate 3D volumes depicting the patient anatomy at each instant within a respiratory cycle (figure 9.1). These techniques usually rely on deformable image registration (DIR) to generate a set of deformable vector fields (DVFs) obtained between different respiratory phases in a 4D dataset. These DVFs are then used to parameterize a motion model relying on B-splines interpolation or principal component analysis (PCA) in function of respiratory surrogates. These motion models are then used to warp a reference 3D image to unseen respiratory phases, thus obtaining time-resolved 3D estimations.

9.2.1.1 Motion modelling techniques with CT

One of the very first studies on motion modelling was that of McClelland *et al* (2006), tested and evaluated on five lung patients treated with conventional radio-therapy. Specifically, to build a motion model, a 4DCT dataset needs to be acquired. By deforming each 4DCT volume to a reference CT (e.g., acquired at end-exhale) a set of DVFs is obtained. The following step consists in acquiring an external surrogate signal, typically mono-dimensional (1D), e.g. with a respiratory belt. A B-spline fitting is then adopted to establish a correlation between the phase of the surrogate signal and the DVFs. Once the correlation is established, a CT volume can be generated at each instant of the 1D surrogate signal acquired in-room during dose

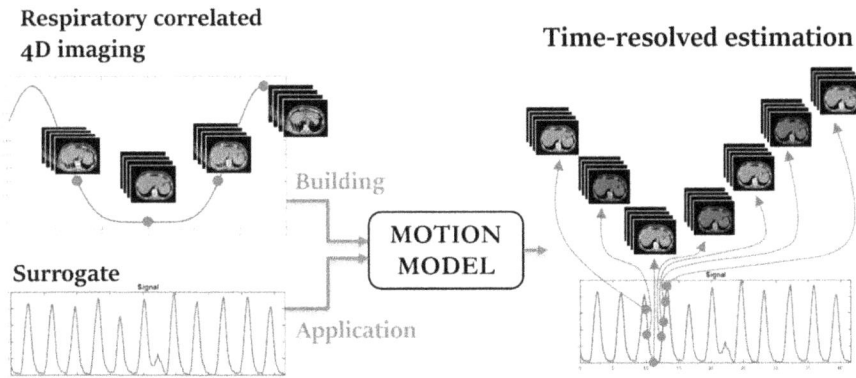

Figure 9.1. Workflow of global respiratory motion modelling.

delivery. In principle this approach is also applicable to 4D Cone Beam CT (CBCT) (Martin *et al* 2013), obtaining predictions directly in the treatment room when an in-room CBCT systems is available.

When adopting multiple respiratory parameters of the 1D external surrogate (i.e., phase and amplitude of respiratory motion), higher prediction accuracy can be achieved with respect to using only a single parameter (Fayad *et al* 2009). Results demonstrate a model error (mean (standard deviation)) of 1.64 (0.28) mm when both parameters are used instead of 3.63 (0.42) mm and 5.08 (0.77) mm for amplitude and phase when used singularly (Fayad *et al* 2012). Nevertheless, 1D external surrogates limit the correlation with internal target motion, thus compromising the performance of the modelling (Trnková *et al* 2018, Bertholet *et al* 2019, Li *et al* 2022).

Motion models exploiting external patient surface as surrogate-based information presented more promising results when compared to models using a simple 1D surrogate signal (Wolfelschneider *et al* 2017). In general, surface information can be extracted from 4DCT data via segmentation and from in-room measurements provided by a time of flight (ToF) camera (Wolfelschneider *et al* 2017, Zhang *et al* 2017). Such models are used to correlate the 3D patient surface information with the internal motion described by the DVFs. The use of surface information would require a multidimensional B-splines fitting, which is computationally more expensive. In this regard, PCA can be used to establish an internal-external correlation model for CT volume estimations. When compared to models using a 1D surrogate signal, surface-based models performed better with a model error of 1.35 (0.21) mm instead of 1.64 (0.28) mm in the thorax (Fayad *et al* 2012).

An intriguing application of motion modelling exploiting external patient surface in PT was proposed by Fassi *et al* (2015). Here, an optical system was used to monitor surface displacement and derive a surrogate signal, from which parameters such as the phase and amplitude (accounting for intra-fraction variations) can be extracted, while baseline shifts (accounting for inter-fraction variations) can be estimated relying on daily 3D CBCT imaging.

Three different experiments were conducted to evaluate the accuracy of the proposed method: (i) the modeling test, to account for inaccuracies for model construction and output estimation, (ii) the rigid alignment test, to simulate the standard clinical procedure for setup error correction, based on the rigid alignment of the patient's anatomy without any organ motion compensation, and (iii) the tracking test, to quantify the effectiveness of the motion modelling approach in compensating for inter-fraction and intra-fraction organ motion. The median absolute variation in WEL within the target volume did not exceed 1.9 mm-WEL for simulated particle beams and a significant improvement was achieved compared with error compensation based on standard rigid alignment (figure 9.2).

This study was extended to a broader patient dataset with a dosimetric analysis being also performed (Wolfelschneider *et al* 2017). The model has demonstrated good accuracy which depended mainly on the quality of the 4DCT dataset, with median 3D distances, measured on hundreds of matching landmarks between estimated and ground truth volumes, of 2.9 (3.0) mm. Negligible dose variations

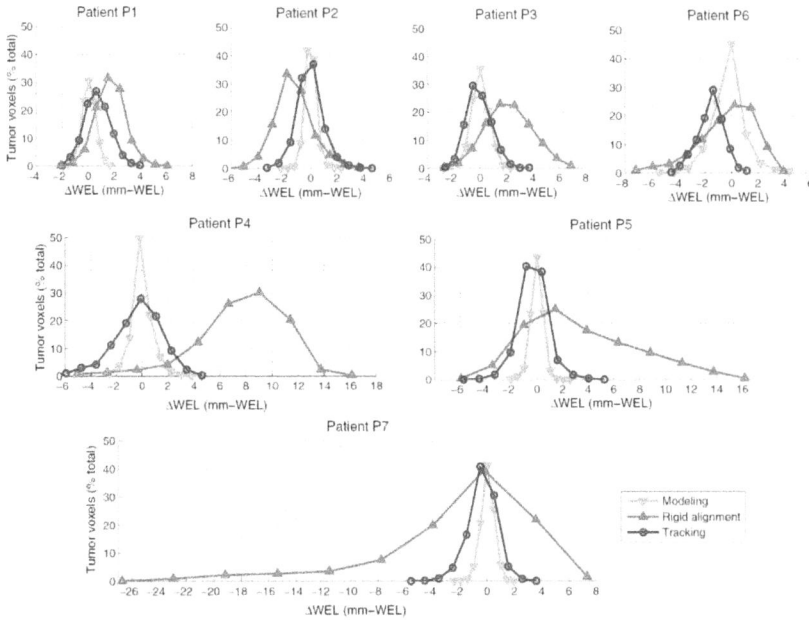

Figure 9.2. Distributions of ΔWEL obtained for each tumor voxel with the particle beam simulated in the ipsilateral direction in (i) modeling test (green), (ii) rigid alignment (red), and (iii) tracking test (blue). Reproduced from Fassi *et al* (2015). © 2015 Institute of Physics and Engineering in Medicine. All rights reserved.

between ground truth and prediction were observed, with a gamma pass rate of 98.9% and a γ-criterion of 2%/2 mm.

These studies demonstrated the model's feasibility to be used as supplementary tool for 4D dose recalculations, and its potential extension for tumor tracking techniques in PT treatments, as it allows for the dynamic localization of all anatomical structures scanned in the planning CT, thus providing complete information on density and WEL variations required for particle beam range adaptation.

The same model was also adopted to evaluate the residual motion within the gating window in the treatment of abdominal tumors with carbon ions, although exploiting the 1D signal derived from a respiratory belt; the study confirmed the effectiveness of the gating procedure implemented at the National Center for Oncological Hadrontherapy (CNAO, Pavia, Italy; Meschini *et al* 2017).

Correlation between an external breathing surrogate and anatomical deformations of the planning 4DCT has been also investigated by Duetschler *et al* (2023). Using motion trajectories of a surface marker acquired during the dose delivery by an optical tracking system, deformable motion fields were retrospectively reconstructed and used to generate time-resolved synthetic 4DCTs by warping a reference CT to perform 4D dose reconstruction for pencil beam scanned proton therapy.

When a beams eye view (BEV) imaging system is available in the treatment room, as present at the Paul Scherrer Institute (PSI, Villigen, Switzerland), 2D x-ray images in fluoroscopy mode can be acquired during treatment delivery, thus providing internal anatomo-pathological information instead of external surrogate-based motion description. To derive 3D information, Zhang *et al* (2013) proposed a method by which 3D deformable motions can be estimated from surrogates obtained using an imaging system. In this study, the authors generated a set of simulated 4DCT data, from which time-resolved digitally reconstructed radiographs (DRRs) were calculated using the BEV geometry for different treatment fields. From these DRRs, surrogate motions from implanted fiducial markers or the diaphragm was used as a predictor to estimate 3D motion in the liver region, relying on a PCA model built on different breathing cycles derived from 4DMRI data. The potential effectiveness of this method for tumor tracking in PT has been also investigated (Zhang *et al* 2014) by comparing different beam tracking scenarios (2D, 2D deformable and 3D) in liver motion cases, with mean magnitudes ranging from 10 to 20 mm. The results showed that, without beam tracking, large interplay effects were observed for all motion cases, resulting in CTV D5%–95% values of 34.9%/58.5%/79.4% for the three scenarios, respectively. These can be reduced to 16.9%/18.8%/29.1% with 2D tracking, to 15.5%/17.9%/23.3% with 2D deformable tracking and to 15.1%/17.8%/21.0% with 3D tracking based on the proposed motion model.

Population-based models have been also proposed in the literature as a possible alternative to patient-specific models to avoid non-therapeutic radiation dose of 4DCT to each patient. The population-based approach allows the inclusion of additional variabilities whilst building the model, and thus can simulate intra- and inter-fraction motion, making the model more robust in the estimation of such variations. Such models are created from 4DCT datasets acquired from previous patients (Fayad *et al* 2009, Fayad *et al* 2018). Once the model is constructed, it can be adapted to a new patient using two CT images, acquired *a priori* for the individual patient, and respiratory synchronized patient-surface information acquired via a ToF camera during treatment. Given the information from the external surrogate as input, the model can predict new CT volumes at each instant of the respiratory cycle using only two static CT volumes. This can eliminate the need for a 4DCT acquisition and the excess dose delivered to the patient.

9.2.1.2 Motion modelling techniques with MRI

The principle for building a motion model from 4DMRI is the same as that for 4DCT (i.e., deriving DFVs between 4DMRI respiratory phases and then relate them with information acquired in-room; King *et al* 2012). Such models, however, provide many advantages over CT-based models, stemming from the intrinsic properties of MRI (Paganelli *et al* 2018c, Keall *et al* 2022). First, in contrast with 4DCT, MRI's radiation-free nature allows dynamic and extended acquisitions of multiple breathing cycles, making MRI-based models able to capture motion variability occurring within or between different breathing cycles. Additionally, these models provide the advantage of using time-resolved MR images (e.g., 1D navigators or 2D cine-MRI) as surrogate: the internal anatomical information available on the 2D images presents more detailed and correlated information than a (1D) external surrogate signal (Paganelli *et al* 2015).

All the CT-based models presented in the previous section can be also extended to MRI, by extracting surrogate information directly from time-resolved 2D images.

To fully exploit the anatomical information contained in the time-resolved 2D data, models have been specifically proposed in the context of MRI guidance. An in-silico study by Paganelli *et al* (2019) provided a comparison among a group of these motion models. Specifically, in Harris *et al* (2016), the motion field derived from cine-MRI data was embedded into the PCA model built on 4DMRI to update the DVF and estimate time-resolved volumes, whereas an optimization framework, which looked at the best estimation according to a similarity measure computed between the estimated volume and the coronal 2D cine-MRI slice, was proposed by Stemkens *et al* (2016). A regional adaptation of the model was instead proposed by Garau *et al* (2019), in which the model built on 4D imaging was updated based on the motion extracted from different regions of interest within interleaved sagittal/coronal 2D cine-MRI frames. This latter approach has demonstrated to provide better performance with respect to the corresponding models using the whole 2D surrogate image information, because it considers a regional adaptation to specific anatomies rather than computing a global similarity measure. Although these models have been specifically implemented for applications with MRI-linacs, they can be potentially adopted offline in PT to evaluate treatment robustness or be embedded in an MRI-guided PT workflow when it is available in the future.

One of the main drawbacks of the motion modelling techniques described until now is the construction of the model on *a priori* 4D imaging datasets, which makes the model sensitive to inter-and intra-fraction changes. To overcome this limitation, it has been proposed to implement population-based models, similarly to those presented for CT-based motion models (Fayad *et al* 2012). Alternatively, time-resolved 3D MRI data can be derived offline from extended 4DMRI acquisition, by retrospectively sorting 4D datasets for each breathing cycle (Zhang *et al* 2013, 2014, Dolde *et al* 2018, 2019, Peteani *et al* (2023)), or from an explicit dictionary of motion states. For the latter case, the method proposed by Feng *et al* (2020) allows for offline learning of a database of possible 3D motion states and corresponding motion signature ranges as well as an online matching of new motion signatures acquired in real time with pre-learned motion states; the online matching can be fast to support real-time applications (in the order of 300 ms). However, for these strategies the derived motion states are those depicted only in the dictionary and re-acquisition of the respiratory-correlated 4D-MRI might be required if a change in motion patterns is detected (Feng 2023).

A simpler and faster solution with respect to global motion modelling techniques that can directly estimate 3D motion without the need of *a priori* 4D imaging is the so-called propagation approach (Paganelli *et al* 2018a). The idea is to deformably register corresponding 2D slices between a 3D volume and 2D cine-MRI, and then propagate the derived motion field in the three anatomical directions. This approach provided promising results, being validated on both computational (Paganelli *et al* 2018a) and physical phantoms (Rabe *et al* 2021), obtaining errors within the maximum MRI voxel resolution.

To calculate the dose on 3D volumes estimated through respiratory motion modelling, electron density information is required. This is directly possible on CT-based motion models, whereas, when modelling is performed relying on MRI,

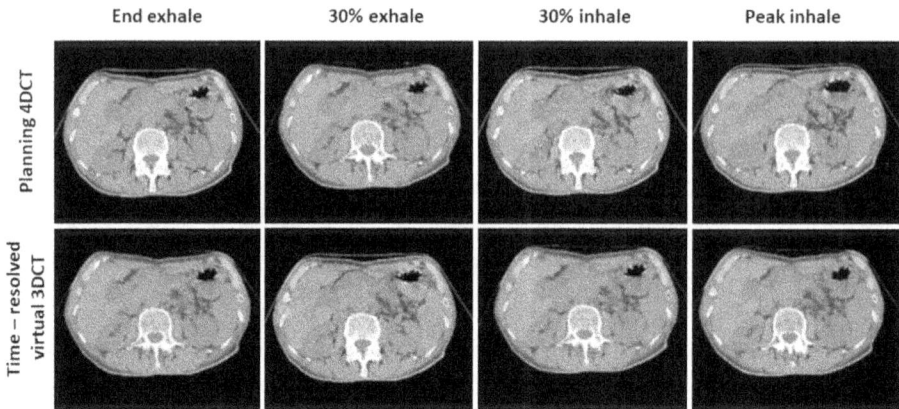

Figure 9.3. Four retrospectively reconstructed phases of a planning 4DCT acquired from a pancreatic cancer patient treated with Carbon Ion Radiotherapy at the National Center for Oncological Hadrontherapy (CNAO, Pavia, Italy) and time-resolved virtual 3D CT generated as proposed by Meschini *et al* (2022).

strategies to derive virtual 4DCT should be applied. The deformation of the planning CT (planning end-exhale CT) with the motion derived from 4DMRI has been heavily investigated in the literature for different PT applications (Boye *et al* 2013, Bernatowicz *et al* 2016, Dolde *et al* 2018, 2019, Meschini *et al* 2020b, Annunziata *et al* 2023). Alternatively, time-resolved virtual 3D CT can be created from cine-MRI data (Meschini *et al* 2022) by combining the virtual 4DCT generation method (Meschini *et al* 2020b) with the propagation approach (Paganelli *et al* 2018a; figure 9.3). Specifically, a reference virtual CT is generated by deforming a reference end-exhale planning CT to the end-exhale phase of MRI. Cine-MRI frames are deformably registered to a reference end-exhale cine frame to generate 2D-DVFs, with the latter reconstructed into 3D-DVFs. Time-resolved virtual CTs (TRvCTs) are then created by warping the reference virtual CT to the resulting 3D-DVFs. Geometric and dosimetric applications of this approach on pancreatic cancer patients treated with carbon ions showed limited inter-fraction motion with corresponding dose variations below 5%, thus demonstrating robust target coverage. Concerning intra-fraction variations, the gating technique was effective in limiting tumor displacement (1.35 mm median gating motion) and corresponding dose variations (-3.9% median D95% variation). The larger exposure of organs at risk (duodenum and stomach) was caused by inter-fraction motion.

It should be also noted that the derivation of the electron density information from MRI data can be also derived through synthetic CT-based on deep learning (DL), which are deeply discussed in chapter 8. Among these approaches, very few applications have been proposed for anatomical sites affected by respiratory motion (Liu *et al* 2019, Cusumano *et al* 2020, Qian *et al* 2020, Florkow *et al* 2020, Olberg *et al* 2021, Parrella *et al* 2023), due to their anatomical complexity. Up to now, most of these DL strategies were mainly implemented to estimate static synthetic volumes, with a limited number of implementations including motion (Thummerer *et al* 2022).

With the recent advent of in-room MRI-linacs in conventional radiotherapy, different attempts have been also made on reconstructing time-resolved 3D MRI data relying on peculiar sampling of the k-space (Paganelli *et al* 2018c), but the trade-off between spatial and temporal resolution is still a limit. These approaches typically have limited real-time capability since they require long acquisition times over multiple respiratory cycles and/or complex iterative image reconstruction that increases overall latency. Nevertheless, some studies proposed the use of k-space MRI data as respiratory surrogate rather than 1D navigators or 2D cine-MRI to derive a time-resolved volumetric dataset (Huttinga *et al* 2021). The idea at the basis of these approaches is to relate a motion-free reference image, typically reconstructed relying on k-space-based sorting, with a respiratory signal extracted from online dynamic sampling of the k-space. The integration of these strategies with factorization or matching of estimated/pre-learned 3D motion fields allows for rapid generation of 3D images (in the order of ms). Such methods are promising, but require customized MR sequences and access to k-space data; this is not as widely available on clinical scanners as those currently available in PT.

9.2.1.3 Motion modelling techniques with US

Another candidate modality that captures internal motion information which is correlated to the organ motion of interest, exposes the patient to no additional radiation dose, and can provide multidimensional surrogate signals, is abdominal US imaging. The motion of the liver and diaphragm can be captured in real time and provides 2D internal information (Preiswerk *et al* 2014, Giger *et al* 2018). Due to physical constraints, direct US imaging of lung tissue is instead not possible. However, with the help of respiratory motion models, motion characteristics extracted from liver US can be used in principle to perform motion modelling of the abdomen or to estimate lung tumor motion (Mostafaei *et al* 2018) and lung deformation (Giger *et al* 2018).

In a recent study proposed by Giger *et al* (2020), a motion model based on PCA and Gaussian process regression (GP; Rasmussen and Williams 2006) was employed to estimate the respiratory motion during dose delivery in PT, by inferring the corresponding DVF of the lungs given as input for the acquired US image. The study relied on motion characteristics extracted from hybrid US and 4DMRI datasets of five healthy volunteers acquired under free respiration that were fused with the anatomical CT data of two lung cancer patients, and 4D dose calculations for scanned proton therapy were then performed using the estimated and the corresponding ground truth respiratory motion. Median geometrical estimation errors were below 2 mm for all datasets and maximum dose differences >5% and >10% were found in 43.2% and 16.3%, respectively, of the different motion entities investigated, demonstrating the feasibility of the proposed US-based motion modelling approach for its application in scanned proton therapy of lung tumors.

The study was also tested in a tumor tracking scenario (Krieger *et al* 2021). Two-field proton beam scanning plans were optimized on the reference CTs, and 4D dose calculations were used to simulate dose delivery for unmitigated motion and 2D and 3D tracking. Model-guided tracking retrieved clinically acceptable target dose homogeneity, as seen in a substantial reduction of the D5%–D95% compared to the non-mitigated simulation. In some cases, however, the tracked deliveries resulted in a shift towards higher or lower dose levels, leading to unacceptable target over- or under-coverage, suggesting that tracking based on 2D US alone may not always effectively mitigate motion effects, making it necessary to combine it with other techniques such as rescanning.

Up to now the works presented in the literature consisted mainly of simulation studies; the integration of US imaging with PT technology should be further investigated and could benefit from the experience gained in conventional RT applications (Al-Badri *et al* 2017, Grimwood *et al* 2018, Ipsen *et al* 2019).

9.2.2 AI-based motion modelling techniques

The construction of the motion modelling techniques described in the previous sections relied mainly on DIR and statistical models. Nonetheless, recent advancements in the field of AI, and especially deep learning (DL), have paved a new path for motion modelling techniques, presenting the capability of using large datasets for training (thus covering a significant variety of breathing patterns) and enabling fast predictions (Mylonas *et al* 2021). Different approaches have been proposed for AI-prediction of target position as alternative to conventional local internal-external prediction models (Hirai *et al* 2019, Mylonas *et al* 2021); however, in this section we will focus on AI-based algorithms for monitoring changes in the full 3D anatomy.

Volumetric patient data can be derived directly from 2D projections of anatomy, without the need of DVFs computation. Specifically, a structured training process within an autoencoder configuration introducing a feature-space transformation among 2D x-ray projections and 3D CT images, was proposed to generate volumetric CT data (Shen *et al* 2019). The encoder part is used to learn important features of input 2D x-ray projections, whereas the decoder generates corresponding 3D CT patient images using the learned features derived from the encoder. Such a network has been validated on abdominal and thoracic patients, with a mean absolute error of 0.018 and 0.025, respectively, between ground truth and generated CT volumes. This method could be potentially used for image-guidance purposes, especially when in-room 2D x-ray images are available throughout the treatment, or even combined with external surrogates to sporadically check the motion model performance.

Other AI-based motion modelling techniques are mainly flourishing for applications in MRI guidance. As an example, a conditional generative adversarial net (cGAN) can be used for the creation of motion models that use navigator-based MRI datasets for the prediction of MRI patient volumes throughout the course of radiotherapy treatment (Frangi *et al* 2018). The model was trained on patient-specific 4DMRI data, reconstructed with navigator slices, and US images acquired simultaneously before treatment, to establish a correspondence between the acquired US images and the DVFs computed among navigator frames. During dose delivery, US images continuously acquired were then used as input to the trained network to generate DVFs that can be used to reconstruct 3D MRI volumes at each respiratory instant.

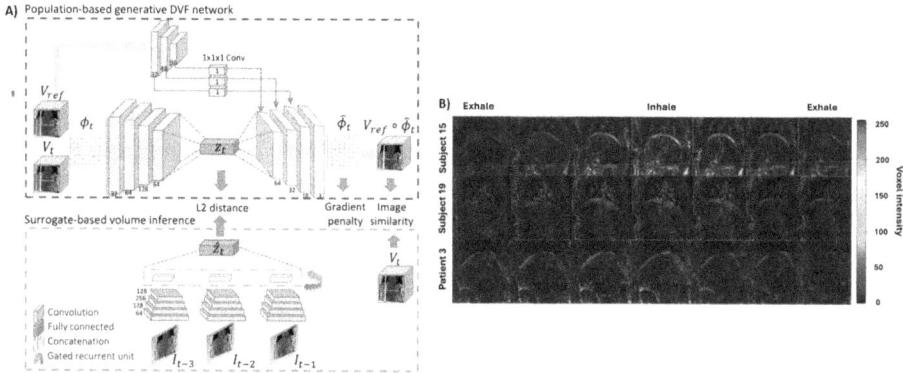

Figure 9.4. (A) Architecture for intra-treatment volume prediction from partial 2D observations and a static 3D reference volume. (B) Difference maps between ground-truth and predicted MRI volumes for two volunteers and one patient in the MRI datasets. Reprinted from Romaguera *et al* (2021). Copyright (2021), with permission from Springer.

An unsupervised network was instead proposed by Romaguera and colleagues (Romaguera *et al* 2021) starting from population-based 4D datasets (e.g., 4DMRI or 4DUS), which were acquired and reconstructed to cover a significant variety of breathing patterns (figure 9.4). Specifically, during training, the model learns how to map volume deformations at different respiratory phases to a low-dimensional space and how to recover the dense deformation. This is performed by an autoencoder network, where the encoder part of the network produces a low-dimensional representation of the input dataset and the decoder part maps this representation back into the original dimensionality of the input, thus producing a motion estimation. To relate the internal motion information in its compact form with partial 2D surrogate observations (cine-MRI or US), a second network is used. Specifically, an image sequence of N 2D slices are given as input in a stack of N encoders, producing an embedding vector. The two compact representations of the 4D and 2D datasets are resembled using a distance similarity loss function. To make the prediction more robust and patient-specific, another independent encoder can be added that plays the role of a feature extraction function, which extracts anatomical information from a patient-specific reference 3D volume. This information is communicated to the autoencoder network through compressed skip connections. A variation of this autoencoder architecture is the conditional variational autoencoder (Romaguera *et al* 2021). In this network, an encoder is used to produce a low-dimensional representation of the input volume deformations at different respiratory phases. Instead of having an embedding vector produced by N encoders, surrogate information can be included by feeding 2D cine-MRI data to a single, independent recurrent encoder-decoder configuration producing an output feature vector. Accordingly, to feed the network with patient-specific information, the reference 3D volume can be given as input in an independent auxiliary encoder. The output feature vectors of each branch combined can generate a latent space sample, relating the internal motion as described by the DVFs with the 2D surrogates, while also considering the anatomy of a specific patient. This latent space sample can be fed into a decoder configuration to predict new reconstructed DVFs. To apply the overall trained network, the only needed inputs are the patient-specific reference volume and the in-room acquired 2D cine-MRI. The output yields new DVFs at each instant of a respiratory cycle, which are used to warp the reference volume and derive new volumes.

Instead of using image surrogates and patient-specific reference volumes to support network training and prediction, estimations of DVFs can be obtained by only feeding acquired 4DMRI datasets (Terpstra *et al* 2021). This network, called TEMPEST, uses retrospectively under sampled 4DMRI data to generate DVFs with high spatiotemporal resolution, capable of being used in real-time. TEMPEST is a multiresolution CNN where each layer operates at different resolutions. In each layer a static and a time-resolved 3D MRI from the acquired 4D dataset are down sampled at different resolutions and the DVF between the volumes is estimated. This approach has been validated on both a computational and physical motion phantom. It was also validated on a test set of 5 patients along with ground truth DVFs obtained from a 4DMRI dataset with conventional registration strategies. It can estimate DVFs with high accuracy (error < 2 mm), in a fast manner (200 ms along with image acquisition) capable of supporting real-time applications and high spatiotemporal resolution.

Solutions have been also recently proposed to reconstruct real-time 3D MRI data from cine-MRI without the need of a 4DMRI dataset, since using combined 4DMRI and cine-MRI data for training can cause an overfitting problem during the 3D reconstruction (Wei *et al* 2022). This could occur due to inconsistencies in intensity between the two images when acquired with different parameters (field strength, imaging time, sampling method). Only a reference 3D MRI is instead required for training along with 3D sparse volumetric images generated from preprocessing cine-MRI data. Specifically, each 3D volume is given as input into separate encoders, respectively, with their outputs then combined and fed to the decoder network, to estimate DVFs describing breathing motion. When applying the network, cine-MRI can be fed as input and obtain corresponding DVFs. The reference 3D MRI can be then warped to the obtained DVFs to reconstruct real-time 3D MRI data. The reconstructing 3D MRI were compared with corresponding phase-sorted cine-MRI using the Dice Similarity Coefficient, with results presenting a mean (standard deviation) value of 96.1% (1.3%), while the reconstruction time was approximately 100 ms.

9.3 Dose variations models

In PT, conventional treatment planning systems rely on an imaging representation of the irradiated region to compute the dose. For irregular breathing, when an imaging dataset describing the actual motion is not available, image-based motion modelling techniques can be used to generate time-resolved 3D CT for dose recalculation or, alternatively, a different method for dose estimation is needed.

An interesting approach to evaluate the dosimetric effect of irregular breathing was proposed in the work by Phillips *et al* (2014) from the Massachusetts General

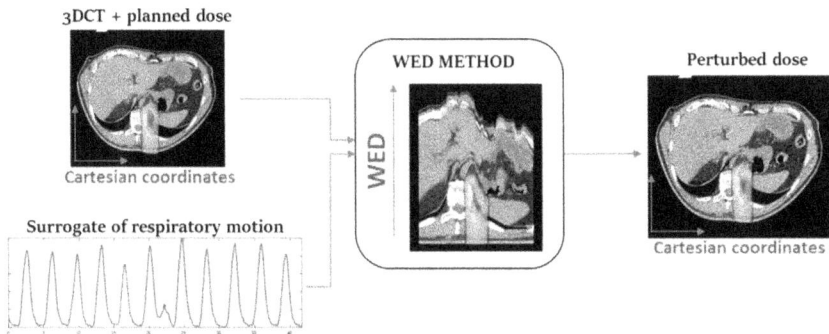

Figure 9.5. Workflow of the WED method.

Hospital (MGH, Boston, Massachusetts, USA). The method entails motion simulation in a patient- and beam-specific water equivalent depth (WED) space, which yields the estimation of dose alterations during un-imaged respiratory states (figure 9.5). Specifically, the method uses a reference CT image for dose calculation of the treatment plan, and a measure or surrogate of tumor motion to estimate the physical dose delivered to a moving target. The CT and the corresponding dose map are converted into the beam-specific WED space, where the beam is considered to interact with a homogeneous water equivalent medium. As deformations associated with target displacement are unknown, the motion is approximated to a translation in the WED space. Therefore, the accuracy of the WED space method estimations is expected to decrease with increasing tissue deformation and consequent density variations within the beam path. The transformation back into the CT coordinates yields to the perturbed dose distribution.

The method was tested on in-silico phantoms where known motion was applied and on a lung patient data simulating a passively-scattered proton treatment, with gamma analysis between the ground truth and estimated doses exhibiting pass rate of 97.8% without motion, 95.7% for 2 cm sinusoidal motion, and 95.7% with 3 cm drift in the phantom (2 mm, 2%), and 90.8% (3 mm, 3%) for the patient data.

The method was also tested for the estimation of physical dose variations in gated carbon ion treatments (Meschini *et al* 2019) and further extended to embed radiobiological models within the WED space, which are crucial when heavy particles such as carbon ions are used (Meschini *et al* 2020a). Specifically, both the planning end-exhale CT and the radiosensitivity alpha/beta maps were transformed in the WED space and translated according to tumor motion. The transformation back in physical coordinates yielded to the desired perturbed maps, which were then combined considering the RBE formulation to obtain the estimated radiobiological weighted dose maps. This approach was tested in a controlled scenario where different motion patterns where simulated, regular and irregular (figure 9.6); it presented proper accuracy within the clinical tolerances for tumors and most of the organs at risks, but the accuracy decreased if the soft tissue deformation increased, mainly due to the intrinsic approximation of the respiratory motion to a rigid translation.

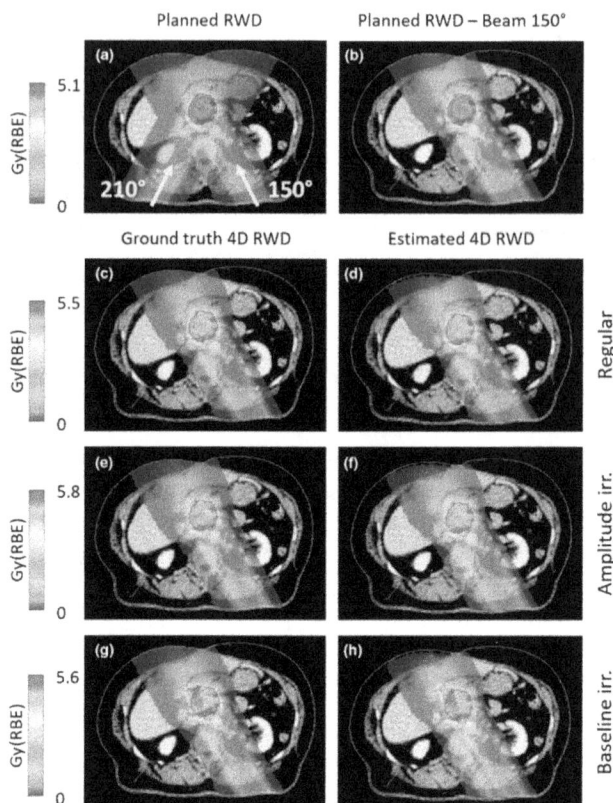

Figure 9.6. Modeling RBE-weighted dose variations. (a) Total planned dose (red contour is the PTV): the beam directions (150° and 210°) are indicated by yellow arrows. (b) Planned dose associated to the 150° beam. Examples of ground truth and estimated 4D RBE-weighted dose (RWD) for the 150° beam for the regular breathing (c and d, respectively), amplitude irregularity (e and f) and baseline irregularity (g and h) simulations. Figure taken with permission from Meschini *et al* (2020b). John Wiley & Sons. © 2020 American Association of Physicists in Medicine.

9.4 Conclusions and future perspectives

In the past few decades, several efforts have been made to implement motion models able to predict motion states not depicted directly in 4D imaging, as a way to support robust treatment planning, offline treatment verification and adaption and on-line tumour tracking in both conventional and particle therapy. In the context of PT, the availability of time-resolved 3D imaging is crucial to account for tumour motion and variations of the radiological path length in organs that moves as a function of respiration. Global motion models designed to predict the entire 3D anatomo-pathological configuration at different respiratory phases are not yet clinically applied, though PT treatments could potentially gain great benefit from them to account for inter- and intra-fraction motion.

Among the different limitations preventing a clinical implementation of image-based motion modelling strategies is the need of 4D imaging as prior, which is not able to compensate for intra-treatment conditions that are different from treatment planning. Different solutions have been reported in the literature, including the exploitation of population-based models, the adoption of multiple breathing cycles from respiratory-correlated 4DMRI, the propagation of the DVFs from static 3D data and the implementation of dose variations models, but a gold standard approach is not yet defined.

Additionally, the definition of the optimal surrogate to be used in prediction models is still under investigation. The optimal surrogate signal should capture internal motion information, which is correlated to the organ motion of interest, expose the patient to no additional radiation dose, and can provide multidimensional surrogate signals. In this sense, radiation-free 2D MR/US imaging are supposed to be more appropriate surrogates than 1D external surrogates or in-room 2D x-rays acquisitions (e.g. fluoroscopy), although these latter are more compatible with current and conventional technologies adopted in the clinical routine of PT; feasibility studies are currently ongoing on the implementation of hybrid MRI-proton systems with promising perspectives (Hoffmann et al 2020), whereas the potential of US-guided PT is still under investigation.

The other main limitation of image-based motion modelling is that it relies on DIR. Although DIR is a well-established tool for organ motion quantification, the variety of proposed DIR algorithms, combined with the lack of effective quantitative quality control metrics of the registration, still requires an appropriate awareness on related potentials and limitations in terms of geometric and dosimetric accuracy (Brock et al 2017, Paganelli et al 2018b; see chapter 3). Particularly, there is evidence that the quality of motion states prediction models is affected by DIR inaccuracies, which may also depend upon artefacts affecting conventional respiratory-correlated imaging modalities (Fassi et al 2015, Wolfelschneider et al 2017, Meschini et al 2022).

Concerning dose variation models, these can be also adopted in treatment optimization, verification and adaptation. Their main advantage is that they do not rely on 4D imaging and they can be used to directly estimate the dose to be delivered in a specific instant without generating a 3D image, also accounting for the biological dose in case of carbon ion treatments. The current implementation, however, just proposes a rigid translation in the WED space according to the adopted surrogate, without accounting for any organ deformation. This should be taken into consideration in the future to make dose variations models robust against motion.

Image-based and dose variations models are not yet implemented to run in real time, making these models only useful for an offline analysis of plan robustness and treatment evaluation. In case of tumour tracking applications, these models should run in real time, even if the estimation of 3D-DVFs is still computationally demanding. In this context, the adoption of AI-based motion models could overcome this limitation by making 3D motion estimation suitable for real-time adaptation (i.e., 3D estimation in the orders of milliseconds).

Finally, the validation of the proposed models to derive time-resolved 3D data is still a challenge as the ground truth 3D information is missing (i.e. lack of time-resolved 3D imaging). Evaluation of these models mainly relies on phantoms

(Paganelli *et al* 2019, Rabe *et al* 2021) or on the comparison with repeated 4DCT (Wolfelschneider *et al* 2017) or extended 4DMRI data (Zhang *et al* 2013, Meschini *et al* 2021), although common guidelines and patient-specific quality assessment needs to be defined to grant a rigorous geometric and dosimetric evaluation to quantify motion models' performance towards clinical implementation.

References

Al-Badri M, Ipsen S, Böttger S and Ernst F 2017 Robotic 4D ultrasound solution for real-time visualization and teleoperation *Curr. Dir. Biomed. Eng.* **3** 559–61

Annunziata S *et al* 2023 Virtual 4DCT generated from 4DMRI in gated particle therapy: phantom validation and application to lung cancer patients *Phys. Med. Biol.* **68** 145004

Bernatowicz K, Peroni M, Perrin R, Weber D C and Lomax A 2016 Four-dimensional dose reconstruction for scanned proton therapy using liver 4DCT-MRI *Int. J. Radiat. Oncol., Biol., Phys.* **95** 216–23

Bertholet J *et al* 2019 Real-time intrafraction motion monitoring in external beam radiotherapy *Phys. Med. Biol.* **64** 15TR01

Boye D, Lomax T and Knopf A 2013 Mapping motion from 4D-MRI to 3D-CT for use in 4D dose calculations: a technical feasibility study *Med. Phys.* **40** 061702

Brock K K, Mutic S, McNutt T R, Li H and Kessler M L 2017 Use of image registration and fusion algorithms and techniques in radiotherapy: report of the AAPM radiation therapy committee Task Group No. 132: report *Med. Phys.* **44** e43–76

Cusumano D *et al* 2020 A deep learning approach to generate synthetic CT in low field MR-guided adaptive radiotherapy for abdominal and pelvic cases *Radiother. Oncol.* **153** 205–12

Dolde K, Naumann P, Dávid C, Gnirs R, Kachelrieß M, Lomax A J, Saito N, Weber D C, Pfaffenberger A and Zhang Y 2018 4D dose calculation for pencil beam scanning proton therapy of pancreatic cancer using repeated 4DMRI datasets *Phys. Med. Biol.* **63** 165005

Dolde K, Naumann P, Dávid C, Kachelriess M, Lomax A J, Weber D C, Saito N, Burigo L N, Pfaffenberger A and Zhang Y 2019 Comparing the effectiveness and efficiency of various gating approaches for PBS proton therapy of pancreatic cancer using 4D-MRI datasets *Phys. Med. Biol.* **64** 085011

Duetschler A, Huang L, Fattori G, Meier G, Bula C, Hrbacek J, Safai S, Weber D C, Lomax A J and Zhang Y 2023 A motion model-guided 4D dose reconstruction for pencil beam scanned proton therapy *Phys. Med. Biol.* **68** 115013

Durante M, Orecchia R and Loeffler J S 2017 Charged-particle therapy in cancer: clinical uses and future perspectives *Nat. Rev. Clin. Oncol.* **14** 483–95

Fassi A, Schaerer J, Fernandes M, Riboldi M, Sarrut D and Baroni G 2014 Tumor tracking method based on a deformable 4D CT breathing motion model driven by an external surface surrogate *Int. J. Radiat. Oncol. Biol. Phys.* **88** 182–8

Fassi A, Seregni M, Riboldi M, Cerveri P, Sarrut D, Ivaldi G B, De Fatis P T, Liotta M and Baroni G 2015 Surrogate-driven deformable motion model for organ motion tracking in particle radiation therapy *Phys. Med. Biol.* **60** 1565–82

Fayad H, Clément J F, Pan T, Roux C, Cheze Le Rest C, Pradier O and Visvikis D 2009 Towards a generic respiratory motion model for 4D CT imaging of the thorax *IEEE Nuclear Science Symp. Conf. Record.* (Piscataway, NJ: IEEE) 3975–9

Fayad H, Gilles M, Pan T and Visvikis D 2018 A 4D global respiratory motion model of the thorax based on CT images: a proof of concept *Med. Phys.* **45** 3043–51

Fayad H J, Buerger C, Tsoumpas C, Cheze-Le-Rest C and Visvikis D 2012 A generic respiratory motion model based on 4D MRI imaging and 2D image navigators *IEEE Nuclear Science Symp. Conf. Record* (Piscataway, NJ: IEEE) 4058–61

Fayad H, Pan T, Pradier O and Visvikis D 2012 Patient specific respiratory motion modeling using a 3D patient's external surface *Med. Phys.* **39** 3386–95

Fayad H, Pan T, Roux C, Le Rest C C, Pradier O and Visvikis D 2009 A 2D-spline patient specific model for use in radiation therapy *Proc. 2009 IEEE Int. Symp. on Biomedical Imaging: From Nano to Macro, ISBI 2009* (Piscataway, NJ: IEEE) 590–3

Feng L 2023 Live-view 4D GRASP MRI: a framework for robust real-time respiratory motion tracking with a sub-second imaging latency *Magn. Reson. Med.* **90** 1053–68

Feng L, Tyagi N and Otazo R 2020 MRSIGMA: magnetic resonance SIGnature MAtching for real-time volumetric imaging *Magn. Reson. Med.* **84** 1280–92

Florkow M C *et al* 2020 Deep learning-enabled MRI-only photon and proton therapy treatment planning for paediatric abdominal tumours *Radiother. Oncol.* **153** 220–7

Frangi A F, Schnabel J A, Davatzikos C, Alberola-López C and Fichtinger G (ed) 2018 *Medical Image Computing and Computer Assisted Intervention—MICCAI 2018* **vol 11073** (Cham: Springer International Publishing)

Garau N, Via R, Meschini G, Lee D, Keall P, Riboldi M, Baroni G and Paganelli C 2019 A ROI-based global motion model established on 4DCT and 2D cine-MRI data for MRI-guidance in radiation therapy *Phys. Med. Biol.* **64** 045002

Giger A *et al* 2020 Liver-ultrasound based motion modelling to estimate 4D dose distributions for lung tumours in scanned proton therapy *Phys. Med. Biol.* **65** 235050

Giger A, Stadelmann M, Preiswerk F, Jud C, De Luca V, Celicanin Z, Bieri O, Salomir R and Cattin P C 2018 Erratum: Ultrasound-driven 4D MRI (*Phys. Med. Biol.* (2018) 63 (145015) DOI: 10.1088/1361–6560/aaca1d) *Phys. Med. Biol.* **63** 179601

Grimwood A, McNair H A, O'Shea T P, Gilroy S, Thomas K, Bamber J C, Tree A C and Harris E J 2018 *In vivo* validation of Elekta's clarity autoscan for ultrasound-based intrafraction motion estimation of the prostate during radiation therapy *Int. J. Radiat. Oncol. Biol. Phys.* **102** 912–21

Harris W, Ren L, Cai J, Zhang Y, Chang Z and Yin F-F 2016 A technique for generating volumetric Cine-magnetic resonance imaging *Int. J. Radiat. Oncol., Biol., Phys.* **95** 844–53

Hirai R, Sakata Y, Tanizawa A and Mori S 2019 Real-time tumor tracking using fluoroscopic imaging with deep neural network analysis *Phys. Med.* **59** 22–9

Hoffmann A *et al* 2020 MR-guided proton therapy: a review and a preview *Radiat. Oncol.* **15** 129

Huttinga N R F, Bruijnen T, van den Berg C A T and Sbrizzi A 2021 Nonrigid 3D motion estimation at high temporal resolution from prospectively undersampled k-space data using low-rank MR-MOTUS *Magn. Reson. Med.* **85** 2309–26

Ipsen S, Bruder R, García-Vázquez V, Schweikard A and Ernst F 2019 Assessment of 4D ultrasound systems for image-guided radiation therapy—image quality, framerates and CT artifacts *Curr. Dir. Biomed. Eng.* **5** 245–8

Kamino Y, Takayama K, Kokubo M, Narita Y, Hirai E, Kawawda N, Mizowaki T, Nagata Y, Nishidai T and Hiraoka M 2006 Development of a four-dimensional image-guided radio-therapy system with a gimbaled x-ray head *Int. J. Radiat. Oncol., Biol., Phys.* **66** 271–8

Keall P J *et al* 2022 Integrated MRI-guided radiotherapy—opportunities and challenges *Nat. Rev. Clin. Oncol.* **19** 458–70

King A P, Buerger C, Tsoumpas C, Marsden P K and Schaeffter T 2012 Thoracic respiratory motion estimation from MRI using a statistical model and a 2-D image navigator *Med. Image Anal.* **16** 252–64

Krieger M *et al* 2021 Liver-ultrasound-guided lung tumour tracking for scanned proton therapy: a feasibility study *Phys. Med. Biol.* **66** 035011

Kurz C *et al* 2020 Medical physics challenges in clinical MR-guided radiotherapy *Radiat. Oncol.* **15** 93

Li H *et al* 2022 AAPM Task Group Report 290: respiratory motion management for particle therapy *Med. Phys.* **49** e50–81

Liu Y *et al* 2019 MRI-based treatment planning for proton radiotherapy: dosimetric validation of a deep learning-based liver synthetic CT generation method *Phys. Med. Biol.* **64** 145015

Martin J, McClelland J, Yip C, Thomas C, Hartill C, Ahmad S, O'Brien R, Meir I, Landau D and Hawkes D 2013 Building motion models of lung tumours from cone-beam CT for radiotherapy applications *Phys. Med. Biol.* **58** 1809–22

McClelland J R, Blackall J M, Tarte S, Chandler A C, Hughes S, Ahmad S, Landau D B and Hawkes D J 2006 A continuous 4D motion model from multiple respiratory cycles for use in lung radiotherapy *Med. Phys.* **33** 3348–58

McClelland J R, Hawkes D J, Schaeffter T and King A P 2013 Respiratory motion models: a review *Med. Image Anal.* **17** 19–42

Meschini G *et al* 2020a Modeling RBE-weighted dose variations in irregularly moving abdominal targets treated with carbon ion beams *Med. Phys.* **47** 2768–78

Meschini G *et al* 2021 An MRI framework for respiratory motion modelling validation *J. Med. Imaging Radiat. Oncol.* **65** 337–44

Meschini G *et al* 2019 Validation of a model for physical dose variations in irregularly moving targets treated with carbon ion beams *Med. Phys.* **46** 3663–73

Meschini G, Seregni M, Pella A, Ciocca M, Fossati P, Valvo F, Riboldi M and Baroni G 2017 Evaluation of residual abdominal tumour motion in carbon ion gated treatments through respiratory motion modelling *Phys. Med.* **34** 28–37

Meschini G *et al* 2022 Time-resolved MRI for off-line treatment robustness evaluation in carbon-ion radiotherapy of pancreatic cancer *Med. Phys.* **49** 2386–95

Meschini G *et al* 2020b Virtual 4DCT from 4DMRI for the management of respiratory motion in carbon ion therapy of abdominal tumors *Med. Phys.* **47** 909–16

Mori S, Knopf A C and Umegaki K 2018 Motion management in particle therapy *Med. Phys.* **45** e994–e1010

Mostafaei F, Tai A, Gore E, Johnstone C, Haase W, Ehlers C, Cooper D T, Lachaine M and Li X A 2018 Feasibility of real-time lung tumor motion monitoring using intrafractional ultrasound and kV cone beam projection images *Med. Phys.* **45** 4619–26

Mylonas A, Booth J and Nguyen D T 2021 A review of artificial intelligence applications for motion tracking in radiotherapy *J. Med. Imaging Radiat. Oncol.* **65** 596–611

Olberg S, Chun J, Su Choi B, Park I, Kim H, Kim T, Sung Kim J, Green O and Park J C 2021 Abdominal synthetic CT reconstruction with intensity projection prior for MRI-only adaptive radiotherapy *Phys. Med. Biol.* **66** 204001

Olsen J, Green O and Kashani R 2015 World's first application of MR-guidance for radiotherapy *Mo. Med.* **112** 358–60

Paganelli C, Lee D, Kipritidis J, Whelan B, Greer P B, Baroni G, Riboldi M and Keall P 2018a Feasibility study on 3D image reconstruction from 2D orthogonal cine-MRI for MRI-guided radiotherapy *J. Med. Imaging Radiat. Oncol.* **62** 389–400

Paganelli C, Meschini G, Molinelli S, Riboldi M and Baroni G 2018b Patient-specific validation of deformable image registration in radiation therapy: overview and caveats *Med. Phys.* **45** e908–22

Paganelli C, Portoso S, Garau N, Meschini G, Via R, Buizza G, Keall P, Riboldi M and Baroni G 2019 Time-resolved volumetric MRI in MRI-guided radiotherapy: an in silico comparative analysis *Phys. Med. Biol.* **64** 185013

Paganelli C, Seregni M, Fattori G, Summers P, Bellomi M, Baroni G and Riboldi M 2015 Magnetic resonance imaging—guided versus surrogate-based motion tracking in liver radiation therapy: a prospective comparative study *Int. J. Radiat. Oncol., Biol., Phys.* **91** 840–8

Paganelli C et al 2018c MRI-guidance for motion management in external beam radiotherapy: current status and future challenges *Phys. Med. Biol.* **63** 22TR03

Pakela J M, Knopf A, Dong L, Rucinski A and Zou W 2022 Management of motion and anatomical variations in charged particle therapy: past, present, and into the future *Front. Oncol.* **12** 806153

Parrella G et al 2023 Synthetic CT in carbon ion radiotherapy of the abdominal site *Bioengineering* **10** 250

Peteani G, Paganelli C et al 2023 Retrospective reconstruction of four-dimensional magnetic resonance from interleaved cine imaging – A comparative study with four-dimensional computed tomography in the lung. *Phys Imaging Radiat. Oncol.* **27** 100529

Phillips J, Gueorguiev G, Shackleford J A, Grassberger C, Dowdell S, Paganetti H and Sharp G C 2014 Computing proton dose to irregularly moving targets *Phys. Med. Biol.* **59** 4261–73

Preiswerk F, De Luca V, Arnold P, Celicanin Z, Petrusca L, Tanner C, Bieri O, Salomir R and Cattin P C 2014 Model-guided respiratory organ motion prediction of the liver from 2D ultrasound *Med. Image Anal.* **18** 740–51

Qian P, Xu K, Wang T, Zheng Q, Yang H, Baydoun A, Zhu J, Traughber B and Muzic R F 2020 Estimating CT from MR abdominal images using novel generative adversarial networks *J. Grid Comput.* **18** 211–26

Raaymakers B W et al 2017 First patients treated with a 1.5 T MRI-Linac: clinical proof of concept of a high-precision, high-field MRI guided radiotherapy treatment *Phys. Med. Biol.* **62** L41–50

Rabe M et al 2021 Porcine lung phantom-based validation of estimated 4D-MRI using orthogonal cine imaging for low-field MR-Linacs *Phys. Med. Biol.* **66** 055006

Rasmussen C E and Williams C K I 2006 *Gaussian Processes for Machine Learning* **vol 2** (Cambridge, MA: MIT Press)

Riboldi M, Orecchia R and Baroni G 2012 Real-time tumour tracking in particle therapy: technological developments and future perspectives *Lancet Oncol.* **13** 383–91

Romaguera L V, Mezheritsky T, Mansour R, Carrier J F and Kadoury S 2021 Probabilistic 4D predictive model from in-room surrogates using conditional generative networks for image-guided radiotherapy *Med. Image Anal.* **74**

Romaguera L V, Mezheritsky T, Mansour R, Tanguay W and Kadoury S 2021 Predictive online 3D target tracking with population-based generative networks for image-guided radiotherapy *Int. J. Comput. Assist. Radiol. Surgery* **16** 1213–25

Seregni M et al 2013 Tumor tracking based on correlation models in scanned ion beam therapy: an experimental study *Phys. Med. Biol.* **58** 4659–78

Shen L, Zhao W and Xing L 2019 Patient-specific reconstruction of volumetric computed tomography images from a single projection view via deep learning *Nat. Biomed. Eng.* **3** 880–8

Shirato H, Oita M, Fujita K, Watanabe Y and Miyasaka K 2004 Feasibility of synchronization of real-time tumor-tracking radiotherapy and intensity-modulated radiotherapy from viewpoint of excessive dose from fluoroscopy *Int. J. Radiat. Oncol. Biol. Phys.* **60** 335–41

Shirato H, Shimizu S, Shimizu T, Nishioka T and Miyasaka K 1999 Real-time tumour-tracking radiotherapy *Lancet* **353** 1331–2

Stemkens B, Tijssen R H N, De Senneville B D, Lagendijk J J W and Van Den Berg C A T 2016 Image-driven, model-based 3D abdominal motion estimation for MR-guided radiotherapy *Phys. Med. Biol.* **61** 5335–55

Terpstra M L, Maspero M, Bruijnen T, Verhoeff J J C, Lagendijk J J W and van den Berg C A T 2021 Real-time 3D motion estimation from undersampled MRI using multi-resolution neural networks *Med. Phys.* **48** 6597–613

Keall P J, Mageras G S, Balter J M, Emery R S, Forster K M, Jiang S B, Kapatoes J M, Low D A, Murphy M J, Murray B R, Ramsey C R, Van Herk M B, Vedam S S, Wong J W and Yorke E 2006 The management of respiratory motion in radiation oncology report of AAPM Task Group 76 *Med Phys.* **33** 3874–900

Thummerer A *et al* 2022 Deep learning–based 4D-synthetic CTs from sparse-view CBCTs for dose calculations in adaptive proton therapy *Med. Phys.* **49** 6824–39

Trnková P *et al* 2018 Clinical implementations of 4D pencil beam scanned particle therapy: report on the 4D treatment planning workshop 2016 and 2017 *Phys. Med.* **54** 121–30

Kilby W, Dooley J R, Kuduvalli G, Sayeh S and Maurer R 2010 The CyberKnife® robotic radiosurgery system in 2010 *Technol. Cancer Res. Treat.* **9** 433–52

Wei R, Chen J, Liang B, Chen X, Men K and Dai J 2022 Real-time 3D MRI reconstruction from cine-MRI using unsupervised network in MRI-guided radiotherapy for liver cancer *Med. Phys.* **50** 3584–96

Wolfelschneider J, Seregni M, Fassi A, Ziegler M, Baroni G, Fietkau R, Riboldi M and Bert C 2017 Examination of a deformable motion model for respiratory movements and 4D dose calculations using different driving surrogates *Med. Phys.* **44** 2066–76

Zhang Y, Huth I, Wegner M, Weber D C and Lomax A J 2017 Surface as a motion surrogate for gated re-scanned pencil beam proton therapy *Phys. Med. Biol.* **62** 4046–61

Zhang Y, Knopf A, Tanner C, Boye D and Lomax A J 2013 Deformable motion reconstruction for scanned proton beam therapy using on-line x-ray imaging *Phys. Med. Biol.* **58** 8621–45

Zhang Y, Knopf A, Tanner C and Lomax A J 2014 Online image guided tumour tracking with scanned proton beams: a comprehensive simulation study *Phys. Med. Biol.* **59** 7793–817

IOP Publishing

Imaging in Particle Therapy
Current practice and future trends
Chiara Paganelli, Chiara Gianoli and Antje Knopf

Chapter 10

Treatment verification in particle therapy

C Gianoli, M De Simoni and A Knopf

10.1 Introduction

During or immediately after treatment delivery, reactive treatment verification techniques can be employed to evaluate the agreement of the delivered dose with respect to the treatment planning scenario. Because of the several weeks of fractionated treatment, unpredictable inter-fractional and intra-fractional anatomical changes, as well as inaccuracies in patient positioning, can occur, thus leading to dosimetric inconsistencies with respect to the treatment planning scenario. In case of relevant disagreements, a decision about possible replanning of the remaining fractions of the treatment can be taken. Different from proactive treatment verification techniques based on in-room tomographic imaging, reactive treatment verification techniques require in general a new treatment planning x-ray CT.

Reactive treatment verification techniques exploit secondary emissions induced by therapeutic radiation. However, the electromagnetic processes underlying the dose distribution are fundamentally different from the nuclear mechanisms inherent to secondary emissions. Due to the space-variant and time-variant relationship between the distribution of the secondary emissions and the dose distribution, they are typically referred to as indirect range verification techniques. For this reason, the range verification paradigm primarily entails the comparison of the measured secondary emissions with a prediction of their distribution based on Monte Carlo simulations of the treatment planning scenario. So far, the clinically investigated range verification techniques are based on positron emitters annihilating in photon pairs (positron emission tomography, PET), prompt photons produced by the de-excitation of the nuclei (prompt gammas, PGs) and, recently, charged secondary particles (mainly protons) produced by nuclear fragmentation. Generally, reactive treatment verification techniques entail the detection of the secondary radiation emerging from the patient produced by the interaction of the therapeutic beam (i.e., the projectile) with the tissue (i.e., the target), as shown in figure 10.1. This definition includes also neutrons, whose feasibility has been investigated but not yet demonstrated (Ytre-Hauge *et al* 2019, Toppi *et al* 2020).

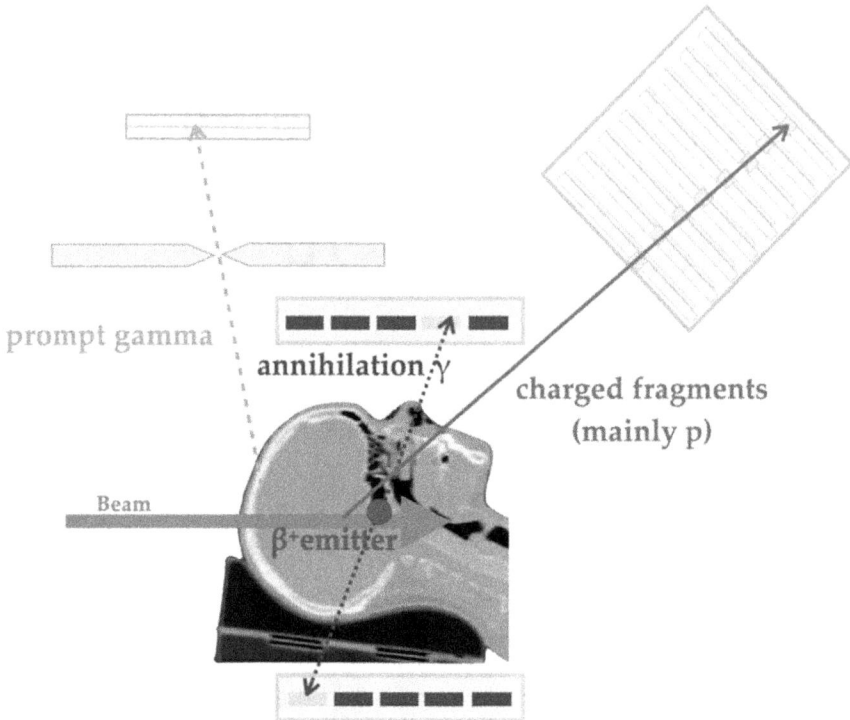

Figure 10.1. Secondary radiation emerging from the patient produced by the interaction of the therapeutic beam (i.e., the projectile) with the tissue (i.e., the target). A schematic representation of a detector configuration relevant to each secondary radiation is depicted. In light blue, the PET detector for the annihilation photon pair from a positron emitter; in orange, a PG detector provided with a collimator system for prompt gammas; in green, a tracking system for charged secondary particles.

As an alternative to the indirect comparison of the measurement with a prediction, the dose distribution can be retrieved from the distribution of the secondary emissions by means of 'dose reconstruction algorithms', based on the forward filtering approach, firstly proposed for PET imaging (Masuda *et al* 2019), and then extended to PG imaging (Schumann *et al* 2016, Pinto *et al* 2020). These include the analytical deconvolution (Parodi and Bortfeld 2006, Remmele *et al* 2011), the evolutionary algorithm (Schumann *et al* 2016, Hofmann *et al* 2019) and the maximum likelihood expectation maximization (ML-EM) algorithm (Masuda *et al* 2019, 2020), whose differences are mainly related to the objective function and its optimization. Approaches based on deep learning have been specifically proposed for dose reconstruction in PET imaging (Hu *et al* 2020, Ma *et al* 2020, Rahman *et al* 2022) and PG imaging (Liu and Huang 2020). However, these approaches have been preliminarily investigated relying on the ground truth distribution of the secondary emission as obtained from simulations, thus not accounting for the detection and the reconstruction of the events. Deep learning has been proposed to close this gap and thus retrieving the PG distribution based on the measurements (Jiang *et al* 2023).

Simulation platforms have been specifically adapted and developed for the investigation of PET and PG imaging. The GATE (Geant4 Application for Tomographic Emission) platform, based on the GEANT4 toolkit, is a Monte Carlo simulation environment that was originally proposed for emission tomography and recently extended to radiation therapy (Jan *et al* 2011, Borys *et al* 2022), provided with the modeling of complex detector and collimation systems. The MEGAlib (Medium-Energy Gamma-ray Astronomy library) platform, also based on the GEANT4 toolkit and originally intended for Compton telescopes in astronomy, has been firstly used in medical imaging for the investigation of the triple coincidence from β+ decaying isotopes emitting a third prompt photon (γ-PET imaging; Lang *et al* 2014). The environment is equipped with capabilities for advanced pre-processing of the raw data and tomographic image reconstruction algorithms for both PET and PG imaging (Liprandi *et al* 2017, Lovatti *et al* 2020). The FLUKA (Fluktuierende Kaskade, or fluctuating cascade) platform is a tool for the simulations of particle transport and interactions with matter for an extended range of applications, including medical physics, with reference to PET imaging as range verification techniques (Sommerer *et al* 2006, Augusto *et al* 2018).

10.2 PET as range verification technique in particle therapy

10.2.1 Physics fundamentals

Nuclear interactions between the projectile and the target produce radioisotopes that emit positrons. The reaction channels, involving both projectile and target, determine the shape of the activity distribution and thus the relationship to the dose distribution (Espana *et al* 2011, Parodi 2012). The positron (β^+), which is the antiparticle of the electron (β^-), annihilates with a tissue electron, thus converting its mass into radiation energy. Due to conservation of momentum and spin, positron–electron annihilation produces two γ-photons, emitted at an energy of 511 keV along opposite directions.

Due to the composition of the tissue, the positron emitters produced are mainly carbon and oxygen isotopes. In particular, ^{11}C, ^{10}C, ^{15}O, ^{13}N and ^{12}N whose half-lives are about 20 min, 19 s, 2 min, 10 min and 11 ms, respectively, are the most abundant (table 10.1) in both proton and carbon ion therapy (Bauer *et al* 2013, Horst *et al* 2019). The former is crucial for PET acquisition after the treatment (i.e., in-room PET and near-room PET), while ^{10}C and ^{15}O are important for PET acquisition during the treatment (i.e., in-beam PET). The activity density for therapeutic ion beams is rather low, about 200 $BqGy^{-1}cm^{-3}$ for carbon ions and about 600 $BqGy^{-1}\,cm^{-3}$ for protons.

At the detector level, the line along which the two γ photons are emitted is called the line of response (LOR). The detection of the two coincident γ-photons along the LOR is referred to as 'count'. The distribution of the counts can then be obtained according to tomographic image reconstruction. However, the count distribution does not coincide with the activity distribution due to the positron range and the half-life of the radioactive decay. The positron range indicates the distance between the position of β^+ decay and the annihilation, which depends on the kinetic energy

Table 10.1. List of the positron emitting isotopes produced in hadron therapy, their half-life, their most probable nuclear reaction channels and threshold energy. The most important nuclear reaction channels are reported in bold. Since the radioactive isotopes (i.e., ^{13}C, ^{15}N and ^{18}O) have very low abundances in the human body, the negligible production nuclear reaction channels are reported in italics. The cross sections of the radioactive capture reaction (p,γ) are typically three orders of magnitude smaller than the main channels.

Radioisotopes	Half-live	Nuclear reaction channel	Threshold energy (MeV)	Reference
^{15}O	2.03 min	**^{16}O(p,pn)^{15}O**	16.79	Zhu and El Fakhri (2013)
		^{16}O(p,d)^{15}O	14.3	Ozoemelam et al (2020)
		^{14}N(p,γ)^{15}O	0	Beebe-Wang et al (2003)
		^{15}N(p,n)^{15}O	3.8	Beebe-Wang et al (2003)
^{14}O	70.6 s	^{16}O(p,t)^{14}O	21.7	Ozoemelam et al (2020)
		^{16}O(p,nd)^{14}O	28.3	Ozoemelam et al (2020)
		^{16}O(p,p2n)^{14}O	30.7	Pönisch et al (2004)
		^{14}N(p,n)^{14}O	6.6	Pönisch et al (2004)
^{11}C	20.38 min	**^{12}C(p,pn)^{11}C**	20.61	Zhu and El Fakhri (2013)
		^{12}C(p,d)^{11}C	17.9	Ozoemelam et al (2020)
		^{14}N(p,2p2n)^{11}C	3.22	Zhu and El Fakhri (2013)
		^{14}N(p,α)^{11}C	3.44	Pönisch et al (2004)
		^{16}O(p,3p3n)^{11}C	59.64	Zhu and El Fakhri (2013)
		^{16}O(p,αpn)^{11}C	27.50	Beebe-Wang et al (2003)
		^{13}C(p,p2n)^{11}C	25.50	Beebe-Wang et al (2003)
		^{15}O(p,αn)^{11}C	14.70	Beebe-Wang et al (2003)
^{10}C	19.3 s	**^{12}C(p,t)^{10}C**	25.3	Ozoemelam et al (2020)
		^{12}C(p,nd)^{10}C	32.1	Ozoemelam et al (2020)
		^{12}C(p,p2n)^{10}C	34.5	Pönisch et al (2004)
		^{16}O(p,3p4n)^{10}C	39.1	Pönisch et al (2004)
		^{14}N(p,nα)^{10}C	17.20	Beebe-Wang et al (2003)
^{13}N	9.97 min	**^{16}O(p,2p2n)^{13}N**	5.66	Zhu and El Fakhri (2013)
		^{16}O(p,α)^{13}N	5.66	Beebe-Wang et al (2003)
		^{14}N(p,pn)^{13}N	11.44	Zhu and El Fakhri (2013)
		^{12}C(p,γ)^{13}N	0	Beebe-Wang et al (2003)
		^{13}C(p,n)^{13}N	3.20	Beebe-Wang et al (2003)
		^{15}N(p,nd)^{13}N	20.40	Beebe-Wang et al (2003)
		^{15}N(p,t)^{13}N	13.80	Beebe-Wang et al (2003)
^{12}N	11 ms	**^{12}C(p,n)^{12}N**	19.6	Ozoemelam et al (2020)
^{17}F	1.07 min	^{16}O(p,γ)^{17}F	0	Beebe-Wang et al (2003)
^{18}F	109.8 min	*^{18}O(p,n)^{17}F*	2.60	Beebe-Wang et al (2003)
^{30}P	2.49 min	^{31}P(p,pn)^{30}P	19.7	Zhu and El Fakhri (2013)
^{38}K	7.63 min	^{40}Ca(p,2p2n)^{38}K	21.2	Zhu and El Fakhri (2013)
^{8}B	770 ms	^{12}C(p,nα)^{8}B	28.3	Ozoemelam et al (2020)
		^{12}C(p,dt)^{8}B	47.4	Ozoemelam et al (2020)

spectrum of the positron, up to the maximum energy of the 'end point', typical of each radioisotope. Since the annihilation cross section is greater at the lower kinetic energies of positrons, the positron range can be up to several millimeters. The half-life indicates the time interval between the production of the positron emitter and the β^+ decay, which is typically modeled by a Poisson distribution.

Treatment verification is based on the comparison of the PET image (i.e., the measured PET) with a Monte Carlo prediction of the PET distribution based on the treatment planning scenario (i.e., the expected PET), in terms of anatomy of the patient and geometry and dosimetry of the irradiation. The prediction requires the mass density and the stoichiometric composition of tissue, along with the timing parameters of irradiation and imaging (i.e., irradiation time, delay between irradiation and imaging, imaging time) as well as the washout estimation. In high perfused tissue, the biological washout of the β^+ emitters degrade the activation level and changes the shape of the activity distribution. The correction of biological washout is based on models designed and characterized on animal studies. The tissue is determined based on thresholds applied to the Hounsfield Units of the treatment planning CT image, thus identifying hard bone, soft bone, fat, muscle and brain. The expected PET is decomposed into three components undergoing fast, medium and slow biological decays. Tissue-specific fractions and biological half-lives are assigned to each of the three components. The β^+ emitter distribution accounting for biological washout is then calculated based on the timing parameters of imaging. The Monte Carlo prediction of the β^+ emitters can be complemented by the γ annihilation, thus explicitly accounting for the positron range and the half-life of the radioactive decay. This way, the effect of tomographic image reconstruction on the count distribution can be predicted.

10.2.2 Quantitative range verification

The quantitative assessment in PET-based treatment verification entails a comparison between the measured PET and the expected PET to identify possible inconsistencies. The expected PET is typically calculated by means of Monte Carlo simulation, but also analytical attempts are reported in literature (Attanasi *et al* 2011). The quantification has been typically based on the distal fall-off of PET image profiles along the beam direction (Parodi *et al* 2007a, 2007b, Knopf *et al* 2008, 2011), which correlates to the particle range. The ranges of both the measured PET and the expected PET are extracted and compared. Different range extraction methods have been proposed, based on different percentages with respect to the activity of individual profiles (80% or 90% of the peaks (Parodi *et al* 2007a)) and global surfaces (2%–8% of the peak (Moglioni *et al* 2022)) or based on the maximization of the cross-correlation of the normalized profiles (Knopf *et al* 2008). However, the extremely low counting statistics in the measured PET is one of the main open challenges.

The measured PET is obtained from tomographic image reconstruction of a few sinogram counts, where the activity emerges from a noisy background in a restricted area in the field of view. The quality of the reconstruction is therefore strongly limited by the noise break-up effect. A possibility to reduce noise is to stop the iterative reconstruction at the first iterations. However, the reconstructed image results far from convergence, and therefore is potentially biased. The bias can be partially reduced by introducing the model of the spatial resolution and the time of flight information within the tomographic image reconstruction (Kurz *et al* 2015) as well as by using basis functions that are extended to regions rather than voxels (Gianoli *et al* 2014). In order to handle the low counting statistics in quantification, indices of agreement between the measured PET and the expected PET relying on the entire activity distribution have been proposed, such as based on the statistical distributions (Pearson's correlation coefficient (Kuess *et al* 2012) or voxel-based morphometry (Kraan *et al* 2022)). The expected PET has been also used not only as a comparison for the measured PET, but also as 'a guide' for the tomographic image reconstruction of the measured PET based on regional basis functions for 3D (three-dimensional) PET-based treatment verification (Gianoli *et al* 2014). Despite the increased robustness to noise and enhanced sensitivity to inconsistencies, the index of agreement provides a relative quantification of such inconsistencies, which is of difficult interpretability since it is not supported by a measure of the displacements between the measured PET and the expected PET. For this reason, the absolute quantification of the range is typically preferred. Recently, a 4D (four-dimensional) ML-EM algorithm, originally presented for cardiac gated PET imaging, has been proposed (Gianoli *et al* 2017). By interpreting the measured PET and the expected PET as two different motion phases of a 4D dataset, the algorithm estimates a measured PET of enhanced image quality, similar to count statistics optimization in motion compensation strategies (Gianoli *et al* 2016), and the deformation field mapping the expected PET onto the measured PET as an absolute measure of the occurred displacements. However, the inaccuracies of the expected PET, especially those due to the modeling of biological washout (i.e., tissue classification in Monte Carlo simulations), translate into biases of the signal distribution, which can be wrongly interpreted as inconsistencies of measured PET. To cope with the inaccuracy of the expected PET, a reference measured PET taken at the beginning of the treatment course can be adopted to assess the reproducibility, instead of the absolute accuracy, of the treatment delivery (Nishio *et al* 2008, Moglioni *et al* 2022).

PET-based treatment verification has been demonstrated as a millimetric range verification technique in low perfusion bony structures of intracranial and cervical spine tumor patients. Patient positioning inaccuracies and anatomical changes have been detected and the treatment has been accordingly adapted for the subsequent treatment fractions. Limitations of this technique have been mainly associated to the extremely low count statistics and high perfusion of tissue, which causes PET activity washout, especially in brain and extra-cranial sites (i.e., abdominopelvic tumours; Parodi *et al* 2007b, Knopf *et al* 2011). In the thoraco-abdominal area, breathing motion represents an additional source of treatment uncertainty. With respect to that, treatment verification of moving targets based on time-resolved PET image acquisition can be accomplished by relying on the whole count statistics image quality, as obtained from the application of 4D PET motion compensation strategies (Knopf *et al* 2014, Gianoli *et al* 2016, Kurz *et al* 2016).

10.2.3 Imaging system configurations

The idea of exploiting PET imaging to verify the particle therapy treatment dates back to 1969, when the proposal of radioactive beam visualization has been put forward at the Lawrence Berkeley Laboratory (Llacer 1988), relying on ^{19}Ne beams. Radioactive beam visualization has been not yet clinically applied but experimental investigations have been conducted at the Heavy Ion Medical Accelerator in Chiba (HIMAC) in Japan (Mohammadi *et al* 2019, 2022) and at the Gesellschaft für Schwerioneneforschung (GSI) in Darmstadt (Boscolo *et al* 2021). Commonly, PET image acquisition for treatment verification makes use of commercial or dedicated PET scanners placed inside the treatment room or in adjacent PET imaging rooms (figure 10.2; Shakirin *et al* 2011). Accordingly, three different PET-based treatment verification techniques are defined: near-room PET, in-room PET and in-beam PET. Extensive clinical experiences have been reported in recent years, starting with the GSI with an in-beam PET prototype, followed by the Massachusetts General Hospital (MGH) in Boston with near-room and in-room PET systems, and most recently, the University Hospital of Heidelberg in collaboration with the Heidelberg Ion beam Therapy centre (HIT) in Germany based on near-room PET systems.

10.2.3.1 Near-room PET
To acquire near-room PET images for treatment verification, patients are typically moved to a dedicated imaging room after the treatment is delivered, where a commercial PET/CT scanner is installed. The combined PET/CT scanner allows for co-registration of the images, as the repositioning of the patient for the near-room PET acquisition can be a source of misalignments with respect to the treatment planning CT image. The time delay between the end of the treatment and the beginning of the PET acquisition strongly influences the quality of the PET image due to the effects of biological washout and the decrease of the count statistics. In particular, the time required to collect meaningful statistics for image acquisition can be up to ~30 min, exacerbating the effects of biological washout and substantially prolonging the image acquisition time, and thus patient discomfort.

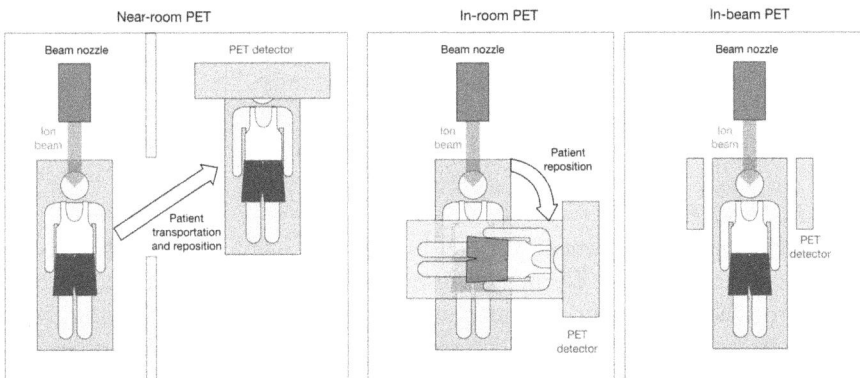

Figure 10.2. PET-based treatment verification techniques: near-room PET (left), in-room PET (center), in-beam PET (right).

The first clinical attempt based on a commercial PET/CT scanner (SET-2300W scanner, Shimadzu Corporation) has been done at the Hyogo Ion Beam Treatment System in Japan (Hishikawa *et al* 2002). The first pilot study reporting near-room PET/CT imaging has been performed at the MGH (Parodi *et al* 2007b), where a conventional cyclotron coupled to passive beam shaping system is installed. A commercial PET/CT scanner (Siemens Biography Sensation 16) has been used for proton therapy verification of 23 patients. The PET/CT images have been acquired at the department of radiology, at more than 10 min walking distance from the proton therapy center. Patients have been transported from the treatment room to the imaging room after the treatment delivery. The time delay has ranged from ~15 to ~30 min, during which time the short-lived radioisotopes, most importantly ^{15}O, have decayed. Other important near-room PET studies have been conducted at HIMAC for proton therapy verification (based on the PET/CT scanner GE Medical System, Discovery ST; Nishio *et al* 2008) and at the proton therapy facility of the University of Florida (based on the PET/CT scanner Philips GEMINI; Hsi *et al* 2009). The University Hospital of Heidelberg in collaboration with HIT conducted a large-scale clinical trial, namely the MIRANDA study (Monitoring of Patients treated with Particle Therapy using Positron-Emission-Tomography) based on a commercial PET/CT scanner (Siemens Biograph mCT 40) after proton and carbon ion beam therapy (Combs *et al* 2012).

10.2.3.2 In-room PET

Following the first experience with near-room PET/CT imaging, MGH has proposed a clinical trial based on a commercial neurological PET scanner (NeuroPET, Photo Diagnostic Systems) mounted on wheels for in-room PET imaging shortly after the patient treatment. In-room PET is commonly performed with a full-ring PET scanner positioned in the treatment room, but not directly on the beam line. The patient couch is rotated and translated directly into the imaging position for the PET acquisition, thus reducing the time delay between the treatment and the image acquisition (approximately 2–3 min) and the repositioning issues compared to near-room PET. Furthermore, image acquisition can be performed in about 5 min, significantly reducing the image acquisition time compared to near-room PET (Zhu and El Fakhri 2013). However, biological washout and count statistics loss remain a problem and, more importantly, the clinical workflow is slowed down by the image acquisition performed after the treatment, as the treatment room is not available for other treatments during imaging.

10.2.3.3 In-beam PET

In-beam PET enables treatment verification during irradiation, without slowing down the clinical workflow. Dedicated in-beam PET systems, designed to be fully integrated into the treatment room, are currently considered the optimal solution for PET-based treatment verification. The most promising aspect of an in-beam PET system is the possibility of acquiring counts while treatment is still in progress, thus minimizing count statistics loss and biological washout. The count statistics increase until the end of treatment and then starts to decrease due to the decay. Compared to in-room PET and near-room PET, in-beam PET is therefore able to acquire the best part of the signal. However, the integration of the in-beam PET system in the treatment room is geometrically limited in the beam direction. This imposes an opening in the detector geometry, thus causing degradation of the spatial resolution due to data truncation (Ferrero *et al* 2019). For this reason, different from near-room and in-room PET systems, treatment verification based on in-beam PET systems is typically based on the projection of the counts onto the central plane along the beam direction, according to 2D imaging.

The first clinical in-beam PET system for treatment verification has been installed at the carbon ion beam therapy facility at the GSI (Pawelke *et al* 1997, Enghardt *et al* 2004). Approximately 400 patients, treated with scanned carbon ion beams, mostly for head and neck tumors, have been daily imaged. The PET imaging system has been constructed from components of the commercial Siemens ECAT EXACT PET scanner, made of bismuth germanium oxide (BGO) coupled with photo multiplier tubes (PMT). The prototype has been designed as a dual-head configuration mounted at the treatment site, above and below the patient couch to avoid interference with the horizontal beam line. At this synchrotron-based facility, pulsed pencil beams are delivered, and counts are collected during the beam extraction pauses and continue after treatment. The counts collected during the beam pulse are distinguished from those acquired during the pauses by synchronizing the imaging system with the control unit of the accelerator (i.e., an ionization chamber). At the proton therapy center in Kashiwa, a planar in-beam PET system manufactured by Hamamatsu Photonics K. K. has been mounted on the rotating gantry (Nishio *et al* 2006, 2010). At the National Centre of Oncological Hadron therapy in Pavia (CNAO, Centro Nazionale di Adroterapia Oncologica), a prototype made of a planar dual-head PET system provided with a tracker for secondary protons has been adopted for a clinical trial. The prototype has been developed by the INSIDE (INnovative Solution for In-beam DosimEtry in hadron therapy) collaboration as an innovative bimodal imaging system for the verification of both proton (Fiorina *et al* 2021) and carbon ion treatments (Toppi *et al* 2021). The PET system, used for proton therapy, has been made of lutetium yttrium orthosilicate (LYSO) crystals coupled with silicon photo multipliers (SiPM), providing the advantage of better energy and time resolution, as well as a compact solution for a reduced detector load. The combined tracker, which has been used for carbon ion therapy, is based on eight orthogonal pairs of square plastic scintillator fibres and represents so far, the only clinically investigated detector for charged fragments[1].

---

[1] The charged fragments produced at $60°-90°$ with respect to the direction of the incoming beam are mainly protons, with a low contamination of deuterons and tritons (less than 10%). For ions heavier than protons, charged secondary particles are mostly generated from the projectile fragmentation, as dominant compared to target fragmentation and those emitted at large angles are sufficient to be correlated with the beam range (Muraro *et al* 2016). Furthermore, the detection of charged fragments, when compared to the photon detection, can be carried out in a nearly background free environment and can be performed with high efficiency. On the other hand, the main disadvantages are that, unlike photons, the fragments suffer from nuclear interactions and multiple scattering in matter and that, at a greater angle to the beam direction, the number of fragments is lower.

10.3 PG detection as range verification technique in particle therapy

10.3.1 Physics fundamentals

Due to the inelastic interaction between the projectile and the target, prompt gamma photons (PGs) of a few MeV energy (from 1 to 2 MeV up to about 7 MeV) are emitted within 1 ns, thus instantaneously providing information about their production point in the patient without interacting with the surrounding tissue (Wrońska 2020). After the first proposal (Stichelbaut and Jongen 2003) and the first proof of principle for proton beams of different energies in water (Min *et al* 2006), several experimental and simulation studies have been conducted to measure the PG emission yield (i.e., the number of PGs per projectile, unit of field of view, and unit of solid angle), energy and spatial distributions as a function of different materials of the target and different projectiles (i.e., particles and beam energies; Pinto *et al* 2014).

The yield, integrated along the entire beam path, depends on the range but the yield per millimeter is not strongly dependent on the energy of the projectile (Krimmer *et al* 2018). A slight decrease of the yield along the beam path is due to the beam attenuation. The yield has an increasing distribution, due to an enhancement of the yield towards lower energies of the primary beam, up to the Bragg peak, where the primary beam does not have sufficient energy to exceed the energy threshold of nuclear reactions. Afterwards, the yield undergoes a rapid fall-off close to the beam range. For beams with 15 cm range in water, the yields per incident ion is 0.05 counts and 0.3 counts, for protons and carbon ions respectively. For instance, in a typical ion beam therapy treatment fraction, the number of delivered ions is around 10^8 for protons and 10^6 for carbon ions. The fall-off of the yield is more correlated to the Bragg peak for carbon ions than for protons (figure 10.3). Moreover, the fall-off for carbon ions is sharper than for protons. However, secondary interactions beyond the Bragg peak are more relevant for carbon ions than for protons.

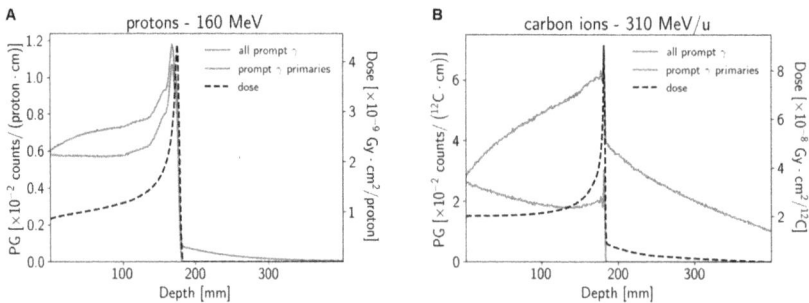

Figure 10.3. PG profiles (energy range 1–10 MeV) obtained from Monte Carlo simulations in Geant4 (v.10.07. p03) of a Gaussian beam (standard deviation of the beam spot size equal to 7 mm) incident at the center of a $15 \times 15 \times 40$ cm^3 water phantom with a source to phantom distance of 1 cm. Initial energies set to 160 MeV and 310 MeV/u (energy spread not included) and number of particles to 2×10^8 and 5×10^6, for protons (A) and carbon ions (B), respectively. Courtesy of Beatrice Foglia and Dr Marco Pinto from the Ludwig Maximilian University of Munich.

The energy spectrum is characterized by a continuum in the few MeV range with some discrete lines corresponding to nuclei transitions from the first excited levels to their ground levels. In particular, the discrete energy at 4.44 and 6.13 MeV are due to the de-excitation of ^{12}C and ^{16}O, respectively, while the discrete energy at 2.2 MeV results from the de-excitation of deuterium after neutron capture by hydrogen and is not correlated with the range. The correlation between the Bragg peak and the yield has been measured for different components of the spectrum (Verburg *et al* 2013). The photons at 4.4 MeV have the highest spatial correlation with the Bragg peak and their line is therefore the most suitable spectrum component for the range verification.

Different reaction channels produce the same discrete energy photons (table 10.2; Verburg *et al* 2012, Ready 2016). In addition to PGs emitted directly following a nuclear interaction, there are contributions from β^+ delayed gamma rays. Depending on the half-life of the β^+ decay, the gamma rays emitted as a result of these reaction channels cannot be distinguishable from the PGs.

Compared to PET, PG is characterized by higher gamma production rates (from 10 times when compared to in-beam PET up to 80 times when compared to near-room PET) and transmission efficiency (about 5 times for prompt gammas). The detection efficiency is lower due to the higher energy photons and, depending on the detector configuration, due to smaller solid angle acceptance (Moteabbed *et al* 2011). The main advantage of prompt gammas as a treatment verification technique are the instantaneous emission, and thus the absence of washout effects, that comes however with a background of secondary radiation, including neutrons.

Similar to PET, the treatment verification based on PG detection is based on the comparison between the measured and the predicted distributions, in accordance with the treatment planning, as simulated based on either Monte Carlo platforms or analytical codes (Sterpin *et al* 2015) accounting for detection and reconstruction of the events.

Table 10.2. Reaction channels producing the most prominent discrete gamma energies (i.e., 4.44 MeV and 6.13 MeV). The most important nuclear reaction channels are reported in bold.

Target	Reaction channel	PG energy (keV)	Half-life
C	**$^{12}C(p,p')^{12}C$**	4443	45 fs
	$^{13}C(p,d)^{12}C$	4443	45 fs
	$^{12}C(p,n)^{12}N$	4443	11 ms ($\beta^+ \rightarrow {}^{12}C*$)
	$^{13}C(p,2p)^{12}N$	4443	11 ms ($\beta^+ \rightarrow {}^{12}C*$)
N	$^{14}N(p,p')^{14}N$	1635	4.8 fs
	$^{14}N(p,n)^{14}O$	1635	71 s ($\beta^+ \rightarrow {}^{14}N*$)
	$^{14}N(p,p')^{14}N$	2313	68 fs
	$^{14}N(p,n)^{14}O$	2313	71 s ($\beta^+ \rightarrow {}^{14}N*$)
	$^{14}N(p,2pn)^{12}C$	4443	45 fs
O	**$^{16}O(p,p\alpha)^{12}C$**	4443	45 fs
	$^{16}O(p,n\alpha)^{12}N$	4443	11 ms ($\beta^+ \rightarrow {}^{12}C*$)
	$^{16}O(p,d)^{15}O$	5241	122 s ($\beta^+ \rightarrow {}^{15}N*$)
	$^{16}O(p,2p)^{15}N$	5270	17 fs
	$^{16}O(p,p')^{16}O$	6129	18 ps

10.3.2 PG techniques and detector configurations

PG detection includes several techniques for treatment verification as different physical properties of the emitted photons can be correlated with the beam range, such as the spatial distribution of the emission with the Prompt Gamma Imaging (PGI) technique, the temporal distribution or time-of-flight (TOF) of the PG with the Prompt Gamma Timing (PGT) and Prompt Gamma Timing Imaging (PGTI) techniques and the energy distribution or spectrum of the PG with the Prompt Gamma Spectroscopy (PGS) technique.

The PG imaging techniques, including PGTI and PGS techniques, require spatial localization of the production point based on mechanical or electronic collimation systems combined with an absorption detector. Spatial localization relays on the back-projection of the detected PG along the photon direction, as determined by the collimator. The 1D collimation system is usually placed along the beam direction, so that the spatial localization is performed along a profile, as 1D imaging. The detected PG is projected onto the beam direction according to the shortest distance of the photon direction to the beam direction (i.e., the common perpendicular). For a 2D collimation system, the detected PG is projected onto the surface parallel to the modules across the beam direction. This is typically referred to as 2D imaging (Min *et al* 2011). Image reconstruction algorithms are needed to reconstruct the statistical PG distribution, yielding to 3D imaging (Draeger *et al* 2018).

10.3.2.1 Prompt gamma imaging

10.3.2.1.1 Mechanical collimation systems
The main challenge for the mechanical collimation is the inverse dependency between spatial resolution and efficiency for a wide energy spectrum. The most-used mechanical collimation systems are made of high density materials (i.e., lead and tungsten) and are based on pinhole, linear slit or multiple slit cameras (Smeets *et al* 2016, Park *et al* 2019).

The slit camera is the basic approach, providing 1D imaging of parallel PGs. The pinhole camera, or knife-edge slit camera, represents a variation of the slit camera, that, inspired by the classical optics, enables 1D imaging of PGs whose directions intersect at the pinhole (figure 10.4(a)). Feasibility studies have been performed by several groups (Smeets *et al* 2012, Perali *et al* 2014, Lopes *et al* 2015) and the first clinical application of a slit camera for relative range verification (i.e., inter-fractional range variations) has been carried out by the Dresden group, composed of scientists from the National Center for Radiation Research in Oncology (OncoRay), the Technische Universität Dresden and the Helmholtz–Zentrum Dresden–Rossendorf, in collaboration with Ion Beam Applications (IBA; Richter *et al* 2016) in passive beam delivery. Inter-fractional range variations within ±2 mm have been detected and the precision of ±2 mm has been subsequently confirmed also in pencil beam delivery.

The first clinical trial of prompt gamma range verification during a whole treatment has been performed with a knife-edge slit camera from IBA at Philadelphia, in pencil beam delivery (Xie *et al* 2017). The prototype has been proposed for an active beam delivery system, enabling the measurement with open and closed collimators for the

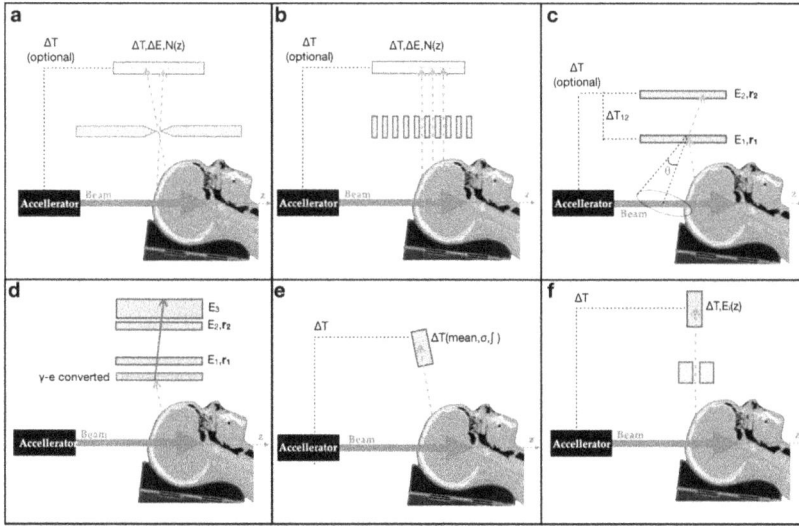

Figure 10.4. PG detector configurations based on mechanical collimation: (a) linear slit camera or knife-edge slit camera; (b) multi-parallel slit camera. The spatial distribution $N(z)$ is used to retrieve information about the range whereas temporal (ΔT) and energy (ΔE) of individual count are used to suppress background. PG detector configuration based on electronic collimation: (c) Compton camera where the direction of the scattered photon ($\mathbf{r}_{1,2}$) and energy depositions ($E_{1,2}$) in the two detector modules describe the cone of possible emission directions while timing information (ΔT and ΔT_{12}) are used for background suppression; (d) three-stage hodoscope where the direction of the scattered electron ($\mathbf{r}_{1,2}$) and energy depositions ($E_{1,2}$) in the two detector modules uniquely describe the emission direction. Pattern of energy depositions in the detector modules is used to suppress background. PG detector configuration requiring no collimation: (e) PGT and PGPI, based on the analysis of the temporal distribution; (f) PGS based on the analysis of the energy distributions where the time information is used to suppress background.

removal of the background. Range variations of up to 1–2 mm have been detected (Nenoff *et al* 2017). A prototype based on a knife-edge slit camera has been constructed based on a collaboration between IBA and Politecnico di Milano. This knife-edge slit camera has been compared with a multi-slit camera of the same weight (Park *et al* 2019). The multi-slit camera represents an extension of the slit camera (Pinto *et al* 2014, Smeets *et al* 2012), enabling 1D imaging but on an extended field of view (FOV; figure 10.4(b)). The design of both collimators has been optimized based on Monte Carlo simulations. The efficiency in PG detection of the knife-edge slit camera has been proved superior but the smaller FOV provided imaging of the Bragg peak region only, while a multi-slit camera allowed imaging of the entire beam path. A collimator system based on multiple knife-edge slit cameras, forming a 2D pattern along the beam direction has been also studied to enable 2D imaging (Ready *et al* 2016). Higher efficiency and precision of about 1 mm have been reported.

10.3.2.1.2 Electronic collimation systems

As an alternative to collimation systems, Compton cameras rely on Compton scattering to determine the direction of the prompt-gamma emission (Krimmer *et al*

2018). This solution has been studied by several groups (Roellinghoff *et al* 2011, Aldawood *et al* 2015, Krimmer *et al* 2015, McCleskey *et al* 2015, Llosá *et al* 2016, Hueso-González *et al* 2016a, Golnik *et al* 2016, Rohling *et al* 2017, Barrio *et al* 2018) thanks to the potential synergism with single photon emission tomography in nuclear medicine applications.

Compton cameras typically consist of low-Z material for the scatterer and high-Z material for the absorber in order to maximize the probability of Compton scattering in the scatterer and the photoelectric absorption of the scattered photon in the absorber. These detection stages can be based on different technologies. The scatterer is typically made of position-sensitive scintillators such as gadolinium aluminium gallium garnet (GAGG) or lanthanum bromide (LaBr$_3$) crystals read out by silicon photo multipliers. The crystals can be either monolithic or pixelated (Muñoz *et al* 2017). Silicon strip detectors can be also adopted (Thirolf *et al* 2016). The absorber component can be made of either monolithic or pixelated scintillators such as lanthanum bromide (LaBr$_3$), lutetium oxyorthosilicate (LSO) or bismuth germanium oxide (BGO) crystals combined with either photo multipliers (PMTs) or silicon photo multipliers (SiPMs; Hueso-González *et al* 2015a).

There are two fundamental configurations of a Compton camera, requiring at least two photon interactions in time coincidence, and thus, relying on two or three detection stages. In the double-scatter configuration, the primary photon scatters once in the first detection stage (i.e., scatterer) and is then fully absorbed in the second detection stage (i.e., absorber; figure 10.4(c)). The Compton interaction is tracked, and the deposited energy is recorded and thus, the energy of the primary photon is determined. As full absorption of high energy photons can be difficult, spectral reconstruction algorithms have been proposed, jointly estimating the energy and the spatial distribution of the primary photons (Muñoz *et al* 2020). In the triple-scatter configuration, the primary photon scatters in the first and second detection stages (i.e., double scatterer), where the Compton interaction is tracked and the deposited energy is recorded, followed by a third position-recording stage (i.e., Compton, photoelectric, or pair production). The energy of the primary photon is uniquely determined by the energies of the two Compton interactions. The advantage of the triple-scatter configuration is that it does not require the full absorption at the third stage. The emission direction of the primary photon can be narrowed down till the Compton cone with the apex defined by the point of Compton interaction in the first detection stage, the axis defined by the direction of the scattered photon (between the first and the second detection stages) and the opening angle equal to the scattering angle, as determined by the Compton scattering kinematics. The production point can be determined by the intersection of the Compton cone with the beam direction, according to 1D imaging. Relying on tomographic image reconstruction algorithms, a Compton camera also enables the 3D imaging of the PG distribution relying on multiple intersecting Compton cones (Draeger *et al* 2018). The production point is therefore indirectly localized. As the accuracy of the reconstructed image depends on the energy and spatial resolution of the detectors, machine learning has been proposed to improve the spatial resolution in the absorber (Kawula *et al* 2021).

Experimental configurations of a Compton camera relying (also) on electron tracking have been proposed. The gamma electron vertex imaging consists of the use of a three-stage hodoscope where a converter is used to produce electrons via Compton scattering and two thin trackers are used to track the electron and a calorimeter is used to fully absorb the energy of the electron (Kim *et al* 2018; figure 10.4(d)). The tracking of the secondary Compton-scattered electron combined with a double-scatter configuration of the Compton camera enables the determination of the direction of the primary photon also from incompletely absorbed photon events, thus increasing detection efficiency (Aldawood *et al* 2015). Alternatively, the pair production mechanism is exploited to track both the electron and the positron (Rohling *et al* 2015, Toppi *et al* 2021).

Despite the limited counting rate capabilities that currently limit clinical applications of Compton cameras under therapeutic conditions, the electronic collimation has the potential advantage of higher detection efficiency when compared to mechanical collimation (Krimmer *et al* 2015). However, the spatial localization of the production point conveys more uncertainty (i.e., the Compton cone) than mechanical collimation (i.e., the PG direction), which in turn imposes higher efficiencies to attain comparable signal to noise ratio (SNR). In general, triple-scatter configuration have a detection efficiency at least one order of magnitude lower of the double-scatter configuration but a more efficient background suppression achieved by demanding a triple coincidence and imposing cuts on energy depositions in each detector stage (Krimmer *et al* 2018). To this purpose, neural networks have been proposed for coincidence identification (Munoz *et al* 2021). In addition to the high temporal resolution required for detection in coincidence through different stages, Compton cameras have to be characterized by high spatial and energy resolution (Rohling *et al* 2017), as both contribute to the accuracy required for range verification in particle therapy.

10.3.2.1.3 *Prompt-gamma spectroscopy*

The PGS technique is based on the analysis of the energy resolved yields ratios of PGs. Cross sections of the PG emissions from different reactions channels (^{12}C(p, pγ4.44 MeV)^{12}C and ^{16}O(p, pγ6.13 MeV)^{16}O; table 10.2) depend on the proton energy. This dependency is specific for each PG energy. The ratio of the spectral lines is exploited to estimate the ratio of the cross sections of the different reaction channels, thus deducing the beam energy (and thus, the range) and the elementary composition of the traversed tissue (Verburg and Seco 2014). The PGS technique requires the measurement of the PG distribution by means of a spectroscopic detector (figure 10.4(f)). This technique has been firstly proposed at MGH in Boston and the prototype has been developed and refined in order to cope with the low detection efficiency due to mechanical collimation in the perspective of clinical applications (Hueso-González *et al* 2018).

10.3.3 Prompt-gamma timing

The PGT technique is based on the correlation between the time of the PG emission and the beam range due to the finite transit time (i.e., time-of-flight, TOF) of the particles (about 1–2 ns in case of proton beams with a 5–20 cm range). As the PG emission is assumed to be instantaneous, the detection time coincides with the stopping time of the particles. The mean and the width of the TOF distribution are calculated. As the transit time is a function of the particle range, the features of the TOF distribution change in presence of range variations (Golnik *et al* 2014), as well as in function of changes of the beam energy. The PGT distribution shifts by 50 ps for a range variation of 1 cm (Hueso-González *et al* 2015b). The PGT technique relies on a single monolithic detector with excellent timing resolution and no collimation, synchronized with the accelerator or with a beam monitoring system (Golnik *et al* 2014, Petzold *et al* 2016; figure 10.4(e)). The TOF distribution results blurred by the time width of the accelerated bunches, in addition to the time resolution of the detector. As a consequence, the PGT technique is applicable only in those facilities characterized by a specific micro-time structure, with short bunches as delivered by cyclotrons (Hueso-González *et al* 2016b). Initial tests of PGT technique in clinical scenario have shown promising results (Werner *et al* 2019) but the detection efficiency in function of the beam intensity and the time resolution remain challenges for clinical applications. An extension of the PGT technique is the PG peak integral (PGPI; Krimmer *et al* 2017), that adds the peak integral of the TOF distribution to the PGT features (i.e. the mean and the width).

10.3.3.1 Prompt-gamma timing imaging

The PGTI technique has been recently proposed to extend the idea behind the PGT technique to obtain the PG distribution from the exclusive measurement of particle TOF (Jacquet *et al* 2021, 2023; figure 10.4(e)). By measuring the TOF between the beam monitoring system and the detection, the PG distribution is reconstructed by solving the analytical equation describing the kinematics of the photon intersecting with the beam direction, according to 1D imaging.

10.4 Emerging range verification techniques

Other range verification techniques have been proposed and explored, either based on secondary emissions or secondary phenomena. In addition to neutron beams (Ytre-Hauge *et al* 2019, Toppi *et al* 2020), imaging of the secondary electron *bremsstrahlung* has been also preliminary investigated for carbon ion (Yamaguchi *et al* 2018) and proton (Yamaguchi *et al* 2016) beams. With respect to physics-related phenomena, the ion-acoustic signal (Lehrack *et al* 2020) as well as the electromagnetic signal (Rädler *et al* 2021, 2023) induced in the Bragg peak have been characterized in realistic dose delivery scenarios to determine the signal-to-noise limits. High beam intensities are generally required to detect those signals. Short pulse duration is fundamental in ion acoustics, thus making this range verification technique promising within the context of FLASH radiotherapy. However, nowadays ultrasound transducers are not capable of detecting the ion-acoustic signal from FLASH radiotherapy. On the other hand, long pulse duration is preferable in magnetrometry. Finally, magnetic resonance imaging (MRI) has been investigated as a treatment verification technique based on biology-related phenomena, by imaging tissue changes induced by the therapeutic radiation relying on MRI contrast agents (Yuan *et al* 2013) or due to paramagnetic species that change the relaxation times (Wancura *et al* 2023) or because of convection in fluids (Schieferecke *et al* 2023, Gantz *et al* 2023).

References

Aldawood S, Castelhano I, Gernhäuser R, Van Der Kolff H, Lang C, Liprandi S and Thirolf P G 2015 Comparative characterization study of a LaBr3 (Ce) scintillation crystal in two surface wrapping scenarios: absorptive and reflective *Front. Oncol.* **5** 270

Attanasi F, Knopf A, Parodi K, Paganetti H, Bortfeld T, Rosso V and Del Guerra A 2011 Extension and validation of an analytical model for *in vivo* PET verification of proton therapy—a phantom and clinical study *Phys. Med. Biol.* **56** 5079

Augusto R S, Bauer J, Bouhali O, Cuccagna C, Gianoli C, Kozłowska W S and Ferrari A 2018 An overview of recent developments in FLUKA PET tools *Phys. Med.* **54** 189–99

Barrio J, Etxebeste A, Granado L, Muñoz E, Oliver J F, Ros A and Llosá G 2018 Performance improvement tests of MACACO: a Compton telescople based on continuous crystals and SiPMs *Nucl. Instrum. Methods Phys. Res., Sect.* A **912** 48–52

Bauer J, Unholtz D, Kurz C and Parodi K 2013 An experimental approach to improve the Monte Carlo modelling of offline PET/CT-imaging of positron emitters induced by scanned proton beams *Phys. Med. Biol.* **58** 5193

Beebe-Wang J, Vaska P, Dilmanian F A, Peggs S G and Schlyer D J 2003 Simulation of proton therapy treatment verification via PET imaging of induced positron-emitters *2003 IEEE Nuclear Science Symp. Conf. Record* (Piscataway, NJ: IEEE) 2496–500

Borys D, Baran J, Brzeziński K, Gajewski J, Chug N, Coussat A and Rucinski A 2022 ProTheRaMon—a GATE simulation framework for proton therapy range monitoring using PET imaging *Phys. Med. Biol.* **67** 224002

Boscolo D, Kostyleva D, Safari M J, Anagnostatou V, Äystö J and Bagchi SSuper-FRS Experiment Collaboration 2021 Radioactive beams for image-guided particle therapy: the BARB experiment at GSI *Front. Oncol.* **11** 737050

Combs S E, Bauer J, Unholtz D, Kurz C, Welzel T, Habermehl D and Parodi K 2012 Monitoring of patients treated with particle therapy using positron-emission-tomography (PET): the MIRANDA study *BMC Cancer* **12** 1–6

Draeger E, Mackin D, Peterson S, Chen H, Avery S, Beddar S and Polf J C 2018 3D prompt gamma imaging for proton beam range verification *Phys. Med. Biol.* **63** 035019

Enghardt W, Crespo P, Fiedler F, Hinz R, Parodi K, Pawelke J and Poenisch F 2004 Charged hadron tumour therapy monitoring by means of PET *Nucl. Instrum. Methods Phys. Res., Sect.* A **525** 284–8

Espana S, Zhu X, Daartz J, El Fakhri G, Bortfeld T and Paganetti H 2011 The reliability of proton-nuclear interaction cross-section data to predict proton-induced PET images in proton therapy *Phys. Med. Biol.* **56** 2687

Ferrero V, Pennazio F, Cerello P, Fiorina E, Garbolino S, Monaco V and Rafecas M 2019 Evaluation of in-beam PET treatment verification in proton therapy with different reconstruction methods *IEEE Trans. Radiat. Plasma Med. Sci.* **4** 202–11

Fiorina E, Ferrero V, Baroni G, Battistoni G, Belcari N, Camarlinghi N and Bisogni M G 2021 Detection of interfractional morphological changes in proton therapy: a simulation and *in vivo* study with the INSIDE in-beam PET *Front. Phys.* **8** 578388

Gantz S, Karsch L, Pawelke J, Schieferecke J, Schellhammer S, Smeets J and Hoffmann A 2023 Direct visualization of proton beam irradiation effects in liquids by MRI *Proc. Natl Acad. Sci.* **120** e2301160120

Gianoli C, Bauer J, Riboldi M, De Bernardi E, Fattori G, Baselli G and Baroni G 2014 Regional MLEM reconstruction strategy for PET-based treatment verification in ion beam radiotherapy *Phys. Med. Biol.* **59** 6979

Gianoli C, De Bernardi E, Ricotti R, Kurz C, Bauer J, Riboldi M and Parodi K 2017 First clinical investigation of a 4D maximum likelihood reconstruction for 4D PET-based treatment verification in ion beam therapy *Radiother. Oncol.* **123** 339–45

Gianoli C, Kurz C, Riboldi M, Bauer J, Fontana G, Baroni G and Parodi K 2016 Clinical evaluation of 4D PET motion compensation strategies for treatment verification in ion beam therapy *Phys. Med. Biol.* **61** 4141

Golnik C, Bemmerer D, Enghardt W, Fiedler F, Hueso-González F, Pausch G and Kormoll T 2016 Tests of a Compton imaging prototype in a monoenergetic 4.44 MeV photon field—a benchmark setup for prompt gamma-ray imaging devices *J. Instrum.* **11** P06009

Golnik C, Hueso-González F, Müller A, Dendooven P, Enghardt W, Fiedler F and Pausch G 2014 Range assessment in particle therapy based on prompt γ-ray timing measurements *Phys. Med. Biol.* **59** 5399

Hishikawa Y, Kagawa K, Murakami M, Sakai H, Akagi T and Abe M 2002 Usefulness of positron-emission tomographic images after proton therapy *Int. J. Radiat. Oncol. Biol. Phys.* **53** 1388–91

Hofmann T, Pinto M, Mohammadi A, Nitta M, Nishikido F, Iwao Y and Parodi K 2019 Dose reconstruction from PET images in carbon ion therapy: a deconvolution approach *Phys. Med. Biol.* **64** 025011

Horst F, Adi W, Aricò G, Brinkmann K T, Durante M, Reidel C A and Schuy C 2019 Measurement of PET isotope production cross sections for protons and carbon ions on carbon and oxygen targets for applications in particle therapy range verification *Phys. Med. Biol.* **64** 205012

Hsi W C, Indelicato D J, Vargas C, Duvvuri S, Li Z and Palta J 2009 *In vivo* verification of proton beam path by using post-treatment PET/CT imaging *Med. Phys.* **36** 4136–46

Hu Z, Li G, Zhang X, Ye K, Lu J and Peng H 2020 A machine learning framework with anatomical prior for online dose verification using positron emitters and PET in proton therapy *Phys. Med. Biol.* **65** 185003

Hueso-González F, Biegun A K, Dendooven P, Enghardt W, Fiedler F, Golnik C and Pausch G 2015a Comparison of LSO and BGO block detectors for prompt gamma imaging in ion beam therapy *J. Instrum.* **10** P09015

Hueso-González F, Enghardt W, Fiedler F, Golnik C, Janssens G, Petzoldt J and Pausch G 2015b First test of the prompt gamma ray timing method with heterogeneous targets at a clinical proton therapy facility *Phys. Med. Biol.* **60** 6247

Hueso-González F, Fiedler F, Golnik C, Kormoll T, Pausch G, Petzoldt J and Enghardt W 2016b Compton camera and prompt gamma ray timing: two methods for *in vivo* range assessment in proton therapy *Front. Oncol.* **6** 80

Hueso-González F, Pausch G, Petzoldt J, Römer K E and Enghardt W 2016a Prompt gamma rays detected with a BGO block Compton camera reveal range deviations of therapeutic proton beams *IEEE Trans. Radiat. Plasma Med. Sci.* **1** 76–86

Hueso-González F, Rabe M, Ruggieri T A, Bortfeld T and Verburg J M 2018 A full-scale clinical prototype for proton range verification using prompt gamma-ray spectroscopy *Phys. Med. Biol.* **63** 185019

Jacquet M, Ansari S, Gallin-Martel M L, André A, Boursier Y, Dupont M and Marcatili S 2023 A high sensitivity Cherenkov detector for prompt gamma timing and time imaging *Sci. Rep.* **13** 3609

Jacquet M, Marcatili S, Gallin-Martel M L, Bouly J L, Boursier Y, Dauvergne D and Testa É 2021 A time-of-flight-based reconstruction for real-time prompt-gamma imaging in proton therapy *Phys. Med. Biol.* **66** 135003

Jan S, Benoit D, Becheva E, Carlier T, Cassol F, Descourt P and Buvat I 2011 GATE V6: a major enhancement of the GATE simulation platform enabling modelling of CT and radiotherapy *Phys. Med. Biol.* **56** 881

Jiang Z, Polf J C, Barajas C A, Gobbert M K and Ren L 2023 A feasibility study of enhanced prompt gamma imaging for range verification in proton therapy using deep learning *Phys. Med. Biol.* **68** 075001

Kawula M, Binder T M, Liprandi S, Viegas R, Parodi K and Thirolf P G 2021 Sub-millimeter precise photon interaction position determination in large monolithic scintillators via convolutional neural network algorithms *Phys. Med. Biol.* **66** 135017

Kim C H, Lee H R, Kim S H, Park J H, Cho S and Jung W G 2018 Gamma electron vertex imaging for in-vivo beam-range measurement in proton therapy: experimental results *Appl. Phys. Lett.* **113** 114101

Knopf A, Nill S, Yohannes I, Graeff C, Dowdell S, Kurz C and Bert C 2014 Challenges of radiotherapy: report on the 4D treatment planning workshop 2013 *Phys. Med.* **30** 809–15

Knopf A, Parodi K, Paganetti H, Bortfeld T, Daartz J, Engelsman M and Shih H 2011 Accuracy of proton beam range verification using post-treatment positron emission tomography/computed tomography as function of treatment site *Int. J. Radiat. Oncol. Biol. Phys.* **79** 297–304

Knopf A, Parodi K, Paganetti H, Cascio E, Bonab A and Bortfeld T 2008 Quantitative assessment of the physical potential of proton beam range verification with PET/CT *Phys. Med. Biol.* **53** 4137

Kraan A C, Berti A, Retico A, Baroni G, Battistoni G, Belcari N and Bisogni M G 2022 Localization of anatomical changes in patients during proton therapy with in-beam PET monitoring: a voxel-based morphometry approach exploiting Monte Carlo simulations *Med. Phys.* **49** 23–40

Krimmer J, Angellier G, Balleyguier L, Dauvergne D, Freud N, Hérault J and Zoccarato Y 2017 A cost-effective monitoring technique in particle therapy via uncollimated prompt gamma peak integration *Appl. Phys. Lett.* **110** 154102

Krimmer J, Dauvergne D, Létang J M and Testa É 2018 Prompt-gamma monitoring in hadrontherapy: a review *Nucl. Instrum. Methods Phys. Res., Sect.* A **878** 58–73

Krimmer J, Ley J L, Abellan C, Cachemiche J P, Caponetto L, Chen X and Zoccarato Y 2015 Development of a Compton camera for medical applications based on silicon strip and scintillation detectors *Nucl. Instrum. Methods Phys. Res., Sect.* A **787** 98–101

Kuess P, Birkfellner W, Enghardt W, Helmbrecht S, Fiedler F and Georg D 2012 Using statistical measures for automated comparison of in-beam PET data *Med. Phys.* **39** 5874–81

Kurz C, Bauer J, Conti M, Guérin L, Eriksson L and Parodi K 2015 Investigating the limits of PET/CT imaging at very low true count rates and high random fractions in ion-beam therapy monitoring *Med. Phys.* **42** 3979–91

Kurz C, Bauer J, Unholtz D, Richter D, Herfarth K, Debus J and Parodi K 2016 Initial clinical evaluation of PET-based ion beam therapy monitoring under consideration of organ motion *Med. Phys.* **43** 975–82

Lang C, Habs D, Parodi K and Thirolf P G 2014 Sub-millimeter nuclear medical imaging with high sensitivity in positron emission tomography using $\beta^+\gamma$ coincidences *J. Instrum.* **9** P01008

Lehrack S, Assmann W, Bender M, Severin D, Trautmann C, Schreiber J and Parodi K 2020 Ionoacoustic detection of swift heavy ions *Nucl. Instrum. Methods Phys. Res., Sect. A* **950** 162935

Liprandi S, Takyu S, Aldawood S, Binder T, Dedes G, Kamada K and Thirolf P G 2017 Characterization of a Compton camera setup with monolithic LaBr 3 (Ce) absorber and segmented GAGG scatter detectors *2017 IEEE Nuclear Science Symp. and Medical Imaging Conf. (NSS/MIC)* (Piscataway, NJ: IEEE) 1–4

Liu C C and Huang H M 2020 A deep learning approach for converting prompt gamma images to proton dose distributions: a Monte Carlo simulation study *Phys. Med.* **69** 110–9

Llacer J 1988 Positron emission medical measurements with accelerated radioactive ion beams *Nucl. Sci. Appl.* **3** 111–31

Llosá G, Trovato M, Barrio J, Etxebeste A, Muñoz E, Lacasta C and Solevi P 2016 First images of a three-layer Compton telescope prototype for treatment monitoring in hadron therapy *Front. Oncol.* **6** 14

Lopes P C, Clementel E, Crespo P, Henrotin S, Huizenga J, Janssens G and Schaart D R 2015 Time-resolved imaging of prompt-gamma rays for proton range verification using a knife-edge slit camera based on digital photon counters *Phys. Med. Biol.* **60** 6063

Lovatti G, Nitta M, Safari M, Gianoli C, Pinto M, Zoglauer A and Parodi K 2020 An advanced simulation and reconstruction framework for a novel In-Beam PET scanner for Pre-clinical proton irradiation *2020 IEEE Nuclear Science Symp. and Medical Imaging Conf. (NSS/MIC)* (Piscataway, NJ: IEEE) 1–3

Ma S, Hu Z, Ye K, Zhang X, Wang Y and Peng H 2020 Feasibility study of patient-specific dose verification in proton therapy utilizing positron emission tomography (PET) and generative adversarial network (GAN) *Med. Phys.* **47** 5194–208

Masuda T, Nishio T, Kataoka J, Arimoto M, Sano A and Karasawa K 2019 ML-EM algorithm for dose estimation using PET in proton therapy *Phys. Med. Biol.* **64** 175011

Masuda T, Nishio T, Sano A and Karasawa K 2020 Extension of the ML-EM algorithm for dose estimation using PET in proton therapy: application to an inhomogeneous target *Phys. Med. Biol.* **65** 185001

McCleskey M, Kaye W, Mackin D S, Beddar S, He Z and Polf J C 2015 Evaluation of a multistage CdZnTe Compton camera for prompt γ imaging for proton therapy *Nucl. Instrum. Methods Phys. Res., Sect. A* **785** 163–9

Min C H, Kim C H, Youn M Y and Kim J W 2006 Prompt gamma measurements for locating the dose falloff region in the proton therapy *Appl. Phys. Lett.* **89** 183517

Min C H, Lee H R and Kim C H 2011 Two-dimensional prompt gamma measurement simulation for *in vivo* dose verification in proton therapy: a Monte Carlo study *Nucl. Technol.* **175** 11–5

Moglioni M, Kraan A C, Baroni G, Battistoni G, Belcari N, Berti A and Bisogni M G 2022 In-vivo range verification analysis with in-beam PET data for patients treated with proton therapy at CNAO *Front. Oncol.* **12** 3469

Mohammadi A, Tashima H, Iwao Y, Takyu S, Akamatsu G, Nishikido F and Yamaya T 2019 Range verification of radioactive ion beams of 11C and 15O using in-beam PET imaging *Phys. Med. Biol.* **64** 145014

Mohammadi A, Tashima H, Takyu S, Iwao Y, Akamatsu G, Kang H G and Yamaya T 2022 Feasibility of triple gamma ray imaging of 10C for range verification in ion therapy *Phys. Med. Biol.* **67** 165001

Moteabbed M, Espana S and Paganetti H 2011 Monte Carlo patient study on the comparison of prompt gamma and PET imaging for range verification in proton therapy *Phys. Med. Biol.* **56** 1063

Muñoz E, Barrientos L, Bernabéu J, Borja-Lloret M, Llosá G, Ros A and Oliver J F 2020 A spectral reconstruction algorithm for two-plane compton cameras *Phys. Med. Biol.* **65** 025011

Muñoz E, Barrio J, Etxebeste A, Ortega P G, Lacasta C, Oliver J F and Llosá G 2017 Performance evaluation of MACACO: a multilayer compton camera *Phys. Med. Biol.* **62** 7321

Munoz E, Ros A, Borja-Lloret M, Barrio J, Dendooven P, Oliver J F and Llosá G 2021 Proton range verification with MACACO II Compton camera enhanced by a neural network for event selection *Sci. Rep.* **11** 1–12

Muraro S, Battistoni G, Collamati F, De Lucia E, Faccini R, Ferroni F and Patera V 2016 Monitoring of hadrontherapy treatments by means of charged particle detection *Front. Oncol.* **6** 177

Nenoff L, Priegnitz M, Janssens G, Petzoldt J, Wohlfahrt P, Trezza A and Richter C 2017 Sensitivity of a prompt-gamma slit-camera to detect range shifts for proton treatment verification *Radiother. Oncol.* **125** 534–40

Nishio T, Miyatake A, Inoue K, Gomi-Miyagishi T, Kohno R, Kameoka S and Ogino T 2008 Experimental verification of proton beam monitoring in a human body by use of activity image of positron-emitting nuclei generated by nuclear fragmentation reaction *Radiol. Phys. Technol.* **1** 44–54

Nishio T, Miyatake A, Ogino T, Nakagawa K, Saijo N and Esumi H 2010 The development and clinical use of a beam ON-LINE PET system mounted on a rotating gantry port in proton therapy *Int. J. Radiat. Oncol. Biol. Phys.* **76** 277–86

Nishio T, Ogino T, Nomura K and Uchida H 2006 Dose-volume delivery guided proton therapy using beam on-line PET system *Med. Phys.* **33** 4190–7

Ozoemelam I, Van der Graaf E, Van Goethem M J, Kapusta M, Zhang N, Brandenburg S and Dendooven P 2020 Feasibility of quasi-prompt PET-based range verification in proton therapy *Phys. Med. Biol.* **65** 245013

Park J H, Kim S H, Ku Y, Lee H S, Kim C H, Shin D H and Jeong J H 2019 Comparison of knife-edge and multi-slit camera for proton beam range verification by Monte Carlo simulation *Nucl. Eng. Technol.* **51** 533–8

Parodi K 2012 PET monitoring of hadrontherapy *Nucl. Med. Rev.* **15** 37–42

Parodi K and Bortfeld T 2006 A filtering approach based on Gaussian–powerlaw convolutions for local PET verification of proton radiotherapy *Phys. Med. Biol.* **51** 1991

Parodi K, Paganetti H, Cascio E, Flanz J B, Bonab A A, Alpert N M and Bortfeld T 2007a PET/CT imaging for treatment verification after proton therapy: a study with plastic phantoms and metallic implants *Med. Phys.* **34** 419–35

Parodi K, Paganetti H, Shih H A, Michaud S, Loeffler J S, DeLaney T F and Bortfeld T 2007b Patient study of *in vivo* verification of beam delivery and range, using positron emission tomography and computed tomography imaging after proton therapy *Int. J. Radiat. Oncol. Biol. Phys.* **68** 920–34

Pawelke J, Enghardt W, Haberer T, Hasch B G, Hinz R, Kramer M and Sobiella M 1997 In-beam PET imaging for the control of heavy-ion tumour therapy *IEEE Trans. Nucl. Sci.* **44** 1492–8

Perali I, Celani A, Bombelli L, Fiorini C, Camera F, Clementel E and Vander Stappen F 2014 Prompt gamma imaging of proton pencil beams at clinical dose rate *Phys. Med. Biol.* **59** 5849

Petzoldt J, Roemer K E, Enghardt W, Fiedler F, Golnik C, Hueso-Gonzalez F and Pausch G 2016 Characterization of the microbunch time structure of proton pencil beams at a clinical treatment facility *Phys. Med. Biol.* **61** 2432

Pinto M, Bajard M, Brons S, Chevallier M, Dauvergne D, Dedes G and Testa M 2014 Absolute prompt-gamma yield measurements for ion beam therapy monitoring *Phys. Med. Biol.* **60** 565

Pinto M, Dauvergne D, Freud N, Krimmer J, Létang J M, Ray C and Testa E 2014 Design optimisation of a TOF-based collimated camera prototype for online hadrontherapy monitoring *Phys. Med. Biol.* **59** 7653

Pinto M, Kröniger K, Bauer J, Nilsson R, Traneus E and Parodi K 2020 A filtering approach for PET and PG predictions in a proton treatment planning system *Phys. Med. Biol.* **65** 095014

Pönisch F, Parodi K, Hasch B G and Enghardt W 2004 The modelling of positron emitter production and PET imaging during carbon ion therapy *Phys. Med. Biol.* **49** 5217

Rädler M, Buizza G, Kawula M, Palaniappan P, Gianoli C, Baroni G and Riboldi M 2023 Impact of secondary particles on the magnetic field generated by a proton pencil beam: a finite-element analysis based on Geant4-DNA simulations *Med. Phys.* **50** 1000–18

Rädler M, Gianoli C, Palaniappan P, Parodi K and Riboldi M 2021 Electromagnetic signal of a proton beam in biological tissues for a potential range-verification approach in proton therapy *Phys. Rev. Appl.* **15** 024066

Rahman A U, Nemallapudi M, Chou C Y, Lin C H and Lee S C 2022 Direct mapping from PET coincidence data to proton-dose and positron activity using a deep learning approach *Phys. Med. Biol.* **67** 185010

Ready J 2016 Development of a multi-knife-edge slit collimator for prompt gamma ray imaging during proton beam cancer therapy *Doctoral Dissertation* (UC Berkeley)

Ready J, Negut V, Mihailescu L and Vetter K 2016 Prompt gamma imaging with a multi-knife-edge slit collimator: evaluation for use in proton beam range verification *Med. Phys.* **43** 3717–7

Remmele S, Hesser J, Paganetti H and Bortfeld T 2011 A deconvolution approach for PET-based dose reconstruction in proton radiotherapy *Phys. Med. Biol.* **56** 7601

Richter C, Pausch G, Barczyk S, Priegnitz M, Keitz I, Thiele J and Baumann M 2016 First clinical application of a prompt gamma based *in vivo* proton range verification system *Radiother. Oncol.* **118** 232–7

Roellinghoff F, Richard M H, Chevallier M, Constanzo J, Dauvergne D, Freud N and Walenta A H 2011 Design of a Compton camera for 3D prompt-γ imaging during ion beam therapy *Nucl. Instrum. Methods Phys. Res., Sect.* A **648** S20–3

Rohling H, Golnik C, Enghardt W, Hueso-González F, Kormoll T, Pausch G and Fiedler F 2015 Simulation study of a combined pair production—Compton camera *for in-vivo* dosimetry during therapeutic proton irradiation *IEEE Trans. Nucl. Sci.* **62** 2023–30

Rohling H, Priegnitz M, Schoene S, Schumann A, Enghardt W, Hueso-González F and Fiedler F 2017 Requirements for a Compton camera for *in vivo* range verification of proton therapy *Phys. Med. Biol.* **62** 2795

Schieferecke J, Gantz S, Hoffmann A and Pawelke J 2023 Investigation of contrast mechanisms for MRI phase signal-based proton beam visualization in water phantoms *Magn. Reson. Med.* **90** 1776–88

Schumann A, Priegnitz M, Schoene S, Enghardt W, Rohling H and Fiedler F 2016 From prompt gamma distribution to dose: a novel approach combining an evolutionary algorithm and filtering based on Gaussian-powerlaw convolutions *Phys. Med. Biol.* **61** 6919

Shakirin G, Braess H, Fiedler F, Kunath D, Laube K, Parodi K and Enghardt W 2011 Implementation and workflow for PET monitoring of therapeutic ion irradiation: a comparison of in-beam, in-room, and off-line techniques *Phys. Med. Biol.* **56** 1281

Smeets J, Roellinghoff F, Janssens G, Perali I, Celani A, Fiorini C and Prieels D 2016 Experimental comparison of knife-edge and multi-parallel slit collimators for prompt gamma imaging of proton pencil beams *Front. Oncol.* **6** 156

Smeets J, Roellinghoff F, Prieels D, Stichelbaut F, Benilov A, Fiorini C and Dubus A 2012 Prompt gamma imaging with a slit camera for real-time range control in proton therapy *Phys. Med. Biol.* **57** 3371

Sommerer F, Parodi K, Ferrari A, Poljanc K, Enghardt W and Aiginger H 2006 Investigating the accuracy of the FLUKA code for transport of therapeutic ion beams in matter *Phys. Med. Biol.* **51** 4385

Sterpin E, Janssens G, Smeets J, Vander Stappen F, Prieels D, Priegnitz M and Vynckier S 2015 Analytical computation of prompt gamma ray emission and detection for proton range verification *Phys. Med. Biol.* **60** 4915

Stichelbaut F and Jongen Y 2003 Verification of the proton beam position in the patient by the detection of prompt gamma-rays emission *39th Meeting of the Particle Therapy Co-Operative Group* vol 16 (San Francisco, CA: PTCOG)

Thirolf P G, Aldawood S, Böhmer M, Bortfeldt J, Castelhano I, Dedes G and Parodi K 2016 A compton camera prototype for prompt gamma medical imaging *EPJ Web Conf.* **117** 05005

Toppi M, Avanzolini I, Balconi L, Battistoni G, Calvi G, De Simoni M and Mattei I 2021 PAPRICA: the pair production imaging chamber—proof of principle *Front. Phys.* **9** 568139

Toppi M, Baroni G, Battistoni G, Bisogni M G, Cerello P, Ciocca M and Sarti A 2021 Monitoring carbon ion beams transverse position detecting charged secondary fragments: results from patient treatment performed at CNAO *Front. Oncol.* **11** 601784

Toppi M, Battistoni G, Bochetti A, De Maria P, De Simoni M, Dong Y and Marafini M 2020 The MONDO tracker: characterisation and study of secondary ultrafast neutrons production in Carbon Ion radiotherapy *Front. Phys.* **8** 567990

Verburg J M, Riley K, Bortfeld T and Seco J 2013 Energy-and time-resolved detection of prompt gamma-rays for proton range verification *Phys. Med. Biol.* **58** L37

Verburg J M and Seco J 2014 Proton range verification through prompt gamma-ray spectroscopy *Phys. Med. Biol.* **59** 7089

Verburg J M, Shih H A and Seco J 2012 Simulation of prompt gamma-ray emission during proton radiotherapy *Phys. Med. Biol.* **57** 5459

Wancura J, Egan J, Sajo E and Sudhyadhom A 2023 MRI of radiation chemistry: first images and investigation of potential mechanisms *Med. Phys.* **50** 495–505

Werner T, Berthold J, Hueso-González F, Koegler T, Petzoldt J, Roemer K and Pausch G 2019 Processing of prompt gamma-ray timing data for proton range measurements at a clinical beam delivery *Phys. Med. Biol.* **64** 105023

Wrońska A 2020 Prompt gamma imaging in proton therapy-status, challenges and developments *J. Phys.: Conf. Ser.* **1561** 012021

Xie Y, Bentefour E H, Janssens G, Smeets J, Vander Stappen F, Hotoiu L and Teo B K K 2017 Prompt gamma imaging for *in vivo* range verification of pencil beam scanning proton therapy *Int. J. Radiat. Oncol. Biol. Phys.* **99** 210–8

Yamaguchi M, Nagao Y, Ando K, Yamamoto S, Sakai M, Parajuli R K and Kawachi N 2018 Imaging of monochromatic beams by measuring secondary electron bremsstrahlung for carbon-ion therapy using a pinhole x-ray camera *Phys. Med. Biol.* **63** 045016

Yamaguchi M, Nagao Y, Ando K, Yamamoto S, Toshito T, Kataoka J and Kawachi N 2016 Secondary-electron-bremsstrahlung imaging for proton therapy *Nucl. Instrum. Methods Phys. Res., Sect.* A **833** 199–207

Ytre-Hauge K S, Skjerdal K, Mattingly J and Meric I 2019 A Monte Carlo feasibility study for neutron based real-time range verification in proton therapy *Sci. Rep.* **9** 2011

Yuan Y, Andronesi O C, Bortfeld T R, Richter C, Wolf R, Guimaraes A R and Seco J 2013 Feasibility study of *in vivo* MRI based dosimetric verification of proton end-of-range for liver cancer patients *Radiother. Oncol.* **106** 378–82

Zhu X, España S, Daartz J, Liebsch N, Ouyang J, Paganetti H and El Fakhri G 2011 Monitoring proton radiation therapy with in-room PET imaging *Phys. Med. Biol.* **56** 4041

Zhu X and El Fakhri G 2013 Proton therapy verification with PET imaging *Theranostics* **3** 731

IOP Publishing

Imaging in Particle Therapy
Current practice and future trends
Chiara Paganelli, Chiara Gianoli and Antje Knopf

Chapter 11

Quantitative imaging in particle therapy

M Zampini*, L Morelli*, G Parrella, G Baroni, G J M Parker[†] and C Paganelli[†]

11.1 Introduction

Medical imaging is a non-invasive tool for visualization, identification, localization, and analysis of pathological tissues. Building on top of imaging for the purpose of visualizing anatomical details, location, and size, new methods have been introduced in radiotherapy (RT) practice to capture and provide information that goes beyond the anatomical, which fall under the term of quantitative imaging (Q-imaging; Gurney-Champion *et al* 2020). Q-imaging is an umbrella term for any biomedical imaging technique with the ability to display pathophysiological features by reporting or quantitatively mapping tissue physical properties (such as water diffusivity), physiological properties (such as blood flow or pH), or metabolic properties (such as oxygen consumption, glucose uptake and metabolite concentration). Q-imaging is often associated with the concept of quantitative imaging biomarkers (Q-imaging) which is 'an objective characteristic derived from an *in vivo* image measured on a ratio or interval scale as an indicator of normal biological processes, pathogenic processes, or a response to a therapeutic intervention' (Kessler *et al* 2015, Sorace *et al* 2020).

In recent years, an increasing number of studies have investigated the potential advantages introduced using Q-imaging in RT settings (Gurney-Champion *et al* 2020). Indeed, the information extracted from Q-imaging can provide a functional description of the tumour allowing identification assistance, staging, and heterogeneity characterization of the target. Considering the lack of routine provision of Q-imaging by vendors, and the general dependence of measurement accuracy and precision on machines and imaging protocols, along with need for accurate patient positioning to replicate treatment set-up (Gurney-Champion *et al* 2020), a consensus on the use of Q-imaging in RT has yet to be defined. This is even more evident in

---

* Both authors contributed equally.
[†] Authors shared co-last

doi:10.1088/978-0-7503-5117-1ch11

particle therapy (PT), where Q-imaging is currently limited, although PT could benefit from Q-imaging to make the most of its physical and radiobiological advantages with respect to conventional RT, as sensitivity to treatment is linked to functional processes such as metabolism, perfusion, angiogenesis, hypoxia, and necrosis (Durante 2020, Schardt 2010, Barker 2015, Tinganelli 2020).

Particle therapy (PT) with protons or carbon ions allows for conformal dose distribution based on the Bragg peak and, especially for heavy ions such as carbon, it shows higher linear energy transfer (LET) and radiobiological effectiveness (RBE), which has provided effective clinical results for deep-seated and radioresistant tumours (Durante and Flanz 2019). Several radiobiological effects are produced by PT, including complex DNA damage, inflammation, inter- and intracellular signaling and increase in reactive oxygen species (ROS) compared to x-rays (Durante *et al* 2017, Byun *et al* 2021), with high-LET beam (i.e., carbon ion) almost independent from oxygen levels, meaning that their RBE is negligibly affected by the oxygen enhancement ratio (OER), in contrast to low-LET particles such as protons. All these effects depend on multiple factors, including the dose, its microscopic distribution and spatial fractionation, as well as the tumour micro-environment complexity and its functional processes, making PT a peculiar treatment where the underlying biological processes are still under investigation.

PET and MRI-based techniques are the most used Q-imaging techniques, while advanced CT-based methods remain less frequently employed. These imaging techniques allow the acquisition of functional images with different contrasts based on the use of different parameters and sequences (in MRI), the use of different radiotracers (in PET) and the attenuation of polychromatic x-ray beams (in CT). In particular, MRI has gained the most attention in clinical research thanks to its tunable contrast and the recent interest in MRI-guided RT/PT (Hoffmann *et al* 2020, Keall *et al* 2022). In addition, unlike other Q-imaging modalities, MRI can provide both anatomical and functional information in a single imaging session, often with improved spatial resolution, which is a valuable feature in the context of clinical applicability (Wang *et al* 2021). Among MRI techniques, quantitative MRI (qMRI) is being widely investigated for an objective and non-invasive tissue characterization, with the end goal to obtain reproducible tissue property maps for the identification of the health state of a tissue, with then less need for histopathological examination. In particular, qMRI encompasses several quantitative functional methods including diffusion-weighted MRI (DWI), diffusion tensor imaging (DTI), as well as perfusion weighted MRI (PWI), magnetic resonance spectroscopy (MRS), and blood-oxygen-level-dependent (BOLD) imaging (Li *et al* 2021).

Thanks to the advantages of Q-imaging, the integration of functional features with high resolution anatomical data has led to the definition of the Biological Target Volume (BTV) (Ling *et al* 2000) as a sub-tumour volume with distinct functional features. On top of target delineation, Q-imaging can be used to improve treatment stratification, dose tailoring, treatment monitoring, early response assessment and local failure prediction. Q-imaging employed at follow-up could provide parameters describing treatment-induced microstructural or metabolic changes in a non-invasive way, allowing for both treatment outcome verification in the target region, and prevention or monitoring of any toxicities induced in structures crossed

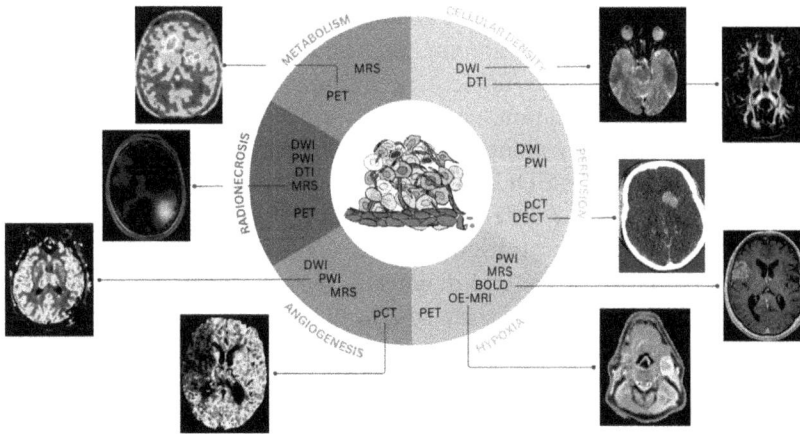

Figure 11.1. Quantitative imaging and the tumour microenvironment: main quantitative imaging techniques employed for investigating tumour biology and microenvironment. DWI, Diffusion Weighted Imaging; PWI, Perfusion Weighted Imaging (Reproduced from Daghighi *et al* (2020). CC BY 4.0.); MRS, MRI Spectroscopy (Reproduced from Chiang *et al* (2018). CC BY 4.0.); DTI, Diffusion Tensor Imaging (Reproduced from Martucci *et al* (2023). CC BY 4.0.); BOLD, Blood-Oxygen-Level-Dependent (Reprinted from Stumpo *et al* (2022), Copyright (2022), with permission from Springer.); OE-MRI, Oxygen-Enhanced MRI (Reproduced from McCabe *et al* (2023). CC BY 4.0.); PET, Positron Emission Tomography (Reproduced from Zhang-Yin *et al* (2022). CC BY 4.0.); pCT, perfusion CT (Reproduced from Haggenmüller *et al* (2023). CC BY 4.0.); DECT, Dual Energy CT (Reproduced from Mangesius *et al* (2021). CC BY 4.0.).

by the treatment beam, including organs at risk (Leibfarth *et al* 2018, O'Connor *et al* 2019, Gurney-Champion *et al* 2020, Li 2021).

This chapter reports the main Q-imaging techniques and related Q-imaging that provide functional information of tissue and healthy organs and that can be exploited in PT (figure 11.1). Similar concepts presented in the review proposed for conventional RT by Gurney-Champion *et al* (2020) can be extended to PT and are hereafter reported. It should be highlighted that in this chapter conventional QIBs that can be directly extracted from Q-imaging are discussed; high dimensional QIBs (e.g., as those derived with radiomics or deep learning) extracted from any image modality (anatomical, quantitative images or more in general volumetric maps, such as dose maps) and related multi-scale modelling revealing macroscopic and microscopic characteristics are reported in chapter 12.

11.2 Quantitative imaging techniques

11.2.1 PET

PET is a functional imaging technique that measures metabolic activity of tissues by means of gamma radiation released indirectly by radiotracers that bind to specific biologically active molecules: the tracers emit positrons that travel a short distance through tissue before annihilating with an electron and emitting back-to-back gamma rays, which leave the body and are captured by rings of detectors. Coincidence detection techniques are employed to acquire signals from the emitted gamma rays in the form of sinograms, which are then reconstructed into images for the assessment of the distribution of the targeted molecule *in vivo*. However, PET imaging remains a low resolution technique and, to overcome this limitation, hybrid PET/CT imaging systems have been developed. These fuse information from both modalities for more accurate tumour localization, viability assessment, and greater staging accuracy than either imaging modality alone, as well as increasing diagnostic confidence.

Fluorodeoxyglucose (^{18}F-FDG) is the most widely used tracer for mapping of glucose uptake, employed to differentiate areas of physiological or non-malignant uptake from those of malignant origin. Indeed, ^{18}F-FDG is taken up by most solid tumours and is therefore of general diagnostic use in cancer: FDG-PET has been used as a marker with an established role in accurate target volume delineation, tumour characterization and staging, treatment monitoring and prognostic evaluation of different cancers such as lung, head and neck and breast cancer (Hirata and Tamaki 2021). In RT, it has been used for treatment planning and response assessment of tumours including brain tumours, head and neck cancer, lung cancer, gastrointestinal tumours and prostate cancer (Unterrainer *et al* 2020).

Other PET tracers of importance are ^{18}F-FMISO, F-FAZA or F-HX4 (Cheney *et al* 2014, Fleming *et al* 2015, Leimgruber *et al* 2020), which allow for direct imaging of tumour hypoxia. Hypoxia is a negative prognostic factor in most solid tumours as it induces radioresistance, especially when low-LET photon or proton irradiation is used. High-LET particles are instead more effective than low-LET beams, but hypoxia can nevertheless affect treatment efficacy (Valable *et al* 2020). Hypoxia is also associated with metastatic potential and with the activation of angiogenesis, thus areas with increased radioresistance must be identified to properly set up dose boosting strategies. Additionally, tracers of low oxygen pressure, or hypoxia, may be of valuable interest for FLASH RT planning. In such a case, hypoxia imaging can be used to guide to the potential benefits from FLASH RT for a particular tumour (El Naqa *et al* 2022), as it is possible that tumour hypoxia imaging could provide insight into the mechanisms of the FLASH effect.

Although PET has been demonstrated to be useful in optimizing the dose as a function of tumour hypoxia in PT (as described in section 12.3.2), tracers of tumour hypoxia are not widely available in most clinical PT centers.

The development of new PET radiopharmaceuticals for higher sensitivity and specificity for characterization, stratification and monitoring still represents a hot research topic (Schuster *et al* 2016). Recent overviews on PET radiotracers used in oncology can be found in Lau *et al* (2020) and Lin *et al* (2022).

PET is also used in PT for *in vivo* range verification, as PET captures the signal contributions of mixed positron emitters that are produced from beam irradiation on the beam path through nuclear fragmentation reactions. Imaging for in-vivo range verification is out of the scope of this chapter; a detailed description of this is instead reported in chapter 10.

11.2.2 MRI: DWI and DTI

DWI uses diffusion sensitizing magnetic field gradients to visualize and quantify the motion of water molecules in biological tissues (Tang and Zhou 2019, Li *et al* 2021).

The diffusion of water molecules is a biophysical phenomenon that can be correlated with the structural characteristics of tissues under both physiological and pathological conditions. The spatial arrangement of membranes and cellular components has an impact on the displacement of water molecules, allowing DWI to be sensitive to microstructural characteristics such as cell density, size, shape, and membrane integrity. In RT, DWI has shown promise for RT outcome prediction, response assessment, as well as for tumour delineation and characterization in several cancer types (Leibfarth *et al* 2018).

Microstructural information is derived from DWI through representations and models of water diffusion: the signal intensity can be fitted using a simple mono-exponential model or more complex models such as Intra-Voxel Incoherent Motion (IVIM), Vascular Extracellular and Restricted Diffusion for Cytometry in Tumours (VERDICT), Restriction Spectrum Imaging (RSI) and others (White *et al* 2013, Panagiotaki *et al* 2014, Novikov *et al* 2018, le Bihan 2019, Tang and Zhou 2019). As the complexity of the diffusion model increases, both the accuracy and the level of detail of microstructural and functional information extracted from the DWI measurements increase, along with the requirements of the data acquisition protocol. The conventional mono-exponential model allows the derivation of the apparent diffusion coefficient (ADC), which is a non-specific measure of tissue diffusion that incorporates multiple effects. These effects can be disentangled (to a degree) by more advanced DWI imaging sequences, which may require long acquisition times, often not feasible with standard protocols in RT/PT settings. For example, IVIM can disentangle the contribution of diffusion and perfusion from the MR signal by interpreting the blood flow in randomly oriented capillaries as a pseudo-diffusion process and by fitting the diffusion signal to a biexponential model (le Bihan *et al* 1986, 2019) extracting quantitative parameters such as diffusion (D), pseudo-diffusion (D*—related to perfusion) and perfusion fraction (f).

When dealing with multi-compartment models, RSI allows for separating the DWI signal into the relative contributions of hindered and restricted signals from the extracellular and intracellular space (White *et al* 2013), whereas VERDICT is able to estimate from the DWI signal three distinct components associated to the extracellular, intracellular and microvasculature compartments (Panagiotaki *et al* 2014).

Diffusion tensor imaging (DTI) follows the same physical principles as DWI but aims to capture information on the orientation of anisotropic diffusion of water molecules in tissues instead of obtaining a single scalar quantification of diffusivity (e.g., as for ADC). Specifically, DTI is used to assess tissue orientation from a set of diffusion-weighted images acquired by applying the diffusion-weighting gradients in multiple directions, thus providing a 3D visualization of anisotropic structures (such as white matter) and deriving descriptors of diffusion directional heterogeneity such as fractional anisotropy (FA), mean diffusivity (MD), and axial and radial diffusivity (AD and RD). Quantification of these parameters in RT settings can provide useful biological information for the minimization of clinical complications (e.g., radionecrosis, ischemia and progressive neurocognitive decline), particularly in the brain; by delineating the anatomy of white matter tracts that are found to be sensitive to radiation damage at the planning phase, and including this information in the therapeutic planning and dose optimization, short-term complications and long-term side-effects in RT can be minimized (Igaki *et al* 2014, Colman *et al* 2022). In addition, DTI has been shown to be a useful tool for more precisely detecting tumour invasion and discriminating radionecrosis from tumour local recurrence (Colman *et al* 2022).

11.2.3 MRI: PWI—DSC, DCE and ASL

In the context of medical imaging, perfusion refers to the capillary blood supply to a tissue, and perfusion weighted imaging (PWI) indicates any imaging sequence able to provide information on the hemodynamic status of a tissue. Perfusion imaging of the brain has been employed to compute maps of hemodynamic parameters such as blood volume, the fraction of the total tissue volume within a voxel occupied by blood, which is a commonly used and robust parameter in neurological and neurooncological perfusion evaluation, a sensitive indicator for evaluating tissue function and viability (Hua *et al* 2019, Li *et al* 2021). In PWI, the most commonly used methods typically use contrast agent. For example, Dynamic Susceptibility Contrast MRI (DSC-MRI) exploits the regional susceptibility-induced MR signal alterations caused by contrast agent transit through the circulation. DSC-MRI and Dynamic Contrast-Enhanced MRI (DCE-MRI—a method that exploits the T1-shortening effects of contrast agents) require the injection of an exogenous contrast agent to discriminate perfused from non-perfused tissues. A further technique, Arterial Spin Labelling (ASL-MRI), does not require any exogenous contrast agent.

In DSC-MRI, after collecting some images at baseline, a bolus of paramagnetic contrast agent (CA, typically a chelate of gadolinium) is injected at a high flow rate. The paramagnetic CA then passes through the circulation causing a locoregional reduction in T2*, which is manifested as a drastic decrease in signal intensity on T2*-weighted images. Therefore, using T2*-weighted sequences, the transit of the CA produces a drop and subsequent recovery of the signal that traces a characteristic curve showing a steeper signal drop in proportion to the vascularization of the structures within the region of interest (McRobbie *et al* 2017, Wang *et al* 2021).

DCE-MRI has become a promising alternative solution for quantifying blood perfusion, particularly when contrast agent leakage from the vasculature has the potential to introduce errors into DSC-MRI (Wang *et al* 2021). In this technique, a gadolinium-based CA reduces the local T1 relaxation time (instead of T2*) and thus, by continuously acquiring T1-weighted images, contrast agent distribution within the patient can be investigated and thus tissue perfusion and capillary permeability can be quantified. In both DSC- and DCE-MRI, some effects of gadolinium deposition have been reported, although no evidence shows any harmful effects from its deposition (Gulani *et al* 2017). DCE-MRI is often used to assess tumour aggressiveness, thanks to its ability to reflect increased or decreased angiogenesis, as in tumour tissue the contrast agent is able to leak from the leaky capillaries of the microcirculation, where it accumulates in the extracellular spaces. The resulting temporal variations in signal intensity allow DCE-MRI to quantify the permeability and perfusion of the tumour microenvironment, features of particular interest, as they are known to influence the RT outcome. Indeed, the tumour microenvironment is characterized by structural (e.g., abnormal architecture of the vasculature) and functional (e.g., changes in microvascular perfusion) alteration in the microvasculature that result in alterations in tumour oxygenation (i.e., hypoxic condition), one of the major determinants of RT response (Zahra *et al* 2007, Matsuo *et al* 2014, Gurney-Champion *et al* 2020).

ASL-MRI is a completely non-invasive technique that uses magnetically labelled protons in the arterial blood supply. The tagging of protons is usually performed by inverting or saturating the signal of water protons in blood water in a region found upstream so that, when the tagged protons flow into the imaged slice, these exchange magnetization with tissue water, thus reducing the MR signal acquired. Subtraction of labeled images from control images eliminates static tissue signal and the remaining signal is a relative measure of perfusion proportional to cerebral blood flow (CBF). With respect to DSC and DCE, ASL has a poorer signal-to-noise ratio and shows sensitivity to patient motion but can be repeated as often as required since gadolinium is not employed and, thus, its potential tissue accumulation is avoided.

ASL perfusion measurement has been successfully employed for tumour characterization, predicting local recurrence, and discriminating it from other radiation-induced effects (e.g., radionecrosis; Chawla *et al* 2007, Detre *et al* 2012, Abdel Razek *et al* 2019).

11.2.4 MRI: MRS

In MR spectroscopy (MRS)—a technique combining mass spectroscopy and magnetic resonance—a volume of tissue is excited, and its free induction decay is recorded and transformed via a Fourier transformation in order to detect the radiofrequency signals generated by specific endogenous and exogenous nuclei (such as ^{1}H, ^{31}P, ^{13}C and ^{19}F) and thus produce a spectrum showing resonance peaks of metabolites or tracers. In this way, MRS can be employed for the detection of the chemical environment of a tumour. Thanks to the metabolic characterization MRS provides, it has shown promise in the diagnosis and monitoring of tumours in the brain, prostate and breast (Kurhanewicz and Vigneron 2008, Horská and Barker 2010, Baltzer and Dietzel 2013).

Specifically for the brain, ^{1}H-MRS is mainly used in clinical routine to detect metabolites such as choline (Cho), N-acetyl aspartate (NAA), lactate (Lac), and creatine (Cr), which can provide information about glial proliferation and membrane synthesis, damage of neuronal tissue, angiogenesis and cellular energy metabolism, respectively (Li et al 2021). ^{1}H-MRS in RT has been shown to improve tumour delineation and normal tissue sparing (Pirzkall *et al* 2001, Narayana *et al* 2007), to potentially generate BTVs for dose painting (Deviers *et al* 2014, Zhou *et al* 2018) and to determine hypoxic regions by exploring the metabolic outcome of tumour hypoxia in breast tumours (Jiang *et al* 2012). Also, the potential of other nuclei such as in hyperpolarized ^{13}C MRI for the *in vivo* description of changes in tumour metabolic pathways by probing lactate metabolism in an active area of investigation but is yet to be studied in PT (Kawai *et al* 2021).

11.2.5 MRI: BOLD and OE-MRI

As previously mentioned, the investigation of tumour oxygenation in radiation oncology is crucial because tumours, due to irregular angiogenesis and high metabolic demand, often have regions of severe oxygen deprivation (i.e., hypoxia) which affect treatment efficacy, especially when low-LET irradiation is used. BOLD-MRI can be an alternative to PET to derive tumour hypoxia; it is a non-invasive functional imaging method that uses endogenous contrast generated by the blood oxygenation level and its effect on the MR signal. The principle of BOLD contrast relies on variations in the magnetic field surrounding red blood cells depending on the oxygen status of hemoglobin. While hemoglobin is diamagnetic (i.e., essentially nonmagnetic) in its fully oxygenated form (oxyhemoglobin), it becomes highly paramagnetic when deoxygenated (deoxyhemoglobin): this paramagnetism causes the generation of local magnetic field gradients, whose strength depends on the concentration of deoxyhemoglobin. Specifically, these local gradients attenuate the T2*-weighted MR signal from blood and tissues containing deoxyhemoglobin, making BOLD imaging able to detect changes in oxygenation within a tissue (McRobbie *et al* 2017). Although the applications are mainly focused on the physiology of functional brain activity or in pathological settings for the investigation of neurological disorders (e.g., stroke, carotid occlusion, aging, dementia), BOLD-MRI has also been employed in oncological applications to identify organs at risk and to investigate tumour oxygenation (Robinson *et al* 2003, Beaton *et al* 2019, Gauthier and Fan 2019).

Oxygen-Enhanced MRI (OE-MRI; also known as Tumour Oxygenation Level Dependent, TOLD) has also been developed as a technique for the quantification and mapping of tumour oxygen delivery (O'Connor *et al* 2016) based on the quantification of the longitudinal relaxation rate R1: as a hyperoxic gas is inhaled, excess molecular oxygen remains dissolved in blood plasma or interstitial tissue fluid in well-oxygenated regions of tissues, thus increasing R1. When combined with MRI perfusion measurements with dedicated acquisition protocols, this approach allows the identification of 'perfused oxygen-refractory' regions that correlate closely with histologically verified regions of hypoxia (O'Connor *et al* 2016). Results on pO_2 measurement based on OE-MRI have been conducted and revealed a great potential in clinical applications aimed at identifying tumour hypoxic sub-regions, spatially mapping hypoxia for RT treatment guidance (e.g., dose painting), and tracking hypoxia changes during RT (Little *et al* 2018, O'Connor *et al* 2019, Salem *et al* 2019).

11.2.6 CT: perfusion CT

Perfusion CT (or dynamic contrast-enhanced CT) employs low molecular weight iodinated contrast agents. When administered as an intravenous bolus, tissue concentration is dependent on vascular flow and interstitial accumulation, resulting in differential attenuation on CT imaging, before recirculation and clearance of the agent by the kidneys, in a manner similar to DCE-MRI. The signal is then fitted by pharmacokinetic models to map parameters related to tumour blood flow and volume, to vascular permeability, used as biomarkers correlated to tumour grade, aggressiveness, and prognosis (Jain 2011).

Tumour vascular perfusion parameters obtained by using perfusion CT (such as the transendothelial volume transfer constant, K^{trans}) have been shown to serve as QIB: perfusion CT measurements have been used for tumour detection, characterization, and staging, along with prediction and monitoring of treatment outcome in RT (Hermans *et al* 2003, Ellika *et al* 2007, Trojanowska *et al* 2012). It was also found to be more sensitive than tumour size for monitoring early and late response to RT (Kambadakone *et al* 2015).

11.2.7 CT: dual-energy CT

Dual-energy CT (and spectral CT), which uses separate x-ray photon energy spectra, provides information about tissues that show unique attenuation profiles when exposed to both low and high-energy polychromatic x-ray beams. Materials have unique attenuation profiles at different energy levels according to their linear attenuation coefficient: indeed, for high and low x-ray energies, small differences in attenuation are observed for materials with low atomic numbers (e.g., water), while materials with high atomic numbers (e.g., iodine) show large differences in attenuation (Hamid *et al* 2021). The detection of iodine, calcium, and uric acid crystals from soft tissues and iodine-containing substances on low-energy images is improved and it is possible to generate virtual unenhanced datasets from contrast-enhanced scans, thus reducing the radiation dose required for further non-enhanced CT. Indeed, whereas conventional single energy CT produces a single image set, dual-energy data can be used to reconstruct material-specific images such as soft tissue, fat and iodine-specific images.

Dual-energy CT (DECT) could potentially be available in-room for PT to ensure accuracy in range and re-planning procedures. Indeed, this technique can be used to overcome the intrinsic restrictions of the Hounsfield Unit look-up table approach, and the reduction of stopping power ratio (SPR) uncertainty represents the main aim of dual-energy CT in PT (details reported in chapter 4). Besides, it provides superior lesion conspicuity and characterization, with improved contrast between normally enhancing parenchyma and hyper-/hypo-vascular lesions (Patel *et al* 2013).

11.3 Applications in PT

11.3.1 Contouring

As in conventional RT settings, most imaging routines in PT employ CT images, which provide the information required for dose planning (i.e., the electronic densities), while less often these are integrated with MRI (mainly anatomical sequences) for determining the position and size of the tumour (Bolsi *et al* 2018). However, especially in cases in which a reduced contrast between tumour tissue and adjacent healthy tissues is found, or where functional information may be of use, Q-imaging could play a key role in overcoming the limitations of conventional imaging routines and ensuring reduced intra- and inter-observer variability (Dirix *et al* 2014) and, thus, safer treatment planning. An increasing number of studies has investigated the advantage derived from integrating Q-imaging (e.g., PET, DWI, DCE-MRI) at the planning stage and specifically at the tumour delineation stage (Dirix *et al* 2014, Paulson *et al* 2015, Gurney-Champion *et al* 2020). For example, in prostate cancer, the ability of DWI and DCE-MRI to successfully discriminate tumour regions from transitional and healthy regions is now widely recognized (Dwivedi and Jagannathan 2022).

In tumours localized in areas close to high-risk healthy structures, tumour coverage based on CT alone is often inadequate, requiring the integration of other imaging modalities (Tan *et al* 2010, Welzel *et al* 2018), and the improvement in the contrast between healthy and tumour tissue provided by Q-imaging can ensure a reduction in the dose delivered to organs at risk (Brændengen *et al* 2011).

11.3.2 Biological target volume and dose painting

A potential strategy for a better dose delivery to the target and a concurrent sparing of the surrounding healthy tissues is the outline of smaller margins, as well as the definition of target sub-volumes. Indeed, the anatomical GTV can be further characterized by identifying sub-GTV volumes based on functional information, which facilitates dose escalation to the target for prescribing an ideal and optimal treatment dose, leading to the definition of the BTV (Ling *et al* 2000).

Locally boosting the tumour irradiation to increase locoregional control based on Q-imaging is generally referred to as dose painting, for which two approaches can be distinguished (van der Heide *et al* 2012, Alonzi 2015). The first approach is dose painting by contours (DPBC) in which a boost volume is created based on a certain threshold which defines the BTV. The voxels with values below this threshold are considered to be at low risk for recurrence and the voxels with values above this threshold are considered to be at high risk. Segmentation of this boost volume can be performed using regular commercial treatment planning software and, subsequently, a boost dose is assigned to the defined boost volume (Chang *et al* 2013, Casares-Magaz *et al* 2016, Her *et al* 2021). The other approach is referred to as dose painting by numbers (DPBN; Bentzen 2005) where a relationship is assumed between the voxel intensity of the quantitative image set in question and the risk of local recurrence in that voxel, thus boosting the dose of a tumour voxel according to the underlying image intensity of this same voxel (Her *et al* 2020). DPBN optimization requires research treatment planning software as commercial packages generally do not allow voxel-based optimization.

In both the approaches, the objective is to map a range of image intensities onto a range of doses. To date, the high accuracy of this mapping is the major limitation and bottleneck for the clinical applicability of dose painting, as safe treatment planning needs to be ensured. However, the use of dose painting starting from maps of tumour hypoxia (e.g., by means of PET, OE-MRI, or BOLD-MRI), cell density (e.g., through DWI), tissue perfusion (e.g., via PWI) and metabolism (e.g., MRS)—all features with a great impact on radiation sensitivity—seems to be a promising approach towards an advanced treatment personalization (Bentzen and Gregoire 2011, van der Heide *et al* 2012, Durante *et al* 2017, Zhou *et al* 2018, Gurney-Champion *et al* 2020, Her *et al* 2020, Her *et al* 2021, Mierzwa *et al* 2022). As an example, dose painting on ADC from DWI was proposed for robust treatment planning to increase tumour control probability in prostate cancer (Grönlund *et al* 2021; figure 11.2) and glioblastoma (Orlandi *et al* 2016).

Specifically in PT, a recent study by Köthe *et al* (2021) investigated the potential of hypoxia-targeted dose escalation in non-small cell lung cancer treated with protons (figure 11.3). Escalated dose levels were simulated in the most hypoxic

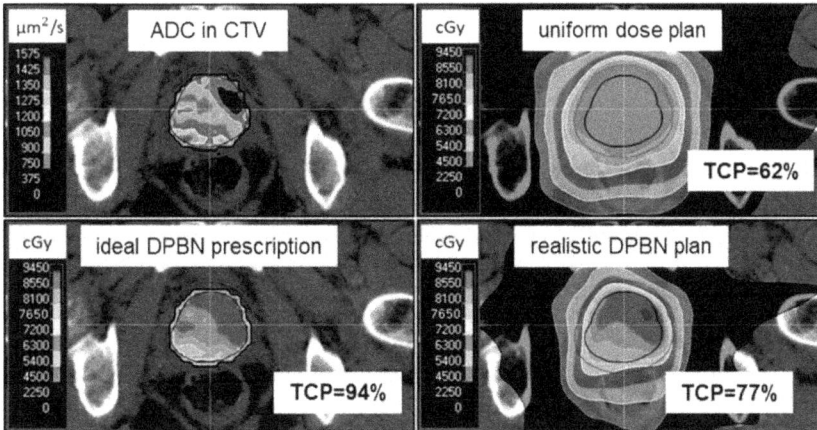

Figure 11.2. Illustration of different dose plans for a CT-image slice of a prostate patient. The blue contour marks the prostate clinical target volume (CTV) and the red contour the planning target volume (PTV) made with a margin of 6mm from the CTV. (Upper left) ADC image data is reported within the CTV. (Lower left) The ideal DPBN prescription shows low-ADC (high cellularity) regions with a prescribed higher dose than the high-ADC regions with a lower dose. (Upper right) A dose plan is optimized to be uniform for the PTV. (Lower right) A DPBN plan is optimized with 15MV photons. Taken and adapted with permission from Grönlund *et al* (2021). Taylor & Francis Ltd. http://tandfonline.com on behalf of © 2021 Acta Oncologica Foundation.

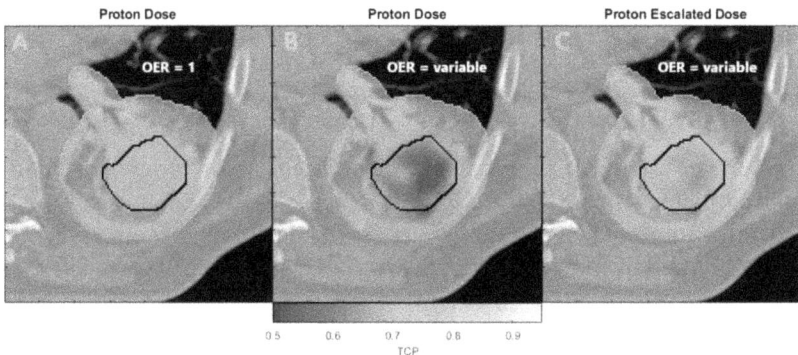

Figure 11.3. Exemplary voxel-wise TCP calculation for a conventional proton plan in non-small cell lung cancer with uniform dose prescription (A, B) and patient-specific escalated dose (22%) to the hypoxic tumour volume (C). PTV contours are in orange, the hypoxic region in black. Taking into account hypoxia information and its influence on TCP, locoregional losses can be observed (B) compared to the planned TCP (A) where OER is assumed to be consistently 1 throughout the target. The dose escalation (C) counteracts the increased radioresistance caused by hypoxia by increasing the dose to the radioresistant area and thus recovers TCP. Reproduced from Köthe *et al* (2021). CC BY 4.0.

region identified by PET imaging of the primary target and its effectiveness in improving locoregional tumour control was assessed, suggesting that the administration of proton therapy for dose escalation to patient-specific regions of tumour hypoxia can mitigate tumour control probability (TCP) reduction due to hypoxia-induced radioresistance, while simultaneously reducing normal tissue complication probability levels. The same approach has been recently tested on 4D imaging to evaluate the impact of organ motion and the application of mitigation strategies on the effectiveness of hypoxia-guided proton therapy (Köthe *et al* 2022).

Studies on hypoxia-targeted dose escalation in proton therapy have been also conducted for esophageal and nasopharyngeal cancers and compared with dose escalation protocols with intensity-modulated RT. These showed that Q-imaging guidance in PT would allow for better treatment outcomes in high-risk target regions (Yasuda *et al* 2018, Zhang *et al* 2022). Clinical trials are currently ongoing (e.g., NCT02802969, NCT03865277), aimed at targeting radioresistant hypoxic areas in head and neck squamous cell carcinomas and chordomas with hypoxia-guided dose painting in PT.

It should be also noted that in addition to physical and biological dose optimization, authors in the literature also introduced LET painting (Bassler *et al* 2010) with the goal of optimizing the LET distribution in PT. Indeed, an additional therapeutic advantage can be achieved with a LET optimization since (i) it is well known that a generic RBE value of 1.1 employed in proton therapy is only an approximation as RBE increases with increasing LET, and (ii) hypoxic tumours can benefit from the low OER of high-LET concentration. Several studies therefore employed LET painting in PT in order to avoid underestimation of NTCP in critical structures (underestimated RBE) and under-dosage in the target (overestimated RBE), as well as to improve TCP by concentrating high-LET radiations in hypoxic sub-regions of the target (Grassberger *et al* 2011, Bassler *et al* 2014, Tinganelli *et al* 2015).

11.3.3 Patient stratification and treatment monitoring

Q-imaging and related QIBs have been demonstrated to be effective in investigating differences in histological subtypes or heterogeneity of properties potentially affecting treatment outcome (e.g., hypoxia, cell density, angiogenesis). Indeed, inter- and intra-tumour heterogeneity is a challenge for personalized RT because needle biopsy underestimates the degree of spatial heterogeneity and is unsuitable for capturing the true extent of temporal heterogeneity, preventing a complete characterization of the tumour (Bedard *et al* 2013, Dagogo-Jack and Shaw 2018). This is particularly relevant for deep-seated and rare tumours typically treated with PT, which are often difficult to reach and characterize.

In an RT/PT workflow, Q-imaging can be also used for early detection of functional and microstructural changes both during and after treatment. Nevertheless, Q-imaging is only marginally employed for disease progression with the only exception of FDG-PET used for the determination of lesion progression (Hirata and Tamaki 2021), and objective response assessment is typically done through tumour endpoints defined in the RECIST (Response Evaluation Criteria in Solid Tumours) criteria, a set of widely adopted guidelines for tumour assessment (Ko *et al* 2021). However, RECIST guidelines are, for example, less appropriate for slow-growing tumours—such as for chordomas, typically treated with PT—because treatment response assessments based on volumetric changes may not be informative of the actual treatment effectiveness, which can be instead assessed by QI. Q-imaging in PT applications, DWI has been investigated as a predictor of histological grading in meningioma tumours (Sacco *et al* 2020, Zampini *et al* 2020), and recent studies were also conducted to monitor and predict PT treatment on both tumours and healthy structures.

Preliminary works have been reported on sacral chordoma patients treated with carbon ions, which suggested that ADC measured from DWI acquisitions can predict treatment outcomes more accurately than RECIST (Preda *et al* 2018, 2020). In a study by Bonekamp *et al* (2016), 92 patients with prostate cancer were evaluated prospectively with DCE-MRI at baseline, day 10 during therapy, and 6 weeks, 6 months and 18 months after treatment completion to monitor primary proton and carbon ion irradiation, showing that DCE parameters changed during therapy within the tumour and in normal appearing contralateral tissue.

As regards normal tissue involvement after PT, ADC and IVIM parameter changes in white matter after proton therapy have also recently been investigated in patients with meningioma tumours (Buizza *et al* 2021), showing trends of decreased ADC and D (i.e., diffusion parameter of IVIM) for white matter regions hit by medium-high [30–40 Gy(RBE)] and high [>40 Gy(RBE)] doses (figure 11.4). This is compatible with diffusion restriction due to radiation-induced cellular injury, which is thought to be caused by radioinduced inflammatory responses including axonal swelling and reactive astrogliosis (Raschke *et al* 2019).

In a study by Uh *et al* (2021), longitudinal DTI data were analyzed to determine the proton dose effect on white matter structures in relation to the irradiated brain volume and baseline age in 90 children and adolescents with craniopharyngioma.

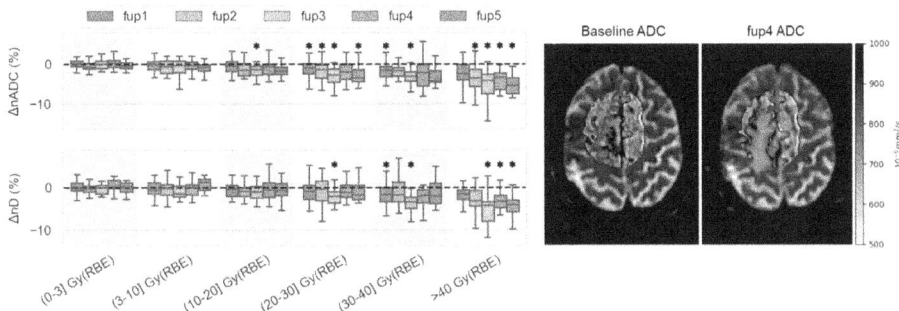

Figure 11.4. Left: Variations of diffusion parameter of IVIM (ADC and D) in white matter with respect to time (different follow-up, fup) and dose levels. Significant changes (α=0.0125) are marked by an *. Right: Example of ADC maps of white matter hit by high doses (>40 Gy(RBE)) superimposed on DWI image acquired at baseline and at the 4th follow-up. Figure adapted from Buizza *et al* (2021). Copyright (2021), with permission from Elsevier.

11.4 Challenges and perspectives

Q-imaging shows promising perspectives for applications in PT to make the most of its physical and radiobiological advantages and push towards more personalized treatments. Escalating the dose according to tumour functional characteristics is expected to improve treatment outcome, while identifying prognostic QIBs would allow patients to be stratified following an optimal treatment strategy by either using baseline information only or by monitoring the response and adjusting the treatment accordingly. For example, QIBs associated with a given prognostic value could guide the selection of treatment features and type as well as the determination of the optimal individual dose. Indeed, the definition of the type of treatment to date is mostly driven by pre-treatment data (e.g., genomic, pathologic, clinical and dosimetric data) along with conventional biomarkers (e.g., molecular or genomic biomarkers), lacking a spatial description of tissue microenvironment. The promising results of QIB-based prognostic and predictive models point towards a key role of QIBs in Q-imaging.

However, Q-imaging still does not find a systematic application in RT and, even more, in PT clinical practice, with clinical protocols often overlooking the potential of functional/metabolic information, and with complex image modalities and advanced models sometimes requiring resources, time, experienced operators, and sophisticated analyses that might be deemed research tools more than clinical ones. Also, while the integration of multi-modal images could bring significant improvements in target delineation and dose optimization, it also adds complexity to the treatment planning phase because of the need for an extremely accurate co-registration with the planning CT (as discussed in chapter 3). As such, optimization and standardization of Q-imaging protocols, as well as quality assurance for the determination of a gold standard practice, must be ensured to allow first a congruous quality of functional information, and then reproducibility of studies and inter-institutional comparison.

The extracted QIBs must ensure high accuracy in order to provide safe and tailored PT treatments, as already discussed in Gurney-Champion *et al* (2020) for conventional RT. To be reliably employed in the clinical routine, Q-imaging must undergo both technical and biological/clinical validation (O'Connor *et al* 2017). Technical validation entails testing for accuracy, repeatability, and reproducibility of the underlying physical measurement, both over time and across sites (Gurney-Champion *et al* 2020). In this sense, the QIB alliance from the Radiological Society of North America (RSNA) aims at improving the value and practicality of QI by evaluating variability across devices, sites, patients and time.

PET and CT are typically more repeatable and reproducible than quantitative MRI (Wang *et al* 2021), although the main drawback is the high radiation dose associated with the repeated imaging; for radiotherapy patients who already are receiving substantial treatment dose, the additional dose may be acceptable. Instead, geometric distortions and uncertainty of diffusion parameters due to non-optimized imaging protocols affect DWI (Leibfarth *et al* 2018) interpretation of perfusion values may result in quite different target volumes for irradiation when using PWI (van der Heide *et al* 2012) and spectral artifacts and lower specificity influence MRS interpretation (Li *et al* 2021) meaning that geometric and quantification robustness is challenging and must be addressed adequately. Thus, technical tolerances related to hardware components should be first identified and then quantified through physical phantoms, by following the available standardized procedures or guidelines and recommendations (Kessler *et al* 2015). At the same time, the analysis of Q-imaging should be carried out through robust software. Computational methods employed to derive clinically useful quantitative parameters should be validated and their quality assessed by making use of phantoms and reliable tools (Keenan *et al* 2018). On the other hand, biological/clinical validation relies on the evaluation of the relationship between imaging and the underlying biophysical parameter of interest. This relationship must be proven to be quantitative, i.e., accurate, repeatable, and reproducible, as well as relevant, specific and consistent (O'Connor *et al* 2017). An increasing number of studies are investigating methods to map the content of images (e.g., MRI) acquired in-vivo onto slices of histo-pathological specimens in order to match the extracted QIB with the corresponding biological ground truth (Her *et al* 2020). Nevertheless, if the clinical validation can be easily performed through clinical scores, challenges are present in PT for biological validation. An optimal biological validation for PT applications should include availability of histological data for tumour characterization and access to experimental beam lines for cells line irradiation, which may be difficult in a PT setting. Monte Carlo simulations of dose deposition could help to overcome this issue, by investigating structural and radiobiological effects at the cellular and DNA level for QIB validation (Kyriakou *et al* 2022).

In conclusion, although effort is still required to translate methods into clinical use, the Q-imaging described in this chapter, together with advanced strategies for QIBs derivation (e.g., radiomics and artificial intelligence) and multi-scale modelling (chapter 12), are expected to describe the in-vivo biological complexity of the pathology and organs at risk on a patient-specific and multi-scale basis, moving us towards biologically-guided treatments in PT.

References

Abdel Razek A A K, Talaat M, El-Serougy L, Abdelsalam M and Gaballa G 2019 Differentiating glioblastomas from solitary brain metastases using arterial spin labeling perfusion- and diffusion tensor imaging-derived metrics *World Neurosurg.* **127** e593–8

Alonzi R 2015 Functional radiotherapy targeting using focused dose escalation *Clin. Oncol.* **27** 601–17

Baltzer P A T and Dietzel M 2013 Breast lesions: diagnosis by using proton MR spectroscopy at 1.5 and 3.0 T—systematic review and meta-analysis *Radiology* **267** 735–46

Barker H E, Paget J T E, Khan A A and Harrington K J 2015 The tumour microenvironment after radiotherapy: Mechanisms of resistance and recurrence *Nat. Rev. Cancer* **15** 409–25

Bassler N, Jäkel O, Søndergaard C S and Petersen J B 2010 Dose- and LET-painting with particle therapy *Acta Oncol.* **49** 1170–6

Bassler N, Toftegaard J, Lühr A, Sorensen B S, Scifoni E, Krämer M and Petersen J B 2014 LET-painting increases tumour control probability in hypoxic tumours *Acta Oncol.* **53** 25–32

Beaton L, Bandula S, Gaze M N and Sharma R A 2019 How rapid advances in imaging are defining the future of precision radiation oncology *Br. J. Cancer* **120** 779–90

Bedard P L, Hansen A R, Ratain M J and Siu L L 2013 Tumour heterogeneity in the clinic *Nature* **501** 355–64

Bentzen S M 2005 Theragnostic imaging for radiation oncology: dose-painting by numbers *Lancet Oncol.* **6** 112–7

Bentzen S M and Gregoire V 2011 Molecular imaging-based dose painting: a novel paradigm for radiation therapy prescription *Semin. Radiat. Oncol.* **21** 101–10

Bolsi A, Peroni M, Amelio D, Dasu A, Stock M, Toma-Dasu I and Hoffmann A 2018 Practice patterns of image guided particle therapy in Europe: a 2016 survey of the European particle therapy network (EPTN) *Radiother. Oncol.* **128** 4–8

Bonekamp D, Wolf M B, Edler C, Katayama S, Schlemmer H P, Herfarth K and Röthke M 2016 Dynamic contrast enhanced MRI monitoring of primary proton and carbon ion irradiation of prostate cancer using a novel hypofractionated raster scan technique *Radiother. Oncol.* **120** 313–9

Brændengen M, Hansson K, Radu C, Siegbahn A, Jacobsson H and Glimelius B 2011 Delineation of gross tumour volume (GTV) for radiation treatment planning of locally advanced rectal cancer using information from MRI or FDG-PET/CT: a prospective study *Int. J. Radiat. Oncol. Biol. Phys.* **81** e439–45

Buizza G, Zampini M A, Riva G, Molinelli S, Fontana G, Imparato S and Paganelli C 2021 Investigating DWI changes in white matter of meningioma patients treated with proton therapy *Phys. Med.* **84** 72–9

Byun H K, Han M C, Yang K, Kim J S, Yoo G S, Koom W S and Kim Y B 2021 Physical and biological characteristics of particle therapy for oncologists *Cancer Res. Treat.* **53** 611–20

Casares-Magaz O, Van Der Heide U A, Rørvik J, Steenbergen P and Muren L P 2016 Prostate radiotherapy a tumour control probability model for radiotherapy of prostate cancer using magnetic resonance imaging-based apparent diffusion coefficient maps *Radiother. Oncol.* **119** 111–6

Chang J H, Wada M, Anderson N J, Lim Joon D, Lee S T, Gong S J and Scott A M 2013 Hypoxia-targeted radiotherapy dose painting for head and neck cancer using 18F-FMISO PET: a biological modeling study *Acta Oncol.* **52** 1723–9

Chawla S, Wang S, Wolf R L, Woo J H, Wang J, O'Rourke D M and Poptani H 2007 Arterial spin-labeling and MR spectroscopy in the differentiation of Gliomas *AJNR: Am. J. Neuroradiol.* **28** 1683

Cheney M D, Chen Y L, Lim R, Winrich B K, Grosu A L, Trofimov A V and Delaney T F 2014 [18F]-fluoromisonidazole positron emission tomography/computed tomography visualization of tumour hypoxia in patients with chordoma of the mobile and sacrococcygeal spine *Int. J. Radiat. Oncol. Biol. Phys.* **90** 1030–6

Chiang G C, Kovanlikaya I, Choi C, Ramakrishna R, Magge R and Shungu D C 2018 Magnetic resonance spectroscopy, positron emission tomography and radiogenomics-relevance to glioma *Front. Neurol. Front. Media S.A* **9** 33

Colman J, Mancini L, Manolopoulos S, Gupta M, Kosmin M and Bisdas S 2022 Is diffusion tensor imaging-guided radiotherapy the new state-of-the-art? A review of the current literature and technical insights *Appl. Sci. (Switz.)* **12** 816

Daghighi S, Bahrami N, Tom W J, Coley N, Seibert T M, Hattangadi-Gluth J A and McDonald C R 2020 Restriction spectrum imaging differentiates true tumour progression from immune-mediated pseudoprogression: case report of a patient with glioblastoma *Front. Oncol.* **10** 487593

Dagogo-Jack I and Shaw A T 2018 Tumour heterogeneity and resistance to cancer therapies *Nat. Rev. Clin. Oncol.* **15** 81–94

Detre J A, Rao H, Wang D J J, Chen Y F and Wang Z 2012 Applications of arterial spin labeled MRI in the brain *J. Magn. Reson. Imaging : JMRI* **35** 1026–37

Deviers A, Ken S, Filleron T, Rowland B, Laruelo A, Catalaa I and Laprie A 2014 Evaluation of the lactate-to-*N*-acetyl-aspartate ratio defined with magnetic resonance spectroscopic imaging before radiation therapy as a new predictive marker of the site of relapse in patients with glioblastoma multiforme *Int. J. Radiat. Oncol. Biol. Phys.* **90** 385–93

Dirix P, Haustermans K and Vandecaveye V 2014 The value of magnetic resonance imaging for radiotherapy planning *Semin. Radiat. Oncol.* **24** 151–9

Durante M and Loeffler J S 2020 Charged particles in radiation oncology *Nat. Rev. Clin. Oncol.* **7** 37–43

Durante M and Flanz J 2019 Charged particle beams to cure cancer: strengths and challenges *Semin. Oncol.* **46** 219–25

Durante M, Orecchia R and Loeffler J S 2017 Charged-particle therapy in cancer: clinical uses and future perspectives *Nat. Rev. Clin. Oncol.* **14** 483–95

Dwivedi D K and Jagannathan N R 2022 Emerging MR methods for improved diagnosis of prostate cancer by multiparametric MRI *Magma (New York.)* **35** 587–608

El Naqa I, Pogue B W, Zhang R, Oraiqat I and Parodi K 2022 Image guidance for FLASH radiotherapy *Med. Phys.* **49** 4109–22

Ellika S K, Jain R, Patel S C, Scarpace L, Schultz L R, Rock J P and Mikkelsen T 2007 Role of perfusion CT in glioma grading and comparison with conventional MR imaging features *AJNR. Am. J. Neuroradiol.* **28** 1981–7

Fleming I N, Manavaki R, Blower P J, West C, Williams K J, Harris A L and Gilbert F J 2015 Imaging tumour hypoxia with positron emission tomography *Br. J. Cancer* **112** 238–50

Gauthier C J and Fan A P 2019 BOLD signal physiology: models and applications *NeuroImage* **187** 116–27

Grassberger C, Trofimov A, Lomax A and Paganetti H 2011 Variations in linear energy transfer within clinical proton therapy fields and the potential for biological treatment planning *Int. J. Radiat. Oncol. Biol. Phys.* **80** 1559–66

Grönlund E, Almhagen E, Johansson S, Traneus E, Nyholm T, Thellenberg C and Ahnesjö A 2021 Robust treatment planning of dose painting for prostate cancer based on ADC-to-Gleason score mappings—what is the potential to increase the tumour control probability? *Acta Oncol.* **60** 199–206

Gulani V, Calamante F, Shellock F G, Kanal E and Reeder S B 2017 Gadolinium deposition in the brain: summary of evidence and recommendations *Lancet Neurol.* **16** 564–70

Gurney-Champion O J, Mahmood F, Schie M V, Julian R, George B, Philippens M E P and Redalen K R 2020 Quantitative imaging for radiotherapy purposes *Radiother. Oncol.* **146** 66–75

Haggenmüller B, Kreiser K, Sollmann N, Huber M, Vogele D, Schmidt S A and Kloth C 2023 Pictorial review on imaging findings in cerebral CTP in patients with acute stroke and its Mimics: a primer for general radiologists *Diagnostics* **13** 447

Hamid S, Nasir M U, So A, Andrews G, Nicolaou S and Qamar S R 2021 Clinical applications of dual-energy CT *Korean J. Radiol.* **22** 970

Her E J, Haworth A, Reynolds H M, Sun Y, Kennedy A, Panettieri V and Ebert M A 2020 Voxel-level biological optimisation of prostate IMRT using patient-specific tumour location and clonogen density derived from mpMRI *Radiat. Oncol.* **15** 172

Her E J, Haworth A, Sun Y, Williams S, Reynolds H M, Kennedy A and Ebert M A 2021 Biologically targeted radiation therapy: incorporating patient-specific hypoxia data derived from quantitative magnetic resonance imaging *Cancers* **13** 4897

Hermans R, Meijerink M, van den Bogaert W, Rijnders A, Weltens C and Lambin P 2003 Tumour perfusion rate determined noninvasively by dynamic computed tomography predicts outcome in head-and-neck cancer after radiotherapy *Int. J. Radiat. Oncol. Biol. Phys.* **57** 1351–6

Hirata K and Tamaki N 2021 Quantitative fdg pet assessment for oncology therapy *Cancers* **13** 1–12

Hoffmann A, Oborn B, Moteabbed M, Yan S, Bortfeld T, Knopf A and Parodi K 2020 MR-guided proton therapy: a review and a preview *Radiat. Oncol. BioMed Central*

Horská A and Barker P B 2010 Imaging of brain tumours: MR spectroscopy and metabolic imaging *Neuroimaging Clin. N. Am.* **20** 293–310

Hua J, Liu P, Kim T, Donahue M, Rane S, Chen J J and Kim S G 2019 MRI techniques to measure arterial and venous cerebral blood volume *NeuroImage* **187** 17–31

Igaki H, Sakumi A, Mukasa A, Saito K, Kunimatsu A, Masutani Y and Ohtomo K 2014 Corticospinal tract-sparing intensity-modulated radiotherapy treatment planning *Rep. Pract. Oncol. Radiother.* **19** 310–6

Jain R 2011 Perfusion CT imaging of brain tumours: an overview *Am. J. Neuroradiol.* **32** 1570–7

Jiang L, Greenwood T R, Artemov D, Raman V, Winnard P T, Heeren R M A and Glunde K 2012 Localized hypoxia results in spatially heterogeneous metabolic signatures in breast tumour models *Neoplasia (United States)* **14** 732–41

Kambadakone A, Yoon S S, Kim T M, Karl D L, Duda D G, DeLaney T F and Sahani D V 2015 CT perfusion as an imaging biomarker in monitoring response to neoadjuvant bevacizumab and radiation in soft-tissue sarcomas: comparison with tumour morphology, circulating and tumour biomarkers, and gene expression *AJR Am. J. Roentgenol.* **204** W11–8

Kawai T, Brender J R, Lee J A, Kramp T, Kishimoto S, Krishna M C and Camphausen K A 2021 Detection of metabolic change in glioblastoma cells after radiotherapy using hyper-polarized 13C-MRI *NMR Biomed.* **34** e4514

Keall P J, Brighi C, Glide-Hurst C, Liney G, Liu P Z Y, Lydiard S and Whelan B 2022 Integrated MRI-guided radiotherapy—opportunities and challenges *Nat. Rev. Clin. Oncol.* **19** 458–70

Keenan K E, Ainslie M, Barker A J, Boss M A, Cecil K M, Charles C and Zheng J 2018 Quantitative magnetic resonance imaging phantoms: a review and the need for a system phantom *Magn. Reson. Med.* **79** 48–61

Kessler L G, Barnhart H X, Buckler A J, Choudhury K R, Kondratovich M v, Toledano A and Sullivan D C 2015 The emerging science of quantitative imaging biomarkers terminology and definitions for scientific studies and regulatory submissions *Stat. Methods Med. Res.* **24** 9–26

Ko C C, Yeh L R, Kuo Y T and Chen J H 2021 Imaging biomarkers for evaluating tumour response: RECIST and beyond *Biomark. Res.* **9** 1–20

Köthe A, Bizzocchi N, Safai S, Lomax A J, Weber D C and Fattori G 2021 Investigating the potential of proton therapy for hypoxia-targeted dose escalation in non-small cell lung cancer *Radiat. Oncol.* **16**

Köthe A, Lomax A J, Giovannelli A C, Safai S, Bizzocchi N, Roelofs E and Fattori G 2022 The impact of organ motion and the appliance of mitigation strategies on the effectiveness of hypoxia-guided proton therapy for non-small cell lung cancer *Radiother. Oncol.* **176** 208–14

Kurhanewicz J and Vigneron D B 2008 Advances in MR spectroscopy of the prostate *Magn. Reson. Imaging Clin. N. Am.* **16** 697–710

Kyriakou I, Sakata D, Tran H N, Perrot Y, Shin W G, Lampe N and Incerti S 2022 Review of the Geant4-DNA simulation toolkit for radiobiological applications at the cellular and DNA level *Cancers* **14**

Lau J, Rousseau E, Kwon D, Lin K S, Bénard F and Chen X 2020 Insight into the development of PET radiopharmaceuticals for oncology *Cancers*

le Bihan D 2019 What can we see with IVIM MRI? *NeuroImage* **187** 56–67

le Bihan D, Breton E, Lallemand D, Grenier P, Cabanis E and Laval-Jeantet M 1986 MR imaging of intravoxel incoherent motions: application to diffusion and perfusion in neurologic disorders *Radiology* **161** 401–7

Leibfarth S, Winter R M, Lyng H, Zips D and Thorwarth D 2018 Potentials and challenges of diffusion-weighted magnetic resonance imaging in radiotherapy *Clin. Trans. Radiat. Oncol.* **13** 29–37

Leimgruber A, Hickson K, Lee S T, Gan H K, Cher L M, Sachinidis J I and Scott A M 2020 Spatial and quantitative mapping of glycolysis and hypoxia in glioblastoma as a predictor of radiotherapy response and sites of relapse *Eur. J. Nucl. Med. Mol. Imaging* **47** 1476–85

Li M, Zhang Q and Yang K 2021 Role of MRI-based functional imaging in improving the therapeutic index of radiotherapy in cancer treatment *Front. Oncol.* **11** 3244

Lin M, Coll R P, Cohen A S, Georgiou D K and Manning H C 2022 PET oncological radiopharmaceuticals: current status and perspectives *Molecules* **27** 6790

Ling C C, Humm J, Larson S, Amols H, Fuks Z, Leibel S and Koutcher J A 2000 Towards multidimensional radiotherapy (MD-CRT): biological imaging and biological conformality *Int. J. Radiat. Oncol. Biol. Phys.* **47** 551–60

Little R A, Jamin Y, Boult J K R, Naish J H, Watson Y, Cheung S and O'Connor J P B 2018 Mapping hypoxia in renal carcinoma with oxygen-enhanced MRI: comparison with intrinsic susceptibility MRI and pathology *Radiology* **288** 739–47

Mangesius S, Janjic T, Steiger R, Haider L, Rehwald R, Knoflach M and Grams A 2021 Dual-energy computed tomography in acute ischemic stroke: state-of-the-art *Eur. Radiol.* **31** 4138–47

Martucci M, Russo R, Schimperna F, D'Apolito G, Panfili M, Grimaldi A and Gaudino S 2023 Magnetic Resonance Imaging of Primary Adult Brain Tumors: State of the Art and Future Perspectives *Biomedicines* **11** 364

Matsuo M, Matsumoto S, Mitchell J B, Krishna M C and Camphausen K 2014 Magnetic resonance imaging of the tumour microenvironment in radiotherapy: perfusion, hypoxia, and metabolism *Semin. Radiat. Oncol.* **24** 210–7

McCabe A, Martin S, Shah J, Morgan P S and Panek R 2023 T1 based oxygen-enhanced MRI in tumours; a scoping review of current research *Br. J. Radiol.*

McRobbie D W, Moore E A and Graves M J 2017 *MRI from Picture to Proton* 3rd edn (Cambridge: Cambridge University Press)

Mierzwa M L, Aryal M, Lee C, Schipper M, VanTil M, Morales K and Cao Y 2022 Randomized phase II study of physiologic MRI-directed adaptive radiation boost in poor prognosis head and neck cancer *Clin. Cancer Res.* **28** OF1–9

Narayana A, Chang J, Thakur S, Huang W, Karimi S, Hou B and Gutin P H 2007 Use of MR spectroscopy and functional imaging in the treatment planning of gliomas *Br. J. Radiol.* **80** 347–54

Novikov D S, Kiselev V G and Jespersen S N 2018 On modeling *Magn. Reson. Med.* **79** 3172–93

O'Connor J P B, Aboagye E O, Adams J E, Aerts H J W L, Barrington S F, Beer A J and Waterton J C 2017 Imaging biomarker roadmap for cancer studies *Nat. Rev. Clin. Oncol.* **14** 169–86

O'Connor J P B, Boult J K R, Jamin Y, Babur M, Finegan K G, Williams K J and Robinson S P 2016 Oxygen-enhanced MRI accurately identifies, quantifies, and maps tumour hypoxia in preclinical cancer models *Cancer Res.* **76** 787–95

O'Connor J P B, Robinson S P and Waterton J C 2019 Imaging tumour hypoxia with oxygen-enhanced MRI and BOLD MRI *Br. J. Radiol.* **92** 20180642

Orlandi M, Botti A, Sghedoni R, Cagni E, Ciammella P, Iotti C and Iori M 2016 Feasibility of voxel-based dose painting for recurrent glioblastoma guided by ADC values of diffusion-weighted MR imaging *Phys. Med.* **32** 1651–8

Panagiotaki E, Walker-Samuel S, Siow B, Johnson S P, Rajkumar V, Pedley R B and Alexander D C 2014 Noninvasive quantification of solid tumour microstructure using VERDICT MRI *Cancer Res.* **74** 1902–12

Patel B N, Thomas J V, Lockhart M E, Berland L L and Morgan D E 2013 Single-source dual-energy spectral multidetector CT of pancreatic adenocarcinoma: optimization of energy level viewing significantly increases lesion contrast *Clin. Radiol.* **68** 148–54

Paulson E S, Erickson B, Schultz C and Allen Li X 2015 Comprehensive MRI simulation methodology using a dedicated MRI scanner in radiation oncology for external beam radiation treatment planning *Med. Phys.* **42** 28–39

Pirzkall A, McKnight T R, Graves E E, Carol M P, Sneed P K, Wara W W and Larson D A 2001 MR-spectroscopy guided target delineation for high-grade gliomas *Int. J. Radiat. Oncol. Biol. Phys.* **50** 915–28

Preda L, Casale S, Fanizza M, Fiore M R, Viselner G, Paganelli C and Valvo F 2020 Predictive role of apparent diffusion coefficient (ADC) from diffusion weighted MRI in patients with sacral chordoma treated with carbon ion radiotherapy (CIRT) alone *Eur. J. Radiol.* **126**

Preda L, Stoppa D, Fiore M R, Fontana G, Camisa S, Sacchi R and Orecchia R 2018 MRI evaluation of sacral chordoma treated with carbon ion radiotherapy alone *Radiother. Oncol.* **128** 203–8

Raschke F, Wesemann T, Wahl H, Appold S, Krause M, Linn J and Troost E G C 2019 Reduced diffusion in normal appearing white matter of glioma patients following radio(chemo) therapy *Radiother. Oncol.* **140** 110–5

Robinson S P, Rijken P F J W, Howe F A, McSheehy P M J, Van der Sanden B P J, Heerschap A and Griffiths J R 2003 Tumour vascular architecture and function evaluated by non-invasive susceptibility MRI methods and immunohistochemistry *J. Magn. Reson. Imaging* **17** 445–54

Sacco S, Ballati F, Gaetani C, Lomoro P, Farina L M, Bacila A and Preda L 2020 Multi-parametric qualitative and quantitative MRI assessment as predictor of histological grading in previously treated meningiomas *Neuroradiology* **62** 1441–9

Salem A, Little R A, Latif A, Featherstone A K, Babur M, Peset I and O'Connor J P B 2019 Oxygen-enhanced MRI is feasible, repeatable, and detects radiotherapy-induced change in hypoxia in xenograft models and in patients with Non-small cell lung cancer *Clin. Cancer Res.* **25** 3818–29

Schardt D, Elsässer T and Schulz-Ertner D 2010 Heavy-ion tumor therapy: Physical and radiobiological benefits *Rev. Modern Phys.* **82** 383–425

Schuster D M, Nanni C and Fanti S 2016 PET tracers beyond FDG in prostate cancer *Semin. Nucl. Med.*

Sorace A G, Elkassem A A, Galgano S J, Lapi S E, Larimer B M, Partridge S C and Smith A D 2020 Imaging for response assessment in cancer clinical trials *Semin. Nucl. Med.* **50** 488–504

Stumpo V, Sebök M, van Niftrik C H B, Seystahl K, Hainc N, Kulcsar Z and Fierstra J 2022 Feasibility of glioblastoma tissue response mapping with physiologic BOLD imaging using precise oxygen and carbon dioxide challenge *Magn. Reson. Mater. Phys. Biol. Med.* **35** 29–44

Tan J, Lim Joon D, Fitt G, Wada M, Lim Joon M, Mercuri A and Khoo V 2010 The utility of multimodality imaging with CT and MRI in defining rectal tumour volumes for radiotherapy treatment planning: a pilot study *J. Med. Imaging Radiat. Oncol.* **54** 562–8

Tang L and Zhou X J 2019 Diffusion MRI of cancer: from low to high *b*-values *J. Magn. Reson. Imaging* **49** 23–40

Tinganelli W, Durante M, Hirayama R, Krämer M, Maier A, Kraft-Weyrather W and Scifoni E 2015 Kill-painting of hypoxic tumours in charged particle therapy *Sci. Rep.* **5** 1–13

Tinganelli W and Durante M 2020 Carbon ion radiobiology *Cancers* **12** 1–43

Trojanowska A, Trojanowski P, Drop A, Jargiełło T and Klatka J 2012 Head and neck cancer: value of perfusion CT in depicting primary tumour spread *Med. Sci. Monit.* **18** CR112

Uh J, Merchant T E, Conklin H M, Ismael Y, Li Y, Han Y and Hua C 2021 Diffusion tensor imaging-based analysis of baseline neurocognitive function and posttreatment white matter changes in pediatric patients with craniopharyngioma treated with surgery and proton therapy *Int. J. Radiat. Oncol. Biol. Phys.* **109** 515–26

Unterrainer M, Eze C, Ilhan H, Marschner S, Roengvoraphoj O, Schmidt-Hegemann N S and Belka C 2020 Recent advances of PET imaging in clinical radiation oncology *Radiat. Oncol.* **15** 88

Valable S, Gérault A N, Lambert G, Leblond M M, Anfray C, Toutain J and Pérès E A 2020 Impact of hypoxia on carbon ion therapy in glioblastoma cells: modulation by let and hypoxia-dependent genes *Cancers* **12** 1–15

van der Heide U A, Houweling A C, Groenendaal G, Beets-Tan R G H and Lambin P 2012 Functional MRI for radiotherapy dose painting *Magn. Reson. Imaging* **30** 1216–23

Wang C, Padgett K R, Su M Y, Mellon E A, Maziero D and Chang Z 2021 Multi-parametric MRI (mpMRI) for treatment response assessment of radiation therapy *Med. Phys.* **49** 2794–819

Welzel T, Meyerhof E, Uhl M, Huang K, von Deimling A, Herfarth K and Debus J 2018 Diagnostic accuracy of DW MR imaging in the differentiation of chordomas and chondrosarcomas of the skull base: a 3.0-T MRI study of 105 cases *Eur. J. Radiol.* **105** 119–24

White N S, Leergaard T B, D'Arceuil H, Bjaalie J G, Dale A M, NS W and AM D 2013 Probing tissue microstructure with restriction spectrum imaging: histological and theoretical validation *Human Brain Mapp.* **34** 327–46

Yasuda K, Takao S, Matsuo Y, Yoshimura T, Tamura M, Minatogawa H and Shirato H 2018 Intensity-modulated proton therapy with dose painting based on hypoxia imaging for nasopharyngeal cancer *Int J. Radiat. Oncol. Biol. Phys.* **102** e378

Zahra M A, Hollingsworth K G, Sala E, Lomas D J and Tan L T 2007 Dynamic contrast-enhanced MRI as a predictor of tumour response to radiotherapy *Lancet Oncol.* **8** 63–74

Zampini M A, Buizza G, Paganelli C, Fontana G, D'Ippolito E, Valvo F and Baroni G 2020 Perfusion and diffusion in meningioma tumours: a preliminary multiparametric analysis with dynamic susceptibility contrast and intraVoxel incoherent motion MRI *Magn. Reson. Imaging* **67** 69–78

Zhang Y, Fan B, Sun T, Xu J, Yin Y, Chen Z and Hu M 2022 The feasibility of dose escalation using intensity-modulated radiotherapy (IMRT) and intensity-modulated proton therapy (IMPT) with FDG PET/CT guided in esophageal cancer *J. Cancer Res. Therap.* **18** 1261–7

Zhang-Yin J T, Girard A and Bertaux M 2022 What does PET imaging bring to neuro-oncology in 2022? A review *Cancers* **14** 879

Zhou M, Zhou Y, Liao H, Rowland B C, Kong X, Arvold N D and Huang R Y 2018 Diagnostic accuracy of 2-hydroxyglutarate magnetic resonance spectroscopy in newly diagnosed brain mass and suspected recurrent gliomas *Neuro-Oncol.* **20** 1262–71

IOP Publishing

Imaging in Particle Therapy
Current practice and future trends
Chiara Paganelli, Chiara Gianoli and Antje Knopf

Chapter 12

Multi-scale modelling in particle therapy with quantitative imaging biomarkers

L Morelli, G Parrella, G Buizza, G Baroni and C Paganelli

12.1 Introduction

Particle therapy (PT) presents different advantages with respect to conventional x-ray radiotherapy (RT) for the treatment of deep-seated and radioresistant tumours. It allows one to achieve a conformal irradiation of the tumour while efficiently reducing the damage to surrounding healthy tissues. At the same time, clear benefits are brought by increased linear energy transfer (LET) and relative biological effectiveness (RBE), which turns into different effects produced at different scales (e.g., from clinical indications of local control or progression disease to biological DNA and cellular damage; Durante *et al* 2017, Tinganelli and Durante 2020, Byun *et al* 2021).

To define the dosimetric requirements and constraints in RT and PT, clinical trials on populations of patients are generally performed, supported by in-vitro experiments based on cell fraction survival in the context of in-vitro cell irradiation. This allows defining models descriptive of the radiobiological interaction and predictive of treatment outcomes (Brown *et al* 2014). Using the mechanistic linear-quadratic RBE formalism, estimates of the expected gain in tumour control probability (TCP) with respect to the risk of normal tissue complication probability (NTCP) are derived, with limited prediction power when applied prospectively (El Naqa *et al* 2012). This is because the individual tumour microstructure, its radio-sensitivity and the biological basis of its interaction with the radiation beam remain poorly described, especially in PT, and a relationship between different indicators of treatment outcome at a patient-specific level is elusive.

The use of medical imaging to guide RT and treatment decisions has gained an increasing attraction, leading to its development from a diagnostic into a treatment personalization tool. The recent interest in quantitative imaging biomarkers (QIBs) and their combination with mathematical models indeed provide strong evidence

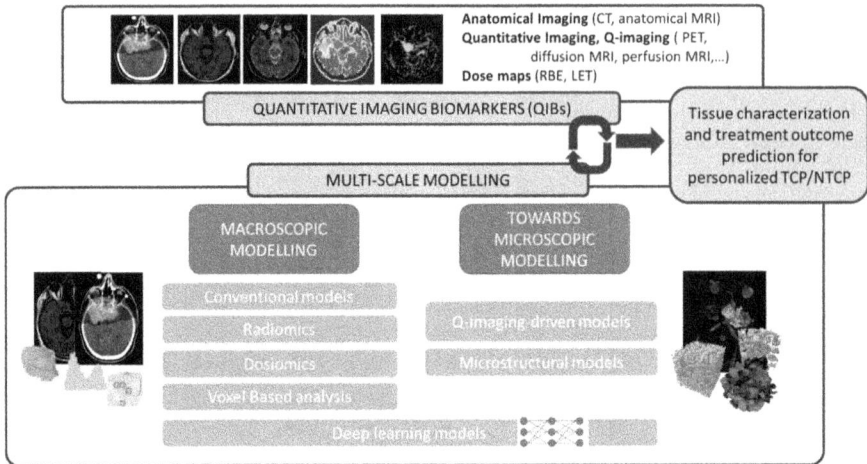

Figure 12.1. Schematic representation of multi-scale modelling with quantitative imaging biomarkers (QIBs).

that quantitative information derived from images can be clinically relevant to characterize tumours and predict their response to treatment (Jaffray 2012, O'Connor *et al* 2017).

In this chapter, we will describe modelling techniques based on QIBs for tissue characterization and treatment outcome prediction in PT, in terms of the spatial scale at which they act, aiming at revealing macroscopic (at the voxel level) and microscopic (at the sub-voxel level) properties on a patient-specific and multi-scale basis (figure 12.1). Hereafter, we will refer to QIBs as features extracted from any image modality (or more generally to any volumetric map, including dose maps), with a specific focus to high-dimensional signatures (e.g., textural radiomic features) with respect to first order statistics (e.g., as described in chapter 11).

12.2 Macroscopic modelling

12.2.1 Conventional models

The most straightforward approach to process quantitative information at the macro-scale consists of using conventional statistical approaches. These can be applied either directly to the imaging content, obtaining data-based QIBs at the macro-scale, or to quantitative imaging (Q-imaging) obtained downstream of modelling the acquired Q-imaging signal (e.g., Apparent Diffusion Coefficient, ADC, computed from diffusion-weighted MRI, DWI), obtaining model-based QIBs at the macro-scale, as those presented in chapter 11.

Typically, statistical approaches involving the use of histogram-based metrics are applied to the volumetric map to identify QIBs descriptive of changes that can be used for tumour characterization or treatment assessment. First-order statistics such as mean, median, extreme values and percentiles are the most widely investigated metrics but parameters capturing features at higher dimensionality like entropy, skewness and kurtosis are more recently being considered. Indeed, several studies are increasingly recognizing these histogram-based heterogeneity parameters to be very promising QIBs, able to better capture clinically valuable tissue characteristics compared to conventional metrics of central tendency (e.g., mean, median; Li *et al* 2022).

The derived QIBs can be then combined with traditional models based on statistics for patient stratification and prognostic factors discovery. Traditional modelling methods have been, however, recently flanked by machine learning approaches, among which Radiomics represents a quantitative paradigm (section 12.2.2). It should be also noted that QIBs directly extracted from Q-imaging can be the starting point to feed mechanistic formulations of TCP/NTCP (section 12.3.1), by exploiting the relationship of QIBs at the macro-scale (voxel level) with that at the micro-scale (sub-voxel).

12.2.2 Radiomics

Radiomics performs the automatic mining of data via extraction, analysis and modelling of medical image features to develop predictive models. The general hypothesis of radiomics is that imaging characteristics reflect physio-pathological tissue information, making it accessible in a quantitative and reproducible way (Lambin *et al* 2017).

The main steps of the radiomic pipeline are: standardized acquisition of imaging data, segmentation of the region of interest (ROI, e.g. tumour, organ at risk—OAR), image pre-processing (e.g., intensity discretization, filtering), extraction of high-dimensional quantitative features, analysis and modelling with respect to a pre-defined target.

The peculiar characteristic of radiomics is the extraction of features that describe multiple high-dimensional radiological characteristics at a macroscopic level, such as shape, intensity and textural patterns. Imaging features are thus expressed in a mineable way, potentially combined with complementary ones (e.g., clinical, demographic), and their relationship to the target outcome is evaluated through traditional statistical models or machine learning models to assist clinical decisions (Lambin *et al* 2017, Beaton *et al* 2019).

The segmentation of the volume of interest is a crucial first step in the radiomic workflow as it defines which voxels within an image are analyzed and thus can affect the derived radiomic features. Typically, manual or semi-automatic approaches are employed but fully automatic approaches performed with deep learning algorithms are emerging in order to overcome intra- and inter-observer variability hindering radiomic features reproducibility (Lambin *et al* 2017, van Timmeren *et al* 2020, Yang *et al* 2020). The second crucial step in the radiomic pipeline is image pre-processing, aimed at homogenizing characteristics of the images such as pixel spacing and grey level intensities. This step significantly affects the features extracted from the images (mostly texture features), and it is therefore essential to explicitly and carefully outline the parameters set in the pre-processing to ensure adequate reproducibility of the extracted QIBs. Among the various imaging modalities, this pre-processing partic-ularly affects modalities such as MRI in which images have arbitrary/relative grey level values (i.e., MR signal intensity), unlike images with defined absolute grey level values (e.g., Hounsfield Units in CT or Standardized Uptake Value in PET imaging; van Timmeren *et al* 2020). In addition, while imaging modalities such as CT and PET are standardized, MRI acquisitions are affected by a great variability in acquisition protocols, which negatively affects the reproducibility and robustness of features and thus makes MRI-based radiomics studies the most challenging (Scalco *et al* 2022). Finally, radiomic workflows typically must embed feature selection methods to reduce features' redundancy. Feature selection methods sometimes require a training phase too, and they typically affect the final performance of the model by defining the relevant subset of features to be used (Parmar *et al* 2015, van Timmeren *et al* 2020).

For any chosen strategy (i.e., statistical, or machine-learning based), a model (e.g., diagnostic, prognostic, or survival model) must undergo two fundamental stages: development and validation. Model development consists of estimating a model's parameters relying on a training dataset, whereas model validation refers to the assessment of the model's performance on unseen data. Internal validation is usually performed during model development by reserving part of the training dataset for validation purposes, usually with cross-validation schemes. Following these schemes, data is repeatedly used for either training or validation and the final performance is given by the aggregated performance over each repetition. External validation, instead, requires an independent dataset for evaluating the model's performance, typically following a hold-out scheme. In this case, an external dataset, acquired independently on the training dataset, is exploited to compute the model's performance and after that the training phase (Collins *et al* 2015) is concluded. It should also be highlighted that various strategies could be applied to sample the training data, balance the classes in the dataset or to augment data in case of a small dataset (Hatt *et al* 2019). As such, the implementation of different methods, and their combination, makes the comparison of different radiomic workflows hard.

Radiomics is widely applied in RT to improve patient stratification, tumour characterization, response assessment, to detect possible disease relapse and for assessing the risk of radiation-induced toxicities (Lambin *et al* 2017, Zhang *et al* 2022), also by adopting the radiomic features to implement personalized TCP/NTCP models. In this regard, a radiomic-based TCP/NTCP is commonly obtained by applying a multivariate logistic regression (e.g., with logit and probit functions) between relevant radiomic features extracted from the ROI, or a combination of them (i.e., radiomic score), and the predicted risk classes (El Naqa *et al* 2018, Desideri *et al* 2020, Coates *et al* 2021, Abdollahi *et al* 2022). An alternative approach would be to perform regression through machine learning approaches, such as Support Vector Machine, defining the TCP as the optimal hyperplane that separates the predicted risk classes (Gulliford 2015).

Very few studies based on radiomics have been reported to date in the literature with application in PT, mainly due to the difficulty of collecting a sufficient number of patient data with a homogenous protocol.

The study presented by Buizza *et al* (2021b) explored the role of multi-parametric radiomic, dosiomic and clinical features as prognostic factors for local recurrence in skull-base chordoma patients undergoing carbon ion radiotherapy. Anatomical

MRI and CT-based radiomic, and dosiomic features of 57 patients were selected and fed to two survival models, singularly or by combining them with clinical factors. Apart from the best model based on dosiomic features (that will be discussed in the following section) which achieved a concordance index (C-index) of 79% in the hold-out test set, multi-parametric radiomic and CT-based models resulted in a C-index above 65%, whereas MRI-based models presented the worst results, probably mainly due to imaging protocol inhomogeneities.

The potential of Q-imaging was also investigated in a preliminary study by Wu and colleagues (Wu *et al* 2019) on a small population of prostate patients treated with carbon ions, to explore the value of the pre-treatment MRI radiomic features in individualized prediction of the therapeutic response. Here, by combining the radiomic features of T2-weighted MRI and ADC maps from DWI, a support vector machine model was implemented and achieved high performance (area-under-curve of 88%).

Radiomic features extracted from anatomical and quantitative MRI have been also investigated in hierarchical networks for the evaluation of intracranial ependymoma patients in response to proton therapy (Dominietto *et al* 2019). Preliminary results showed that the complex network was able to identify the interface between tumour and healthy surrounded tissue, to segment intra-tumoural tissue heterogeneity and to identify effects in response to therapy (relapse or not of ependymoma) based on node hierarchies.

Nevertheless, all these studies are applied on limited datasets, thus further validation is required on wider populations.

12.2.3 Dosiomics

Recently, in addition to conventional imaging modalities, several studies proposed dose-based Radiomics approaches also called Dosiomics. Although dose maps are not properly an imaging modality, they can provide useful quantitative information for the development of prognostic and predictive models. Indeed, dosiomics allows high-dimensional analysis of dose distributions to characterize the delivered treatment via descriptors of spatial patterns in dose maps.

Dosiomics in RT has been successfully applied to predict treatment outcome outperforming both radiomics-based prognostic models (Wu *et al* 2020) and conventional dosimetric-based models (Murakami *et al* 2021) indicating a potential key role in advanced RT plan design. Dosiomics applied in RT also showed to have higher accuracy in the prediction of normal tissue complication probability (NTCP) than conventional clinical and dosimetric features, which do not incorporate spatial information of dose distribution and rely on the conventional point-wise parameters extracted from dose–volume histograms (DVH; Liang *et al* 2019, Lucia *et al* 2021, Puttanawarut *et al* 2021, Yang *et al* 2023).

In PT, dosiomic features from RBE-weighted maps have shown promising results outperforming MRI-based and CT-based Radiomics in terms of performance and generalization abilities when predicting the risk of adverse local control in skull-base chordoma treated with carbon ions (Buizza *et al* 2021b).

More recently, a dosiomics study applied to sacral chordoma treated with carbon ions reported RBE-weighted dose maps and dose-averaged LET distributions (LET_d) as sources of prognostic QIBs that can successfully predict local tumour recurrences, with LET_d-based models being the most predictive with respect to RBE-weighted maps and DVH parameters (Morelli *et al* 2023; figure 12.2). These results are also supported by recent studies based on conventional statistics-based modelling, highlighting LET_d metrics as predictors of local recurrences in chondrosarcoma and sacral chordoma (Matsumoto *et al* 2020, Molinelli *et al* 2021). The increasing evidence of LET_d being a physical quantity that relates well to treatment effectiveness brought to the development of LET-based optimization routines, that aim at maximizing LET within the target, while keeping the traditional constraints on RBE-weighted dose distributions. This approach could be customized to maximize high-LET particles in hypoxic regions moving towards a homogeneous cell killing over the target (i.e., kill-painting; Tinganelli *et al* 2015).

Moreover, the integration of dosiomic features (i.e., dosiomic score) into TCP/NTCP models is a promising approach that may improve their effectiveness for treatment evaluation (Liang *et al* 2019, Murakami *et al* 2021, Wu *et al* 2020), even if the robustness of such data-driven models in PT is still an open issue. Nonetheless, hybrid models including conventional dosimetric parameters (DVH-based) and dosiomic features could represent an effective alternative towards treatment personalization (Lucia *et al* 2021).

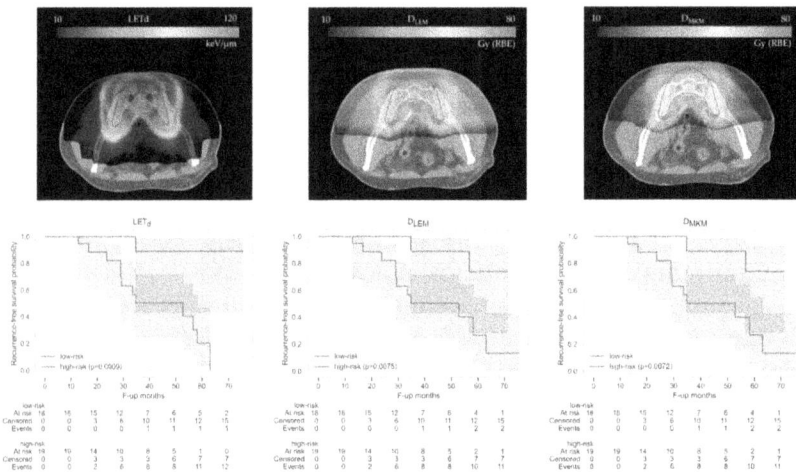

Figure 12.2. Kaplan–Meier survival curves for patients at high-(red) and low-risk (blue) of high dose local recurrences as stratified by r-Cox (Cox proportional hazards model regularized with an elastic net penalty) models using LET_d (left) D_{LEM} (middle—LEM, Local Effect Model), D_{MKM} (right—MKM, Microdosimetric Kinetic Model) features selected by LASSO (Least Absolute Shrinkage and Selection Operator Regression). Shaded areas show curves of 95% confidence intervals and the p-values obtained from the comparison between high- and low-risk patients are reported in the legend. Below the plot, the number of patients belonging to each risk group at specific time points (months) during follow-up (F-up) is reported. Figure adapted from Morelli *et al* (2023).

12.2.4 Voxel-based analysis

Recently, 2D or 3D methods for dose distribution analysis have been proposed to overcome the limitations of a DVH-based analysis on OARs, i.e., DVH implies (i) treating the OAR as a homogeneous entity in its response to radiation, losing its fine-structure biology, and (ii) the application of an organ-based approach that relies on an a-priori definition of the anatomical region involved in a given toxicity outcome. Those methods, collectively referred to as pixel- or voxel-based (VB) methods, evaluate local dose response patterns and go beyond the organ-based philosophy of NTCP modelling. Comprehensive reviews on VB methods in RT are reported by Palma *et al* (2020a) and Ebert *et al* (2021).

A VB analysis consists in the spatial normalization of the different anatomies in the analyzed cohort of patients to a common coordinate system (Palma *et al* 2020a). Spatial normalization is typically performed through Deformable Image Registration (DIR), which outputs a deformation vector field that is used to warp the correspondent dose maps to the common coordinate system, so that they can be directly compared point-by-point. Regions with significant correlations between a clinical outcome and the local dose release are identified by means of statistical inference on the spatial signature of dose response, which can be then incorporated in the NTCP formulation.

First studies on 2D methods for dose distribution analysis in PT were conducted on thoracic cancer patients (Palma *et al* 2020a) and brain tumour patients (Palma *et al* 2020b) treated with scanned proton therapy. In both studies, the relative dose–surface histogram of a tissue of interest (skin and scalp, respectively) was extracted and used for Lyman–Kutcher–Burman NTCP modelling. The 3D VB analysis was instead recently adopted to investigate thoracic dose–response patterns for pericardial effusion and mortality in patients treated for locally advanced non-small-cell lung cancer by intensity-modulated RT (IMRT) or passive-scanning proton therapy (PSPT; Cella *et al* 2021). Local dose differences between patients with and without pericardial effusion and mortality were investigated through the VB approach (figure 12.3). The analysis highlighted largely overlapping clusters significantly associated with pericardial effusion endpoints in the heart and lungs, while no significant dosimetric patterns related to mortality endpoints were found. A mismatch of dose patterns related to radiation-induced cardiac toxicity and the observed organ-based dose–response was also observed between PSPT and IMRT. Indeed, the thoracic regions spared by PSPT poorly overlapped with the areas involved in pericardial effusion development.

This approach has also found applications in PT to evaluate how much the proton RBE variability impacts proton therapy treatments and, in particular, outcome. This is of interest because, although the proton RBE is accounted for by using a fixed value of 1.1 in treatment planning and delivery, the RBE of protons varies depending on a combination of dose, endpoint, tissue radiosensitivity, and LET. A couple of retrospective studies considered post-treatment image changes as a surrogate for biological effect (Garbacz *et al* 2021, Bertolet *et al* 2022). These image changes, e.g., signal intensity variation on post-treatment MRI, were

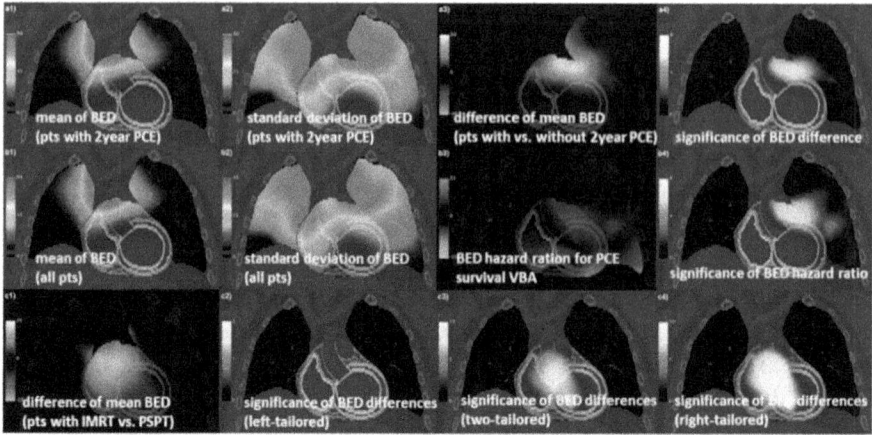

Figure 12.3. CT fused with the results of the voxel-based analyses (VB). Pts, patients; BED, biologically effective dose; PCE, pericardial effusion; IMRT, intensity-modulated radiation therapy; PSPT, passive-scanning proton therapy. Figure taken and adapted with permission from Cella *et al* (2021).

correlated at the voxel level through VB analysis with proton dose as well as LET, and used to model radiation effects. Some of these studies demonstrated a significant effect of dose and LET, while in others the effect was found to be non-significant (Garbacz *et al* 2021, Wagenaar *et al* 2021, Bertolet *et al* 2022), meaning that further investigations are required.

12.3 Towards microscopic modelling

12.3.1 Q-imaging-driven TCP/NTCP models

Appropriate modelling strategies can also leverage Q-imaging data to gain insights at the microscopic level by adopting the knowledge of microscopic tumour characteristics from QIBs to feed conventional mechanistic formulations of tissue-radiation interactions. Radiobiological models strongly depend on dose and radio-sensitivity parameters, as they are mostly derived from the observation of cell cultures response to radiation, with tumour microenvironment also found to have an impact (Webb and Nahum 1993).

Attempts to personalize these mechanistic formulations include using Q-imaging to define the probability of tumour presence and elective volumes as input to TCP models (Thorwarth *et al* 2017), or indirectly linking radiosensitivity to tumour aggressiveness with perfusion weighted MRI (PWI) (G. P. Chen *et al* 2007). However, since tissue radiosensitivity depends on many intertwined factors, a direct in-vivo non-invasive measurement capable of capturing intra- and inter-tumour heterogeneity is yet to be found (Mayo *et al* 2019).

Conventional statistical relationships, such as correlation, have been instead measured between DWI signals (or DWI-derived QIBs such as ADC) and histopathological features like cellularity or cell proliferation index (e.g., Ki-67 index; Ginat *et al* 2012, Surov *et al* 2017, Mayo *et al* 2019).

The information on cellularity distributions has been successfully exploited to obtain patient-specific TCP models in conventional RT (Casares-Magaz *et al* 2016, 2018) and PT (Buizza *et al* 2019). For this latter application, a personalized TCP model in skull-base chordoma patients treated with carbon ions was built by using DWI to infer the initial tumour cellular density. Although further improvement of the proposed model is required in terms of (i) providing a more robust relationship between cellular density and conventional ADC and (ii) considering radiosensitivity parameters of the particle beam, this study was one of the first attempts to derive personalized TCP models in PT and demonstrated that the inclusion of patient-specific DWI information provides a more conservative prediction of tumour control than a conventional approach, thus pushing towards dose escalation or boost strategies. A recent example in this direction was proposed by Köthe *et al* (2021), where hypoxia-based QIBs from PET were used to simulate a hypoxia-driven dose escalation protocol in non-small cell lung cancer patients treated with proton therapy. Results from this study suggest that both TCP and NTCP could benefit from such an approach.

12.3.2 Microstructural models

The adoption of routinely acquired Q-imaging to derive tissue properties by using a simple and conventional statistical approach, however, is constrained to the voxel dimension. More complex approaches, namely microstructural models, have been implemented to describe the biophysical properties of tissue microstructure from imaging data, aiming at estimating sub-voxel parameters, such as intracellular volume fraction or cell sizes. The main idea at the foundation of these models is to derive from the macroscopic scale (i.e., voxel-wise scale) a new layer of structural complexity at a finer scale, typically that of cellular dimensions (i.e., ~ 1–10 μm). These models simulate and then sum up diffusive (or other functional) dynamics over this finer layer, thus deriving the effect over a macroscopic voxel scale. In this way the measured macroscopic signal can be mapped onto the underlying structural complexity. In order to estimate the underlying tissue microstructure, Q-imaging signal representation and biophysical models are combined with assumptions (e.g., no exchange between intra- and extracellular compartments) and structural simplifications (e.g., cells modeled as spheres) that should be carefully chosen and designed because they may bias the estimation of the microstructural model (Afzali *et al* 2021).

Over the years, microstructural models were developed using a multi-compartmental approach in which the MRI signal is described as the sum of the contributions of several compartments, each representing a single structure that makes up the tissue. With multi-compartmental models, microstructural features can be estimated by fitting the biophysical model describing a specific tissue function to the measured MRI signal which can, for example, describe perfusion or diffusion phenomena (Tang and Zhou 2019, Afzali *et al* 2021, Novikov 2021). Multicompartmental models are, for example, applied to PWI, and in particular DCE-MRI, to investigate intra-tumour heterogeneity in terms of tumour vasculature and blood fractional volume (Chen *et al* 2011, Xie *et al* 2021). Similarly, multi-compartment models are implemented with DWI: the two-compartments Intra Voxel Incoherent Motion (IVIM; le Bihan 2019) model can describe free diffusion in the tissue and perfusion in the blood capillary network; VERDICT (Panagiotaki *et al* 2014) instead is a three-compartment model able to discriminate the contribution of water trapped in cells, water in the vascular network and interstitial water in the DWI signal, to estimate tissue properties such as the size and packing density of cells, and vascular as well as extracellular-extravascular space volume fractions (Panagiotaki *et al* 2014, Johnston *et al* 2019, Sen *et al* 2022). Despite the great potential, the greatest limitation of advanced microstructural models like VERDICT or others (e.g., multi-compartmental Restriction Spectrum Imaging) remains the challenging clinical application in RT/PT settings, due to the need for long acquisition time and dedicated MRI sequences that cannot be widely implemented on MR scanners employed for RT/PT.

Besides multi-compartmental approaches for microscopic modelling, recent intriguing developments focused on the use of Monte Carlo (MC) simulations of MRI signals. Specifically, digital synthetic substrates can be generated to reproduce tissue microenvironments. MRI signals can then be generated from them and used to estimate which specific structure provides a given signal at the macroscopic scale. Simplifications of geometries and shapes of the structures (e.g., modeled as cylinders, spheres, ellipsoids) are combined with assumptions on tissue properties (e.g., diffusivity, permeability, and dispersion) to generate realistic synthetic substrates. Most applications of such microstructural models are developed in the context of neurodegenerative diseases (Afzali *et al* 2021, Novikov 2021).

More recently, few studies started to explore these models for tumour character-ization and treatment outcome prediction in PT (Buizza *et al* 2021a, Morelli *et al* 2023). Specifically, they performed MC simulations of conventional DWI from synthetic substrates mimicking a tumour cell packing as an aggregate of spheres and ellipsoids with well-defined density and functional characteristics. Starting from these simulations, machine-learning-based models were proposed to map the signal measured at the macroscopic scale (voxel level) to those simulated from the substrates. Through this mapping, the microstructural features that best matched the simulated signal (on substrates) to the measured signal (on voxels of patients' images) were estimated. Extracted microstructural features describing cell radius, intra/extracellular volume fraction, diffusivity, and cell density were found to be promising QIBs for tumour characterization and prediction of local recurrence after PT (figure 12.4). Overall, microstructural models such as these, employing simu-lations to extract information on tumour microenvironment from conventional MRI sequences, would allow the investigation of microstructural features before, during, and after PT treatment, even in contexts in which more complex imaging acquisitions and multi-compartmental models are not feasible.

In addition to the possibility of characterizing the sub-voxel morphology of the tumour microenvironment, modelling the dynamics of blood microcirculation during RT has recently gained attention. Specifically, a 4D blood flow model was implemented starting from high-resolution T1- and T2-weighted MRI scans of the

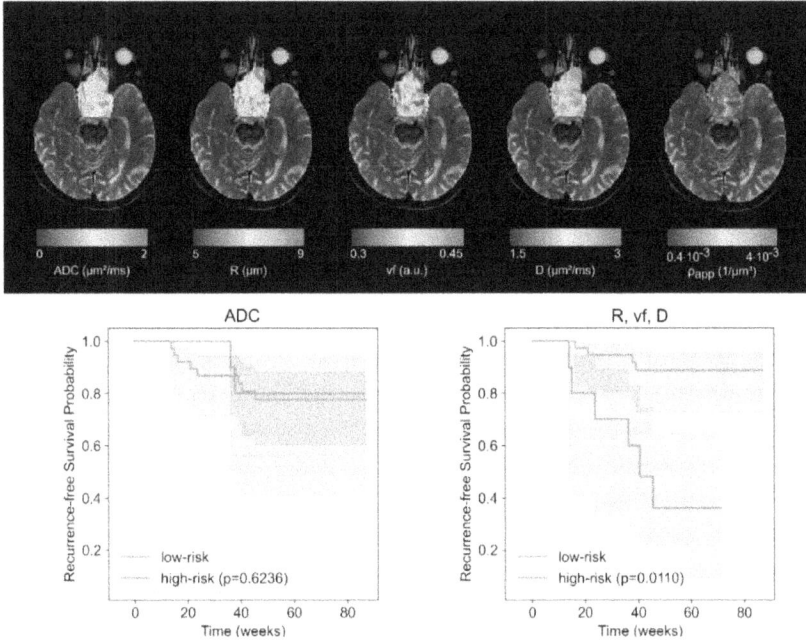

Figure 12.4. Example of microstructural maps (R, vf, D, and ρ_{app}) derived from measured ADC data (top). Kaplan–Meier survival curves for patients at high-(red) and low-risk (green) of a local tumour recurrence as stratified by Cox-Proportional-Hazards models (bottom). Displayed recurrence-free survival curves are estimated from entropy values of ADC (left) and microstructural parameters (R, vf, D, right). Shaded areas show curves 95% confidence intervals and the p-values obtained from the comparison between high- and low-risk patients are reported in the legends. ADC, apparent diffusion coefficient ($\mu m^2/ms$); R, cell radius (μm); vf, intra/extracellular volume fraction (a.u.); D, diffusivity ($\mu m^2/ms$); ρ_{app}, apparent cellularity ($1/\mu m^3$). Adapted from Morelli, *et al* (2023).

brain with the goal of tracking the blood fractional volume circulating during the irradiation and the resulting accumulated dose. The blood flow model has been successfully applied to compare dose accumulation in circulating blood in photon and proton therapy, investigating its impact on radiation-induced lymphopenia under different delivery conditions (Hammi *et al* 2020). Blood flow models such as this could then be employed for a more comprehensive tumour characterization towards tailored treatments, e.g., deriving in-vivo radiosensitivity information of circulating lymphocytes (McCullum *et al* 2023). Another parameter of interest to model is tumour hypoxia, as hypoxia is typically associated to radiosensitivity. An intriguing approach has been proposed by Schiavo *et al* (2022, 2023b), which implemented an in-silico tumour model simulating realistic 3D microvascular structures and related oxygenation maps, featuring regions with different levels and typologies of hypoxia (chronic, acute and anemic). Such model, if integrated into a treatment planning system, could allow evaluations and comparisons of various scenarios when deciding the therapy to administer (Schiavo *et al* 2023a).

12.4 Deep learning modelling

In recent years, a growing interest in deep learning (DL) has shown the potential of this methodology as a way to improve the radiomics' workflow, or speed-up expensive simulation methods such as MC. Indeed, neural networks could be directly fed with raw data and trained to perform end-to-end tasks, replacing the whole radiomics workflow which is often subject to variabilities due to image processing, segmentation and feature extraction (Coates *et al* 2021, Zhang *et al* 2022). Alternatively, DL methods could be integrated into the pipeline to include new DL-based features (Lao *et al* 2017, Cho *et al* 2021), or just standardize the image processing and segmentation steps (Scalco *et al* 2022, Zhang *et al* 2022) as they are able to learn tissue features with powerful characterization capabilities and without human intervention. In this context, the predictive performance of the network could also benefit from the intrinsic nonlinearity of neural networks against the use of linear survival models, such as the widely used Cox-net (i.e., Cox proportional hazard model with elastic net penalty).

DL algorithms are typically network architectures composed of three or more layers, and the actual learning phase takes place in the hidden layers, requiring many training samples to build robust models (Zhang *et al* 2022). Overall, DL algorithms can be classified into generative and discriminative. When using generative algorithms (e.g., generative adversarial networks, GAN), the conditional probabilities of the various output labels are calculated and, from these, the category with the highest probability is selected as the predicted result. Discriminative algorithms (e.g., convolutional neural networks, CNN), instead, are aimed at directly learning the relationship between input and output.

Tumour tissue identification and automatic contouring of target and OAR volumes are two of the widest applications of DL in RT settings (Tong *et al* 2018, Ye *et al* 2020, Zeineldin *et al* 2020). In addition, a large number of DL applications for RT treatment assessment are aimed at predicting local recurrence and radiation-induced toxicities (Men *et al* 2019, Gao *et al* 2020, Huang *et al* 2021, Appelt *et al* 2022, Tanaka *et al* 2022). The inclusion of time-to-event information in DL architectures allowed to move from the sole patient stratification tasks (Hosny *et al* 2018) (i.e., binary classification, prediction) to survival analysis, being able to estimate survival curves and discrete event probabilities on a patient-specific basis (Lombardo *et al* 2021). In this field, increased evidence in the literature shows survival networks to outperform conventional ML survival models (e.g., Cox-net) for head and neck, lung and pancreatic adenocarcinoma (Diamant *et al* 2019, Kim *et al* 2020, Zhang *et al* 2020). Finally, more recent studies are exploring the application of DL to generate optimized dose plans based on a pre-specified trade-off between PTV coverage and OAR sparing (Huang *et al* 2021, Ma *et al* 2021). Up to now, however, a very limited number of studies on DL were applied to PT, with most of them focusing on the generation of synthetic CT for treatment plan optimization and adaptation (as described in chapter 8).

Similarly, microstructural modelling can benefit from the advantages provided by DL, although most of the applications in the literature do not apply to the RT/PT context. For example, in multi-compartmental models in which the MR signal is fitted to estimate certain parameters (e.g., IVIM model), different fitting algorithms may be characterized by variabilities that may bias the final estimates. Specifically, different fitting algorithms (e.g., Bayesian, Least-Squares) may be associated with different fitting times, inter-subject variability, robustness to noise and outliers, precision, and accuracy. For these reasons, authors started to explore the use of neural networks to estimate microstructural parameters, demonstrating superiority over conventional fitting methods and pushing toward greater performance and robustness for clinical applications (Bertleff *et al* 2017, Barbieri *et al* 2020, de Almeida Martins *et al* 2021). In addition, the possibility of integrating previously trained networks directly into MRI scanners could lead toward an almost real-time use of microstructural parameters during (or immediately downstream of) patient acquisition (Barbieri *et al* 2020).

Deep learning can be also applied to bridge the gap between experimental and clinical applications through Image Quality Transfer techniques (Alexander *et al* 2017). These are aimed to map 'low-quality' (e.g., clinical) images onto 'high-quality' (e.g., experimental) images to gain improved features of interest, such as the spatial resolution or the scale of the information content. Indeed, starting from simulated data or dictionaries of high-quality data, authors are investigating the possibility of employing DL to extend microstructural models (e.g., VERDICT or others) to conventional MRI sequences that are fast and compatible with standard clinical protocols (Alexander *et al* 2017, Chiou *et al* 2021).

12.5 Challenges and future perspectives

Integrating patient-specific imaging with advanced mathematical models revealing macroscopic, microscopic and radiobiological information can provide the empowerment of patients' stratification, treatment outcome prediction and subsequent treatment optimization and personalization in PT. However, different challenges still prevent a straightforward implementation of multi-scale modelling with QIBs in clinical practice.

Even if the radiomics paradigm has recently gained noticeable momentum with promising perspectives for personalized TCP and NTCP modelling, variabilities in data acquisition are dominant in RT/PT settings. This aspect could be mitigated by the adoption of quantitative protocols or by post-processing harmonization techniques (Da-ano *et al* 2020), as well as strategies to investigate the impact of imaging parameters on radiomic features (Molina *et al* 2017). At the same time, efforts towards standardization of algorithmic implementations (Zwanenburg *et al* 2020) and transparency in reporting results (Collins *et al* 2015) are required. In this regard, the radiomics quality score (RQS) introduced by Lambin *et al* (2017), which includes criteria to reward and penalize the methodology and analyses, should be assessed in radiomics-based studies towards homogeneous evaluation and reporting guidelines.

Similarly, the dosiomics paradigm needs analogous countermeasures. The results reported up to now, where dosiomics seems to be more promising than radiomics in PT, may be due to the higher standardization of the dose protocol for the investigated patient cohorts than anatomical/quantitative imaging acquisition protocols. However, attention should be paid also to the dose maps on which the analysis is performed, as, for example, different radiobiological models are adopted in different PT centers and a generalization of the results cannot be directly made and should be carefully evaluated (Buizza *et al* 2021b). In this perspective, dosiomics performed on LET could support generalization as LET does not strongly depend on radiobiological models adopted at different facilities, as biological doses do (Morelli *et al* 2023).

Another approach that is put forward to the refinement of the traditional NTCP strategies towards personalized RT plans is that of the VB approach, which consists in the spatial correlation of RT outcomes and delivered dose. This approach already demonstrated promising results, but the underlying mathematical modelling requires proper evaluation, to account for the accuracy of deformable image registration algorithms adopted, the potential overfitting of the statistical analysis and the sensitivity to organ motion (Palma *et al* 2020a).

In this regard, end-to-end analyses with deep learning methods are put forward to overcome most issues of the above-mentioned macroscopic modelling, starting from the variability in image processing and segmentation, to intensity discretization and feature extraction. However, a factor to take into consideration when dealing with radiomics, dosiomics, voxel-based analysis and deep learning, is the need for large high-quality datasets and multi-centric studies, which is already challenging in RT and becomes a huge obstacle in PT. This could be counteracted by data augmentation or transfer learning techniques (Hatt *et al* 2019), which however introduce additional issues.

Also, the thorough validation of high-dimensional features (O'Connor *et al* 2017) and models (Zwanenburg and Löck 2018) is a mandatory step before signatures can be safely adopted in clinical settings, as discussed in chapter 11. A common issue of traditional and machine learning approaches based on radiological imaging, other than the limited power in case of small dataset, is that they do not directly provide an explanation of the underlying biophysical phenomena and may be implemented as accompanying approaches to translational research (Vogelius *et al* 2020). Proper technical, clinical and biological validation is required to adopt imaging features for clinical decision-making (O'Connor *et al* 2017). The integration of molecular information could help bridging the gap between the radiological macroscopic scale and the microscopic level at which genomic phenotyping is defined, but the field of radiogenomics is not yet mature to support clinical applications (Sala *et al* 2017, Coates *et al* 2021).

Adopting QIBs towards microscopic modelling has opened new perspectives for a direct, non-invasive, in-vivo description of tissue at the micro-scale and of its interaction with the radiation beam, but proper validation is required also in this case. To assess the performance of models at the microscopic scale, different approaches can be used, including: (i) numerical analyses to investigate the robustness of parameters under ideal conditions or with different noise levels, (ii) physical phantoms representing a simplified tissues to test the model parameters on an ideal sample that can be investigated by conventional microscopy approaches, (iii) ex-vivo measures that, combined with microscopy, provide a direct microstructure validation (Afzali *et al* 2021).

Other limitations when working at the microscopic scale are the assumptions and simplifications built in the models. As an example, the substrates mimicking cellular packings as a collection of spheres or ellipsoids are not complex enough to simulate a realistic tissue microstructure. To mitigate this, solutions could include to augment cellular packings with more detailed components, such as vessels, incorporate dynamics of blood microcirculation (Hammi *et al* 2020, McCullum *et al* 2023) and tumour hypoxia (Schiavo *et al* 2022, 2023b), and integrate simulations of radiation-tissue interactions. Recent and ongoing efforts in realistic Monte Carlo-based simulations allow modelling radiation-tissue effects from the patient to the DNA scale (e.g., Geant4-DNA (Incerti *et al* 2010), TOPAS-nBio (Schuemann *et al* 2019)), also including radiation-initiated chemical reactions. Such tools enable multi-scale numerical simulations and could couple the current understanding of macroscopic and microscopic radiation-tissue interactions.

In this context, DL could also play a relevant role to support the high computational costs of simulations, to overcome technical limitations of microstructural modelling and to derive useful information at the microscopic scale also when complex and long imaging acquisitions are not available or compatible with clinical protocols.

In conclusion, when proper imaging protocols and well-structured datasets are available in PT, macro-scale and micro-scale modelling together with deep learning strategies are put forward to support PT and boost the development of new technologies, such as FLASH and minibeams (El Naqa *et al* 2022, Schneider 2022, Atkinson *et al* 2023), towards tailored treatment plan design and, thus, improved patients' outcomes (El Naqa *et al* 2012).

References

Abdollahi H, Chin E, Clark H, Hyde D E, Thomas S, Wu J, Uribe C F and Rahmim A 2022 Radiomics-guided radiation therapy: opportunities and challenges *Phys. Med. Biol.* **67** 12TR02

Afzali M, Pieciak T, Newman S, Garyfallidis E, Özarslan E, Cheng H and Jones D K 2021 The sensitivity of diffusion MRI to microstructural properties and experimental factors *J. Neurosci. Methods* **347** 108951

Alexander D C *et al* 2017 Image quality transfer and applications in diffusion MRI *NeuroImage* **152** 283–98

Appelt A L, Elhaminia B, Gooya A, Gilbert A and Nix M 2022 Deep Learning for Radiotherapy outcome prediction using dose data—a review *Clin. Oncol.* **34** e87–96

Atkinson J, Bezak E, Le H and Kempson I 2023 The current status of FLASH particle therapy: a systematic review *Phys. Eng. Sci. Med.* **46** 529–60

Barbieri S, Gurney-Champion O J, Klaassen R and Thoeny H C 2020 Deep learning how to fit an intravoxel incoherent motion model to diffusion-weighted MRI *Magn. Reson. Med.* **83** 312–21

Beaton L, Bandula S, Gaze M N and Sharma R A 2019 How rapid advances in imaging are defining the future of precision radiation oncology *Br. J. Cancer* **120** 779–90

Bertleff M, Domsch S, Weingärtner S, Zapp J, O'Brien K, Barth M and Schad L R 2017 Diffusion parameter mapping with the combined intravoxel incoherent motion and kurtosis model using artificial neural networks at 3 T *NMR Biomed.* **30** e3833

Bertolet A, Abolfath R, Carlson D J, Lustig R A, Hill-Kayser C, Alonso-Basanta M and Carabe A 2022 Correlation of LET with MRI changes in brain and potential implications for normal tissue complication probability for patients with meningioma treated with pencil beam scanning proton therapy *Int. J. Radiat. Oncol. Biol. Phys.* **112** 237–46

Brown J M, Carlson D J and Brenner D J 2014 The tumor radiobiology of SRS and SBRT: Are more than the 5 Rs involved? *Int. J. Radiat. Oncol. Biol. Phys.* **88** 254–62

Buizza G, Molinelli S, D'Ippolito E, Fontana G, Pella A, Valvo F, Preda L, Orecchia R, Baroni G and Paganelli C 2019 MRI-based tumour control probability in skull-base chordomas treated with carbon-ion therapy *Radiother. Oncol.* **137** 32–7

Buizza G, Paganelli C, Ballati F, Sacco S, Preda L, Iannalfi A, Alexander D C, Baroni G, Palombo M and Sciences P 2021a Improving the characterization of meningioma microstructure in proton therapy from conventional apparent diffusion coefficient measurements using Monte Carlo simulations of diffusion MRI *Med. Phys.* **48** 1250–61

Buizza G *et al* 2021b Radiomics and dosiomics for predicting local control after carbon-ion radiotherapy in skull-base chordoma *Cancers* **13** 1–15

Byun H K, Han M C, Yang K, Kim J S, Yoo G S, Koom W S and Kim Y B 2021 Physical and biological characteristics of particle therapy for oncologists *Cancer Res. Treat.* **53** 611–20

Casares-Magaz O, Raidou R G, Rørvik J, Vilanova A and Muren L P 2018 Uncertainty evaluation of image-based tumour control probability models in radiotherapy of prostate cancer using a visual analytic tool *Phys. Imaging Radiat. Oncol.* **5** 5–8

Casares-Magaz O, van der Heide U A, Rørvik J, Steenbergen P and Muren L P 2016 A tumour control probability model for radiotherapy of prostate cancer using magnetic resonance imaging-based apparent diffusion coefficient maps *Radiother. Oncol.* **119** 111–6

Cella L, Monti S, Xu T, Liuzzi R, Stanzione A, Durante M, Mohan R, Liao Z and Palma G 2021 Probing thoracic dose patterns associated to pericardial effusion and mortality in patients treated with photons and protons for locally advanced non-small-cell lung cancer *Radiother. Oncol.* **160** 148–58

Chen G P, Ahunbay E, Schultz C and Li X A 2007 Development of an inverse optimization package to plan nonuniform dose distributions based on spatially inhomogeneous radio-sensitivity extracted from biological images *Med. Phys.* **34** 1198–205

Chen L, Choyke P L, Chan T H, Chi C Y, Wang G and Wang Y 2011 Tissue-specific compartmental analysis for dynamic contrast-enhanced MR imaging of complex tumors *IEEE Trans. Med. Imaging* **30** 2044–58

Chiou E, Valindria V, Giganti F, Punwani S, Kokkinos I and Panagiotaki E 2021 Synthesizing VERDICT maps from standard DWI data using GANs *Lecture Notes in Computer Science (Including Subseries Lecture Notes in Artificial Intelligence and Lecture Notes in Bioinformatics)* **13006 LNCS** 58–67

Cho H H, Lee H Y, Kim E, Lee G, Kim J, Kwon J and Park H 2021 Radiomics-guided deep neural networks stratify lung adenocarcinoma prognosis from CT scans *Commun. Biol.* **4** 1–12

Chang S, Liu G, Zhao L, Dilworth J T, Zheng W, Jawad S, Yan D, Chen P, Stevens C and Kabolizadeh P 2020 Feasibility study: spot-scanning proton arc therapy (SPArc) for left-sided whole breast radiotherapy *Radiat. Oncol.* **15** 1–11

Coates J T T, Pirovano G and El Naqa I 2021 Radiomic and radiogenomic modeling for radiotherapy: strategies, pitfalls, and challenges *J. Med. Imaging* **8** 031902

Collins G S, Reitsma J B, Altman D G and Moons K G M 2015 Transparent reporting of a multivariable prediction model for individual prognosis or diagnosis (TRIPOD) the TRIPOD statement *Circulation* **131** 211–9

Da-ano R *et al* 2020 Performance comparison of modified ComBat for harmonization of radiomic features for multicenter studies *Sci. Rep.* **10** 1–12

de Almeida Martins J P, Nilsson M, Lampinen B, Palombo M, While P T, Westin C F and Szczepankiewicz F 2021 Neural networks for parameter estimation in microstructural MRI: application to a diffusion-relaxation model of white matter *NeuroImage* **244** 118601

Desideri I, Loi M, Francolini G, Becherini C, Livi L and Bonomo P 2020 Application of radiomics for the prediction of radiation-induced toxicity in the IMRT Era: current state-of-the-art *Front. Oncol.* **10** 1708

Diamant A, Chatterjee A, Vallières M, Shenouda G and Seuntjens J 2019 Deep learning in head and neck cancer outcome prediction *Sci. Rep.* **9** 1–10

Dominietto M, Pica A, Safai S, Lomax A J, Weber D C and Capobianco E 2019 Role of complex networks for integrating medical images and radiomic features of intracranial ependymoma patients in response to proton radiotherapy *Front. Med.* **6** 333

Durante M, Orecchia R and Loeffler J S 2017 Charged-particle therapy in cancer: clinical uses and future perspectives *Nat. Rev. Clin. Oncol.* **14** 483–95

Ebert M A, Gulliford S, Acosta O, de Crevoisier R, McNutt T, Heemsbergen W D, Witte M, Palma G, Rancati T and Fiorino C 2021 Spatial descriptions of radiotherapy dose: normal tissue complication models and statistical associations *Phys. Med. Biol.* **66** 12TR01

El Naqa I, Pandey G, Aerts H, Chien J T, Andreassen C N, Niemierko A and ten Haken R K 2018 Radiation therapy outcomes models in the era of radiomics and radiogenomics: uncertainties and validation *Int. J. Radiat. Oncol. Biol. Phys.* **102** 1070–3

El Naqa I, Pater P and Seuntjens J 2012 Monte Carlo role in radiobiological modelling of radiotherapy outcomes *Phys. Med. Biol.* **57** 75–97

El Naqa I, Pogue B W, Zhang R, Oraiqat I and Parodi K 2022 Image guidance for FLASH radiotherapy *Med. Phys.* **49** 4109–22

Gao Y *et al* 2020 Deep learning methodology for differentiating glioma recurrence from radiation necrosis using multimodal magnetic resonance imaging: Algorithm development and validation *JMIR Med. Inform.* **8** e19805

Garbacz M *et al* 2021 Study of relationship between dose, LET and the risk of brain necrosis after proton therapy for skull base tumors *Radiother. Oncol.* **163** 143–9

Ginat D T, Mangla R, Yeaney G, Johnson M and Ekholm S 2012 Diffusion-weighted imaging for differentiating benign from malignant skull lesions and correlation with cell density *Am. J. Roentgenol.* **198** W597–601

Grau C, Baumann M and Weber D C 2018 Optimizing clinical research and generating prospective high-quality data in particle therapy in Europe: introducing the European particle therapy network (EPTN) *Radiother. Oncol.* **128** 1–3

Grau C, Durante M, Georg D, Langendijk J A and Weber D C 2020 Particle therapy in Europe. *Mol. Oncol.* **14** 1492–9

Gurney-Champion O J, Mahmood F, van Schie M, Julian R, George B, Philippens M E, van der Heide U A, Thorwarth D and Redalen K R 2020 Quantitative imaging for radiotherapy purposes *Radiother. Oncol.* **146** 66–75

Gulliford S 2015 Modelling of normal tissue complication probabilities (NTCP): review of application of machine learning in predicting NTCP *Machine Learning in Radiation Oncology* (Cham: Springer International Publishing) pp 277–310

Hammi A, Paganetti H and Grassberger C 2020 4D blood flow model for dose calculation to circulating blood and lymphocytes *Phys. Med. Biol.* **65** 055008

Hatt M, le Rest C C, Tixier F, Badic B, Schick U and Visvikis D 2019 Radiomics: data are also images *J. Nucl. Med.* **60** 38S–44S

Hoffmann A, Oborn B, Moteabbed M, Yan S, Bortfeld T, Knopf A, Fuchs H, Georg D, Seco J and Spadea M F 2020 MR-guided proton therapy: a review and a preview *Radiat. Oncol.* **15** 1–13

Hosny A, Parmar C, Coroller T P, Grossmann P, Zeleznik R, Kumar A, Bussink J, Gillies R J, Mak R H and Aerts H J W L 2018 Deep learning for lung cancer prognostication: a retrospective multi-cohort radiomics study *PLoS Med.* **15** e1002711

https://www.aapm.org/

https://www.ptcog.site/

Huang D, Bai H, Wang L, Hou Y, Li L, Xia Y, Yan Z, Chen W, Chang L and Li W 2021 The application and development of deep learning in radiotherapy: a systematic review *Technol. Cancer Res. Treat.* **20** 15330338211016386

Incerti S *et al* 2010 THE Geant4-DNA project *Int. J. Mod. Simul. Sci. Comput.* **1** 157–78

Jaffray D A 2012 Image-guided radiotherapy: from current concept to future perspectives *Nat. Rev. Clin. Oncol.* **9** 688–99

Johnston E W *et al* 2019 VERDICT MRI for prostate cancer: intracellular volume fraction versus apparent diffusion coefficient *Radiology* **291** 391–7

Keall P J, Brighi C, Glide-Hurst C, Liney G, Liu P Z, Lydiard S, Paganelli C, Pham T, Shan S and Tree A C 2022 Integrated MRI-guided radiotherapy—opportunities and challenges *Nat. Rev. Clinical Oncology* **19** 458–70

Kishan A U, Ma T M, Lamb J M, Casado M, Wilhalme H, Low D A, Sheng K, Sharma S, Nickols N G and Pham J 2023 Magnetic resonance imaging–guided vs computed tomography–guided stereotactic body radiotherapy for prostate cancer: the MIRAGE randomized clinical trial *JAMA Oncol.* **9** 365–73

Kim H, Mo Goo J, Hee Lee K, Kim Y T and Park C M 2020 Preoperative ct-based deep learning model for predicting disease-free survival in patients with lung adenocarcinomas *Radiology* **296** 216–24

Köthe A, Bizzocchi N, Safai S, Lomax A J, Weber D C and Fattori G 2021 Investigating the potential of proton therapy for hypoxia-targeted dose escalation in non-small cell lung cancer *Radiat. Oncol.* **16** 199

Krieger M, Giger A, Salomir R, Bieri O, Celicanin Z, Cattin P C, Lomax A J, Weber D C and Zhang Y 2020 Impact of internal target volume definition for pencil beam scanned proton treatment planning in the presence of respiratory motion variability for lung cancer: a proof of concept *Radiother. Oncol.* **145** 154–61

Lambin P *et al* 2017 Radiomics: the bridge between medical imaging and personalized medicine *Nat. Rev. Clin. Oncol.* **14** 749–62

Lao J, Chen Y, Li Z C, Li Q, Zhang J, Liu J and Zhai G 2017 A deep learning-based radiomics model for prediction of survival in glioblastoma multiforme *Sci. Rep.* **7** 1–8

Lambin P, Leijenaar R T, Deist T M, Peerlings J, De Jong E E, Van Timmeren J, Sanduleanu S, Larue R T, Even A J and Jochems A 2017 Radiomics: the bridge between medical imaging and personalized medicine *Nat. Rev. Clin. Oncol.* **14** 749–62

Landry G and Hua C 2018 Current state and future applications of radiological image guidance for particle therapy *Med. Phys.* **45** e1086–95

Landry G, Kurz C and Traverso A 2023 The role of artificial intelligence in radiotherapy clinical practice *BJR| Open* **5** 0030

le Bihan D 2019 What can we see with IVIM MRI? *NeuroImage* **187** 56–67

Li H H, Sun B, Tan C, Li R, Fu C X, Grimm R, Zhu H and Peng W J 2022 The value of whole-tumor histogram and texture analysis using intravoxel incoherent motion in differentiating pathologic subtypes of locally advanced gastric cancer *Front. Oncol.* **12** 1

Liang B *et al* 2020 Online daily adaptive proton therapy *Br. J. Radiol.* **93** 20190594

Liang B, Yan H, Tian Y, Chen X, Yan L, Zhang T, Zhou Z, Wang L and Dai J 2019 Dosiomics: extracting 3D spatial features from dose distribution to predict incidence of radiation pneumonitis *Front. Oncol.* **9** 269

Lombardo E *et al* 2021 Distant metastasis time to event analysis with CNNs in independent head and neck cancer cohorts *Sci. Rep.* **11** 1–12

Lucia F *et al* 2021 Radiomics analysis of 3D dose distributions to predict toxicity of radiotherapy for cervical cancer *J. Pers. Med.* **11** 398

Ma J, Nguyen D, Bai T, Folkerts M, Jia X, Lu W, Zhou L and Jiang S 2021 A feasibility study on deep learning-based individualized 3D dose distribution prediction *Med. Phys.* **48** 4438–47

Matsumoto S *et al* 2020 Unresectable chondrosarcomas treated with carbon ion radiotherapy: relationship between dose-averaged linear energy transfer and local recurrence *Anticancer Res.* **40** 6429–35

Mayo T, Haderlein M, Schuster B, Wiesmüller A, Hummel C, Bachl M, Schmidt M, Fietkau R and Distel L 2019 Is in vivo and ex vivo irradiation equally reliable for individual radiosensitivity testing by three colour fluorescence in situ hybridization? *Radiat. Oncol.* **15** 1–9

McCullum L *et al* 2023 Predicting severity of radiation induced Lymphopenia in individual proton therapy patients for varying dose rate and fractionation using dynamic 4-dimensional blood flow simulations *Int. J. Radiat. Oncol. Biol. Phys.* **116** 1226–33

Men K, Geng H, Zhong H, Fan Y, Lin A and Xiao Y 2019 A deep learning model for predicting Xerostomia Due to radiation therapy for head and neck squamous cell carcinoma in the RTOG 0522 clinical trial *Int. J. Radiat. Oncol. Biol. Phys.* **105** 440–7

Meijers A, Jakobi A, Stützer K, Guterres Marmitt G, Both S, Langendijk J, Richter C and Knopf A 2019 Log file-based dose reconstruction and accumulation for 4D adaptive pencil beam scanned proton therapy in a clinical treatment planning system: Implementation and proof-of-concept *Med. Phys.* **46** 1140–9

Meschini G, Seregni M, Molinelli S, Vai A, Phillips J, Sharp G C, Pella A, Valvo F, Ciocca M and Riboldi M 2019 Validation of a model for physical dose variations in irregularly moving targets treated with carbon ion beams *Med. Phys.* **46** 3663–73

Meschini G, Vai A, Barcellini A, Fontana G, Molinelli S, Mastella E, Pella A, Vitolo V, Imparato S and Orlandi E 2022 Time-resolved MRI for off-line treatment robustness evaluation in carbon-ion radiotherapy of pancreatic cancer *Med. Phys.* **49** 2386–95

Meschini G, Vai A, Paganelli C, Molinelli S, Fontana G, Pella A, Preda L, Vitolo V, Valvo F and Ciocca M 2020 Virtual 4DCT from 4DMRI for the management of respiratory motion in carbon ion therapy of abdominal tumors *Med. Phys.* **47** 909–16

Morelli L, Parrella G, Molinelli S, Magro G, Annunziata S, Mairani A, Chalaszczyk A, Fiore M R, Ciocca M and Paganelli C 2022 A Dosiomics analysis based on linear energy transfer and biological dose maps to predict local recurrence in sacral chordomas after carbon-ion radiotherapy *Cancers* **15** 33

Morelli L *et al* 2023 Microstructural parameters from DW-MRI for tumour characterization and local recurrence prediction in particle therapy of skull-base chordoma *Med. Phys.* **50** 2900–13

Mori S, Knopf A C and Umegaki K 2018 Motion management in particle therapy *Med. Physics* **45** e994–e1010

Molina D, Pérez-Beteta J, Martínez-González A, Martino J, Velasquez C, Arana E and Pérez-García V M 2017 Lack of robustness of textural measures obtained from 3D brain tumor MRIs impose a need for standardization *PLoS One* **12** e0178843

Molinelli S, Magro G, Mairani A, Allajbej A, Mirandola A, Chalaszczyk A, Imparato S, Ciocca M, Fiore M R and Orlandi E 2021 How LEM-based RBE and dose-averaged LET affected clinical outcomes of sacral chordoma patients treated with carbon ion radiotherapy *Radiother. Oncol.* **163** 209–14

Morelli L *et al* 2023 Microstructural parameters from DW-MRI for tumour characterization and local recurrence prediction in particle therapy of skull-base chordoma *Med. Phys.* **50** 2900–13

Morelli L *et al* 2023 A Dosiomics analysis based on linear energy transfer and biological dose maps to predict local recurrence in Sacral Chordomas after carbon-ion radiotherapy *Cancers* **15** 33

Murakami Y *et al* 2021 Dose-based radiomic analysis (Dosiomics) for Intensity modulated radiation therapy in patients with prostate cancer: correlation between planned dose distribution and biochemical failure *Int. J. Radiat. Oncol. Biol. Phys.* **112** 247–59

Novikov D S 2021 The present and the future of microstructure MRI: from a paradigm shift to normal science *J. Neurosci. Methods* **351** 108947

O'Connor J P B *et al* 2017 Imaging biomarker roadmap for cancer studies *Nat. Rev. Clin. Oncol.* **14** 169–86

O'Connor J P, Aboagye E O, Adams J E, Aerts H J, Barrington S F, Beer A J, Boellaard R, Bohndiek S E, Brady M and Brown G 2017 Imaging biomarker roadmap for cancer studies *Nat. Rev. Clin. Oncol.* **14** 169–86

Palma G, Monti S and Cella L 2020a Voxel-based analysis in radiation oncology: a methodological cookbook *Phys. Med.* **69** 192–204

Palma G, Monti S, Conson M, Xu T, Hahn S, Durante M, Mohan R, Liao Z and Cella L 2020b NTCP models for severe radiation induced dermatitis after IMRT or proton therapy for thoracic cancer patients *Front. Oncol.* **10** 344

Palma G *et al* 2020c Modelling the risk of radiation induced alopecia in brain tumor patients treated with scanned proton beams *Radiother. Oncol.* **144** 127–34

Panagiotaki E, Walker-Samuel S, Siow B, Johnson S P, Rajkumar V, Pedley R B, Lythgoe M F and Alexander D C 2014 Noninvasive quantification of solid tumor Microstructure using VERDICT MRI *Cancer Res.* **74** 1902–12

Parmar C, Grossmann P, Bussink J, Lambin P and Aerts H J W L 2015 Machine learning methods for quantitative radiomic biomarkers *Sci. Rep.* **5** 13087

Paganelli C, Meschini G, Molinelli S, Riboldi M and Baroni G 2018a Patient-specific validation of deformable image registration in radiation therapy: overview and caveats *Med. Phys.* **45** e908–22

Paganelli C, Whelan B, Peroni M, Summers P, Fast M, Van de Lindt T, McClelland J, Eiben B, Keall P and Lomax T 2018b MRI-guidance for motion management in external beam radiotherapy: current status and future challenges *Phys. Med. Biol.* **63** 22TR03

Paganetti H, Botas P, Sharp G C and Winey B 2021 Adaptive proton therapy *Phys. Med. Biol.* **66** 22TR01

Parrella G, Vai A, Nakas A, Garau N, Meschini G, Camagni F, Molinelli S, Barcellini A, Pella A and Ciocca M 2023 Synthetic CT in carbon ion radiotherapy of the Abdominal site *Bioengineering* **10** 250

Peters N, Wohlfahrt P, Hofmann C, Möhler C, Menkel S, Tschiche M, Krause M, Troost E G, Enghardt W and Richter C 2022 Reduction of clinical safety margins in proton therapy enabled by the clinical implementation of dual-energy CT for direct stopping-power prediction *Radiother. Oncol.* **166** 71–8

Puttanawarut C, Sirirutbunkajorn N, Khachonkham S, Pattaranutaporn P and Wongsawat Y 2021 Biological dosiomic features for the prediction of radiation pneumonitis in esophageal cancer patients *Radiat. Oncol.* **16** 220

Sala E, Mema E, Himoto Y, Veeraraghavan H, Brenton J D, Snyder A, Weigelt B and Vargas H A 2017 Unravelling tumour heterogeneity using next-generation imaging: radiomics, radiogenomics, and habitat imaging *Clin. Radiol.* **72** 3–10

Scalco E, Rizzo G and Mastropietro A 2022 The stability of oncologic MRI radiomic features and the potential role of deep learning: a review *Phys. Med. Biol.* **67** 09TR03

Schiavo F, Kjellsson Lindblom E and Toma-Dasu I 2022 Towards the virtual tumor for optimizing radiotherapy treatments of hypoxic tumors: A novel model of heterogeneous tissue vasculature and oxygenation *J. Theor. Biol.* **547** 111175

Schiavo F, Toma-Dasu I and Kjellsson Lindblom E 2023a Hypoxia dose painting in SBRT - the virtual clinical trial approach *Acta Oncol. (Stockholm, Sweden)* **62** 1239–45

Schiavo F, Toma-Dasu I and Kjellsson Lindblom E 2023b The impact of Heterogeneous cell density in Hypoxic tumors treated with radiotherapy *Adv. Exp. Med. Biol.* **1438** 121–6

Schneider T 2022 Technical aspects of proton minibeam radiation therapy: minibeam generation and delivery *Phys. Med.* **100** 64–71

Schuemann J, McNamara A L, Ramos-Méndez J, Perl J, Held K D, Paganetti H, Incerti S and Faddegon B 2019 TOPAS-nBio: an extension to the TOPAS simulation toolkit for cellular and sub-cellular radiobiology *Radiat. Res.* **191** 125–38

Schneider T 2022 Technical aspects of proton minibeam radiation therapy: minibeam generation and delivery *Phys. Med.* **100** 64–71

Sen S *et al* 2022 Differentiating false positive lesions from clinically significant cancer and normal prostate tissue using VERDICT MRI and other diffusion models *Diagnostics* **12** 1631

Surov A, Meyer H J and Wienke A 2017 Correlation between apparent diffusion coefficient (ADC) and cellularity is different in several tumors: a meta-analysis *Oncotarget* **8** 59492–9

Tanaka S, Kadoya N, Sugai Y, Umeda M, Ishizawa M, Katsuta Y, Ito K, Takeda K and Jingu K 2022 A deep learning-based radiomics approach to predict head and neck tumor regression for adaptive radiotherapy *Sci. Rep.* **12** 1–13

Tang L and Zhou X J 2019 Diffusion MRI of cancer: from low to high b-values *J. Magn. Reson. Imaging* **49** 23–40

Thorwarth D, Notohamiprodjo M, Zips D and Müller A C 2017 Personalized precision radiotherapy by integration of multi-parametric functional and biological imaging in prostate cancer: a feasibility study *Z. Med. Phys.* **27** 21–30

Thummerer A, De Jong B A, Zaffino P, Meijers A, Marmitt G G, Seco J, Steenbakkers R J, Langendijk J A, Both S and Spadea M F 2020a Comparison of the suitability of CBCT-and

MR-based synthetic CTs for daily adaptive proton therapy in head and neck patients *Phys. Med. Biol.* **65** 235036

Thummerer A, Zaffino P, Meijers A, Marmitt G G, Seco J, Steenbakkers R J, Langendijk J A, Both S, Spadea M F and Knopf A C 2020b Comparison of CBCT based synthetic CT methods suitable for proton dose calculations in adaptive proton therapy *Phys. Med. Biol.* **65** 095002

Tinganelli W and Durante M 2020 Carbon ion radiobiology *Cancers* **12** 1–43

Tinganelli W, Durante M, Hirayama R, Krämer M, Maier A, Kraft-Weyrather W, Furusawa Y, Friedrich T and Scifoni E 2015 Kill-painting of hypoxic tumours in charged particle therapy *Sci. Rep.* **5** 1–13

Tong N, Gou S, Yang S, Ruan D and Sheng K 2018 Fully automatic multi-organ segmentation for head and neck cancer radiotherapy using shape representation model constrained fully convolutional neural networks *Med. Phys.* **45** 4558–67

van Timmeren J E, Cester D, Tanadini-Lang S, Alkadhi H and Baessler B 2020 Radiomics in medical imaging—'how-to' guide and critical reflection *Insights into Imaging* **11** 91

Vogelius I R, Petersen J and Bentzen S M 2020 Harnessing data science to advance radiation oncology *Mol. Oncol.* **14** 1514–28

Volz L, Sheng Y, Durante M and Graeff C 2022 Considerations for upright particle therapy patient positioning and associated image guidance *Front. Oncol.* **12** 930850

Wagenaar D, Schuit E, van der Schaaf A, Langendijk J A and Both S 2021 Can the mean linear energy transfer of organs be directly related to patient toxicities for current head and neck cancer intensity-modulated proton therapy practice? *Radiother. Oncol.* **165** 159–65

Webb S and Nahum A E 1993 A model for calculating tumour control probability in radiotherapy including the effects of inhomogeneous distributions of dose and clonogenic cell density *Phys. Med. Biol.* **38** 653–66

Wei R, Chen J, Liang B, Chen X, Men K and Dai J 2023 Real-time 3D MRI reconstruction from cine-MRI using unsupervised network in MRI-guided radiotherapy for liver cancer *Med. Phys.* **50** 3584–96

Wu A *et al* 2020 Dosiomics improves prediction of locoregional recurrence for intensity modulated radiotherapy treated head and neck cancer cases *Oral Oncol.* **104** 104625

Wu S, Jiao Y, Zhang Y, Ren X, Li P, Yu Q, Zhang Q, Wang Q and Fu S 2019 Imaging-based individualized response prediction of carbon ion radiotherapy for prostate cancer patients *Cancer Manag. Res.* **11** 9121–31

Xie Y, Zhao J and Zhang P 2021 A multicompartment model for intratumor tissue-specific analysis of DCE-MRI using non-negative matrix factorization *Med. Phys.* **48** 2400–11

Yang F, Simpson G, Young L, Ford J, Dogan N and Wang L 2020 Impact of contouring variability on oncological PET radiomics features in the lung *Sci. Rep.* **10** 1–10

Yang S S *et al* 2023 Dosiomics risk model for predicting radiation induced temporal lobe injury and guiding individual intensity modulated radiation therapy *Int. J. Radiat. Oncol. Biol. Phys.* **115** 1291–1300

Ye Y, Cai Z, Huang B, He Y, Zeng P, Zou G, Deng W, Chen H and Huang B 2020 Fully-automated segmentation of Nasopharyngeal Carcinoma on dual-sequence MRI using convolutional neural networks *Front. Oncol.* **10** 166

Zeineldin R A, Karar M E, Coburger J, Wirtz C R and Burgert O 2020 DeepSeg: deep neural network framework for automatic brain tumor segmentation using magnetic resonance FLAIR images *Int. J. Comput. Assist. Radiol. Surg.* **15** 909–20

Zhang X, Zhang Y, Zhang G, Qiu X, Tan W, Yin X and Liao L 2022 Deep learning with radiomics for disease diagnosis and treatment: challenges and potential *Front. Oncol.* **12** 1

Zhang Y, Lobo-Mueller E M, Karanicolas P, Gallinger S, Haider M A and Khalvati F 2020 CNN-based survival model for pancreatic ductal adenocarcinoma in medical imaging *BMC Med. Imaging* **20** 1–8

Zhang Y, Knopf A, Tanner C and Lomax A J 2014 Online image guided tumour tracking with scanned proton beams: a comprehensive simulation study *Phys. Med. Biol.* **59** 7793

Zwanenburg A and Löck S 2018 Why validation of prognostic models matters? *Radiother. Oncol.* **127** 370–3

Zwanenburg A *et al* 2020 The image biomarker standardization initiative: standardized quantitative radiomics for high-throughput image-based phenotyping *Radiology* **295** 328–38

IOP Publishing

Imaging in Particle Therapy
Current practice and future trends
Chiara Paganelli, Chiara Gianoli and Antje Knopf

Chapter 13

Integration of imaging in clinical protocols of particle therapy

P Trnkova, A Bolsi, A Knopf and A Hoffmann

13.1 Introduction

In this chapter, the contribution of image guidance in particle therapy (PT) is addressed considering the requirements related to the anatomical tumour location, the clinical experience and clinical needs of many particle therapy centres; those needs are currently in the focus of the PT imaging research community. The Particle Therapy Co-Operative Group (PTCOG) is an organisation connecting the research and clinical community of proton, light ion and heavy charged particle radiotherapy, which regularly collects information on all the centres and their clinical and research activities. As of 2023, there were 29 clinically operational particle therapy (PT) centres in Europe, 44 in USA, 24 in Japan and 16 in the rest of the Asia. Out of those, 70% had less than 10 years of experience, 40% less than 5 years. There were large differences among the centres with regards to number of treatment rooms, vendors, and beam delivery technology, as well as academic or clinical settings.

The information in this chapter about the integration of medical imaging in clinical PT protocols is mainly based on several surveys that were conducted between 2016 and 2022. The European Particle Therapy Network (EPTN) collected data from 19 European particle therapy centres in 2016–17 on the assessment of current practice in image-guided particle therapy (IGPT; Bolsi *et al* 2018). A more detailed body site-specific survey on current practice was performed between the years 2019–22. Response data from 20 European PT centres was collected and analysed for brain, prostate, abdomen, cranio-spinal axis irradiation (CSA) and extremities. The Patterns of Practice for Adaptive and Real-Time Particle Therapy (POP ART PT) survey collected answers from 70 worldwide PT centres between July 2020 and June 2021 on establishing the current status of clinical implementation in real-time respiratory motion management (RRMM) and adaptive particle therapy (APT; Trnkova *et al* 2023, Zhang *et al* 2023). The survey additionally explored what the biggest burdens in the clinical implementation of the existing technologies are. In contrast to EPTN surveys, which were fully focussed on imaging in every step of the clinical particle therapy workflow, the POP ART PT survey aimed at RRMM and APT and imaging was only a marginal part of the survey. Results of all surveys are summarized here to highlight the most important site-specific aspects of imaging in clinical proton therapy.

Additional sources of information considered in this chapter were the reports from the yearly 4D workshop (Knopf *et al* 2010, 2014, 2016, Bert *et al* 2014, Trnková *et al* 2018, Czerska *et al* 2021) and PTCOG Clinical Subcommittees Consensus Guidelines for head and neck (Lin *et al* 2021) and thorax (Chang *et al* 2017). The 4D workshop has taken place annually since 2009. During the workshop the status of research and clinical implementation for motion management in PT is addressed. The development of high-quality imaging suitable for PT is regularly discussed. The reports from the workshops were published in peer-reviewed journals. PTCOG Clinical Subcommittees aim at deriving recommendations for specific treatment sites. So far recommendations for head and neck and thorax have been published. In table 13.1, an overview of the source of information per treatment site is provided.

Most of the PT centres in all the performed surveys revealed that they gained their knowledge on the use of imaging and relevant protocols either from already existing centres or from photon therapy clinics. As of 2022, there is still a lack of guidelines for imaging and image guidance in PT. Imaging is currently mainly used for the following steps of the treatment workflow: diagnosis, treatment planning, patient positioning, evaluation of the necessity of the plan adaptation and motion monitoring and follow-up. The POP ART PT survey indicated that most of the 3D imaging modalities are located outside of the PT treatment room (referred to as near-room) and that there is a lack of in-room and in-beam volumetric imaging. As of 2021, depending on the treatment site, in-room and/or in-beam imaging on its own was used only in 18%–32% of APT workflows and in 14%–33% in combination with near-room imaging (Trnkova *et al* 2023).

Table 13.1. Overview of the treatment sites, their workflow specifics and source of information.

Treatment site	Workflow specifics	Source of information
Brain	Static	EPTN Survey
CSA	Static, multi-isocentre	EPTN Survey
Extremities	Static	EPTN Survey
Prostate	Adaptive	EPTN Survey
		POP ART PT Survey
Abdomen	Adaptive, motion management	EPTN Survey
Lung	Adaptive, motion management	POP ART PT Survey
		PTCOG Thorax Subcommittee
Head and neck	Adaptive	POP ART PT Survey
		PTCOG Head&Neck Subcommittee
Breast	Motion management	—

13.2 Imaging for static/rigid treatment sites

The brain, cranio-spinal axis (CSA) and extremities can be considered as static treatment sites for which imaging is required at several steps of the PT workflow (figure 13.1).

In the planning process, the dose calculation is performed based on computed tomography (CT) images. Different CT modalities are used among different institutes: most centres use single-energy CT (SECT), with a CT calibration to proton stopping power procedure in place (Schneider *et al* 1996), whilst a few other centres use direct relative proton stopping power computed from dual-energy CT (DECT; Wohlfahrt and Richter 2020). CT acquisition protocols differ among institutes, and they are specific for each treatment site (Bolsi *et al* 2018). Depending on the specific needs, additional CT imaging with contrast and algorithms for metal artefacts reduction is used in the clinical practice. The benefit and accuracy of those algorithms has been shown in multiple studies (Wei *et al* 2006, Andersson *et al* 2014). Typically, tumour delineation benefits from multi-modal imaging, including magnetic resonance imaging (MRI) and positron emission tomography (PET) combined with CT imaging (PET-CT). Those images are acquired and registered with the planning CT scan, based on rigid registration. Only in a few centres, a near-room MRI scanner is available in the PT department and image acquisition with treatment fixation devices are possible, which results in registration uncertainties. In case patient positioning is the same for all the imaging acquisitions, including the planning CT scan, the uncertainties in the registration process can be minimised.

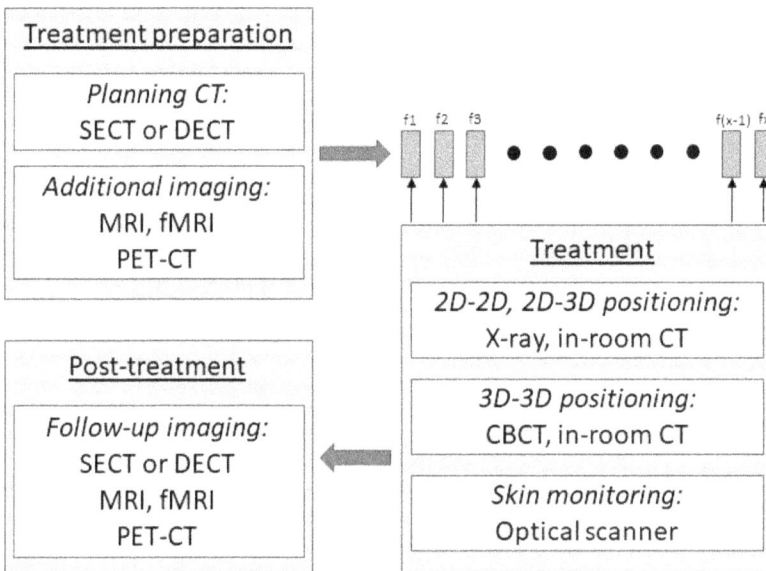

Figure 13.1. Schematic overview of the steps of PT workflow where imaging is performed. 'f' stands for a treatment fraction.

For static target volumes, image guidance for patient positioning verification is mostly 2D IGPT, based on mixed x-ray projections matched with digitally reconstructed radiographs (DRRs) from planning CT scans. For some centres the use of 3D IGPT, either based on in-beam cone-beam CT (CBCT) or on in-room CT, is part of the clinical routine, with reduced frequencies as compared to daily imaging. For both 2D and 3D IGPT, the registration of daily and reference images is focused on accurate bone matching. Volumetric images provide important information related to positioning accuracy/reproducibility and anatomical changes and they might be used as a trigger for the adaptation process. As tumours and anatomical treatment sites are stable over the course of treatment, plan adaptation is rather ad-hoc and it can be triggered by routine 3D image acquisitions, which are mostly based on re-evaluation CT. An example of 2D/2D, 2D/3D and 3D/3D image guidance for patients treated in the head is reported in figure 13.2.

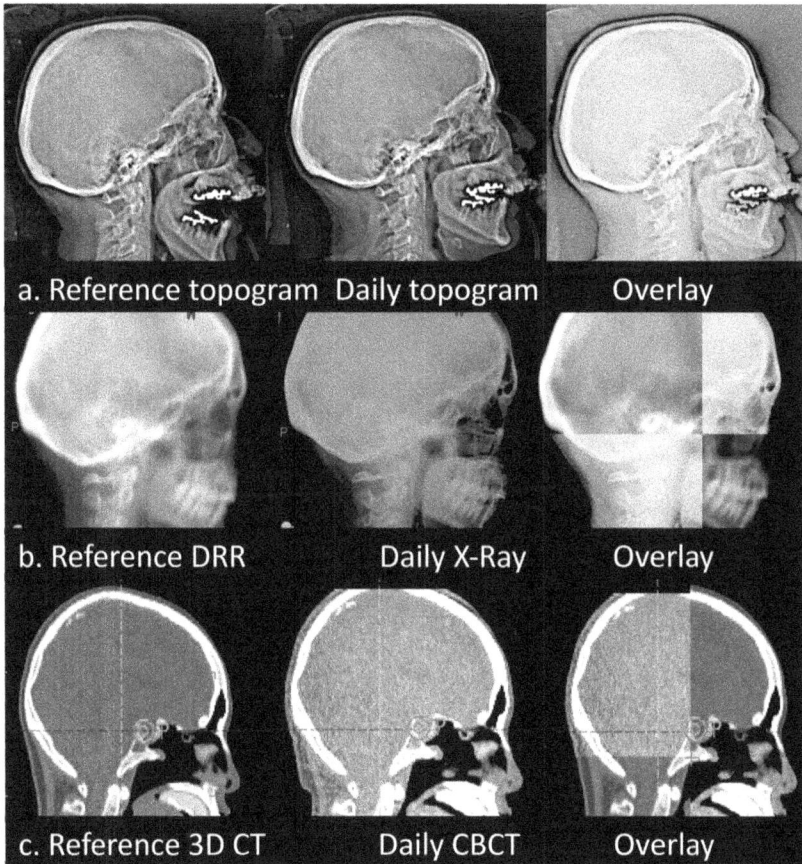

Figure 13.2. Example of different image guidance options for intracranial cases: (a) 2D/2D topogram comparison; (b) 2D/3D comparison between reference DRR and x-ray; and (c) volumetric comparison between planning CT and daily CBCT scans.

CSA irradiations are included among the rigid treatment sites, but they present special challenges mainly due to the extent of the volume to be treated (from top of the head to end of the spinal cord; figure 13.2) and the limited size of the image and treatment fields. Therefore, daily, multiple images need to be taken along the full length of the spine; positioning corrections need to be computed from those different images. To reduce the number of x-ray acquisitions, some centres have introduced optical surface imaging systems which help in the initial setup of the patients (Liu *et al* 2021). Those systems provide the advantage of dose-free images, and they are mainly used for extracranial treatments, especially in case of positioning systems without indexing (i.e. matrasses).

Intracranial tumour patients are generally immobilised with bite blocks or personalised thermoplastic masks, with a patient-specific mould-care pillow or standard neck rest. In those cases, the use of surface imaging is redundant, and therefore not applied.

13.2.1 Brain

The EPTN survey results on brain treatments include feedback of 6 treating PT centres, most of them with extensive experience in such treatments. The clinical IGPT workflow for this body site is based on the specific experience of each centre and on data published in literature (Amelio *et al* 2013). The treatment planning CT scan is generally performed with SECT, as DECT is currently only available and implemented in the clinical workflow in very few centres. MRI is generally used for tumour delineation purposes, based on specific MRI pulse sequences, such as inversion-recovery gradient echo (IR-GRE) and T1-MPRAGE that have been included in the standardized Brain Tumour Imaging Protocol (Ellingson *et al* 2015). The MR images are rigidly registered with the planning CT images. In most cases, the MRI acquisitions are not performed in treatment position, thus increasing the inaccuracy of image registration. Repeated MR imaging during the treatment course can be used to check treatment response and anatomical changes. PET acquisitions are also generally used in the treatment preparation phase; those images are rigidly registered with planning CT ones. Pre-treatment image guidance is generally based on 2D x-ray images matched with DRR (Shafai-Erfani *et al* 2018, Zechner *et al* 2022); only a few centres acquire further in-treatment images. 3D images (CBCT) are currently limited in very few centres, and they are acquired on regular intervals (daily or weekly after the first fraction CBCT acquisition). In most of the centres intra-fractional motion is monitored by the acquisition of post-treatment 2D images. Image guidance in both the treatment planning phase and the positioning verification is performed with specific protocols defined for paediatric patients in 50% of the centres, with the goal of reducing the image guidance delivered dose. The rest of the centres use the same imaging protocols for children and adults.

13.2.2 CSA

Eleven centres treating CSA patients provided feedback in the CSA specific EPTN survey, half of them treating very few patients per year (<10/y) and half of them with larger experience (>10/y or more); and all the information about CSA is based on

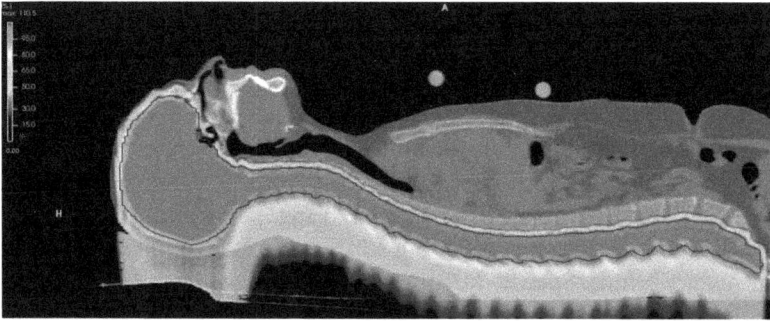

Figure 13.3. Typical dose distribution for CSA treatment, which is followed by a local boost. The cranio-caudal extension of field, depending on the age and height of the patient, can be from 40 cm up to 100 cm. In this case the patient is in supine positioned and treated with two posterior-anterior fields at narrow angles.

unpublished data. In comparison to other treatment sites, the prone position is often used for treatment. As the CSA treatment is usually done in children, paediatric protocols are commonly used for immobilization (i.e. mould-care to shell the whole patient), and patients are treated under anaesthesia. SECT is the main treatment planning imaging modality, with currently very limited clinical implementation of DECT. MRI images are frequently used for delineation purposes. The recommended MRI pulse sequences for CSA imaging were published by the SIOPE-Brain Tumour Group (Ajithkumar *et al* 2018, Wood *et al* 2019).

The most relevant difference to other treatment sites is the use of several isocentres and merged fields as the treatment volume is long (Farace *et al* 2017, Medek *et al* 2019; figure 13.3). For this reason, a daily setup procedure can take up to 45 min. All the centres perform verification imaging before every fraction, and typically images are taken before treating each isocentre. In all centres a 2D IGRT approach is routinely applied, and in some, an additional 3D IGPT strategy is implemented with repeated CT acquisitions. Each centre has developed specific protocols to deal with the registrations of the different merged fields, considering potential discrepancies between the resulting correction offsets.

Surface imaging is getting more and more integrated in clinical routine for the initial patient setup: optical images are used to adjust the patient position before proceeding with x-rays acquisition, thus reducing the number of x-ray acquisitions and thus the non-therapeutic dose.

13.2.3 Extremities

Eight centres provided feedback on the extremities survey, five of which treat extremity patients. Most of the centres are using SECT for treatment planning, and only very few routinely use DECT. For challenging cases, when anatomical changes are detected and re-planning is required, this will be based on repeated CT acquisitions, with the same conditions (CT scanner and protocol settings) of the nominal planning CT scan. MR imaging is used mainly for delineation purposes for most of the centres: in half of the cases the MR acquisition is performed with specific MR sequences for radiation therapy and with the extremities in treatment position, to minimise uncertainties in the registration. For most of the centres daily image guidance is based on 2D x-rays vs. DRR match based on bone anatomy. Surface imaging is rarely used as well as CBCT imaging. Intra-fraction monitoring using post-treatment control images is rarely performed. Treatment of extremities, despite being performed in multiple centres, does not involve a large patient population, which is normally limited to a maximum of 10–20 patients per centre. Specific literature on this topic is scarce. Therefore, most of the centres base their IGPT workflow on their own experience.

13.3 Treatment sites requiring adaptation or motion management

In moving targets or in targets requiring adaptation, imaging is included in several steps of the treatment preparation and delivery phase. In case of a site with large inter-fraction variability (e.g., shrinkage of the tumour in head and neck treatments), the imaging used in treatment preparation, during the treatment and in follow-up is the same as for static targets (section 13.1). However, an additional workflow step is introduced to evaluate the impact of the variation on plan quality (figure 13.4). If the

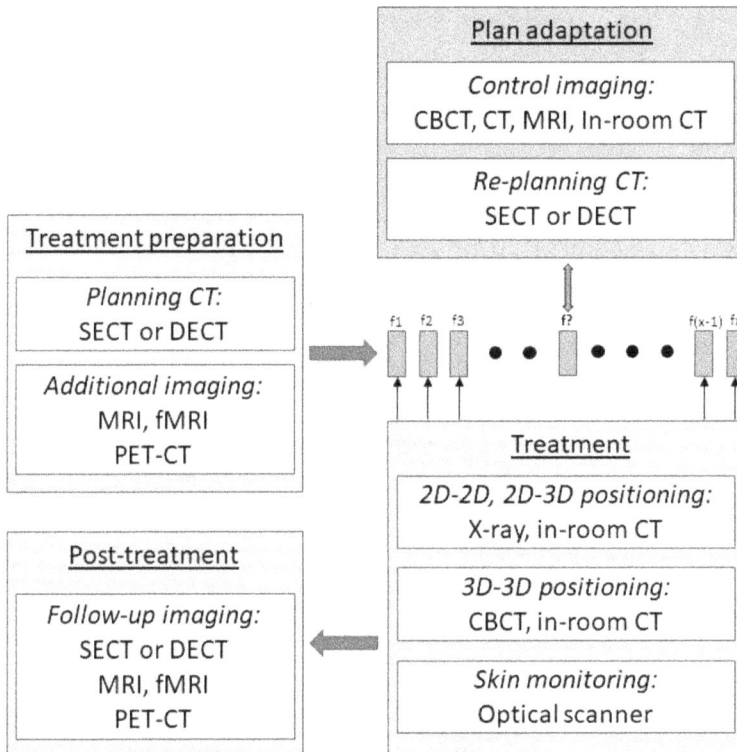

Figure 13.4. Schematic overview of the steps of adaptive PT workflow where imaging is performed. 'f' stands for a fraction.

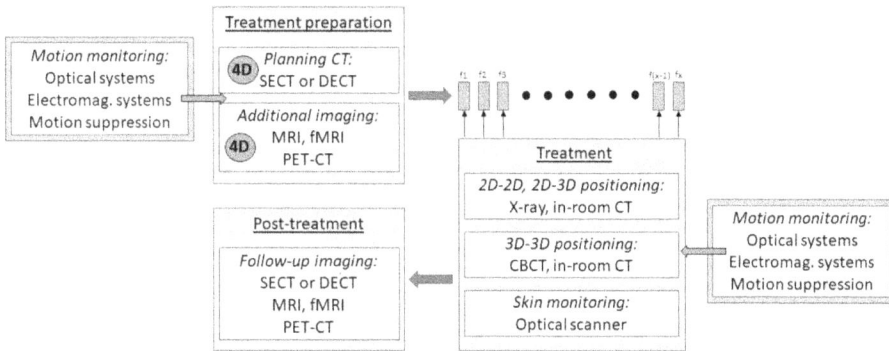

Figure 13.5. Schematic overview of the steps of PT workflow where imaging is performed. 'f' stands for a fraction.

plan quality is compromised and plan adaptation is required, an offline planning CT scan is acquired for a new treatment plan (Trnkova *et al* 2023). The monitoring of plan quality, i.e. for triggering of plan adaptation is performed either with in-beam CBCT, in-room CT or near-room repeated CT or MRI. If the treatment sites are rather stable over the course of treatment, plan adaptation is initialized ad hoc when needed. For treatment sites where anatomical changes are expected, repeated imaging is performed on a regular basis as indicated by institutional protocols.

In the case of treatment sites impacted by breathing (i.e., intra-fraction variability), motion mitigation is necessary for safe treatment delivery (figure 13.5; Keall *et al* 2006, Trnková *et al* 2018). Motion mitigation can either be passive, e.g., application of safety margins or rescanning, or active by motion suppression or irradiation only at certain phases of the motion (Zhang *et al* 2023). For understanding the amplitude and frequency of the motion, 4DCT obtaining images at several phases of breathing motion, eventually supported by 4DMRI, is commonly acquired, which serve as basis for 4D dose calculation or for motion monitoring and integral target volume (ITV) definition (Knopf *et al* 2022). For the acquisition of 4D imaging, motion monitoring is needed and defined as tracking the motion states during or directly before imaging and treatment. External optical or electromagnetic monitoring systems are used to characterize the motion amplitude and to assort the images into individual phases (Fattori *et al* 2017). However, the low temporal resolution, insensitivity to motion variations and off-line acquisition still limit the optimal consideration of 4DCT motion during treatment planning and online motion monitoring (Czerska *et al* 2021).

For the verification of patient positioning, in-beam 2D x-ray or CBCT imaging is used. In some institutes also in-room CT imaging is integrated in the workflow. In case of moving targets, the imaging can be performed statically, with a comparison of the daily imaging to the reference DRR generated from a static CT image. The static CT image can be either an average CT calculated from all 4DCT images, or an image corresponding to a certain phase (i.e. mid-ventilation). For monitoring of the internal motion during the treatment, high-quality 4D imaging like fluoroscopy or

4D CBCT is needed (den Otter *et al* 2020). However, none of these techniques are widely implemented in the clinic so far.

The treatment sites included in this section are prostate, abdomen, lung, head and neck and breast. Oesophagus and lymphomas also belong to this category, however, none of the surveys have explicitly addressed them. The information was collected from EPTN survey and POP ART PT. The treatment sites located in the thorax and abdomen require consideration of both, motion monitoring and plan adaptation as they are impacted by breathing motion. In case of pelvis and head and neck regions, APT is implemented.

The only treatment site that is always immobilised is the head and neck region, where either thermoplastic masks or bite blocks or both are used. Some institutes use thermoplastic masks also for the abdomen region. However, more often, no fixation is used for more caudal treatments. Vacuum cushions, mould cares, hand holders or knee blocks are used to achieve as reproducible a position as possible.

13.3.1 Prostate

The EPTN survey that finished in early 2020 and included data from eight centres treating prostate cancer showed that the number of prostate patients treated with PT in Europe is still low, with the majority of centres treating less than ten patients per year. Mainly actively scanned proton beams are used in combination with implanted fiducial markers. Most centres routinely treat patients in supine position with knee supports and rectum/bladder stabilization procedures. Endorectal balloons are routinely or optionally used by 50% of the centres, whereas rectal spacers are seldomly used. For treatment planning, SECT is in routine use in all centres. DECT imaging is not routinely used in most centres. All centres use MRI for target volume and organ delineation and rigid MRI-to-CT registration is standardly performed. In 50% of the centres, the MRI scan is acquired in treatment position. PET imaging is in use primarily for staging and target volume delineation. For patient positioning, the daily setup procedure is performed predominantly inside the treatment room. Surface scanning is optionally used for surveillance in one centre. All centres acquire repeated CT scans during the course of treatment to evaluate the need for re-planning. Few centres acquire CBCT or MRI scans for re-planning. Re-planning is routinely based on CT imaging or optionally on CBCT imaging. 2D IGPT is routinely used for gantry-based treatments and performed before each treatment fraction. 3D IGPT is seldomly used by few centres. Post-treatment images are not routinely acquired in most centres.

The POP ART PT survey showed that 41% of the centres were users of APT with 75% of them using ad hoc off-line APT and 39% using APT per protocol. Most APT users created more than one treatment plan for less than 5% of the prostate patients. CT was the most used imaging modality for APT. CBCT and 2D x-ray imaging were also used for APT by 21% and 14% of the users, respectively. MRI and surface imaging were sporadically and not at all used, respectively. A combination of the aforementioned imaging modalities was used by 21% of the APT users. The frequency of imaging ranged from 14% prior to each fraction to 46% and 50% for specific number of fractions or ad hoc, respectively.

13.3.2 Abdomen

The EPTN survey collected response data from 11 centres treating various indications (hepatocellular carcinoma, sacral chordoma, soft-tissue sarcoma, osteogenic sarcoma) with proton beams only. A lot of similarities exist with the way prostate cancer patients are treated. The standard patient position is supine, with prone positioning as an option. Most centres routinely use a knee support and procedures for rectum/bladder stabilization. Fiducial markers as well as thermoplastic masks are not in routine use. For treatment planning, SECT imaging is in routine use in most centres, mainly for tumour identification. Most centres do not use DECT imaging for initial treatment planning. All centres use MRI, at least optionally, mainly for contouring, and rigid MRI-to-CT registration is used as standard. In the majority of centres, the MRI scan is acquired in treatment position. PET imaging is mainly as option in use, primarily for staging and target volume delineation. For patient positioning, the daily setup procedure is performed predominantly inside the treatment room. Surface scanning is used, at least optionally, for initial positioning and surveillance is used in about 50% of the centres. The need for re-planning is evaluated by all centres through the acquisition of repeated CT scans. Some centres acquire MRI and CBCT scans for re-planning, the latter being in the minority. Re-planning is routinely based on repeated CT imaging but not on CBCT imaging. 2D IGPT with gantry-based systems is in routine use and performed before each treatment fraction. 3D IGPT is in routine or optional use by about 50% of the centres. Post-treatment control images are not routinely acquired in most centres.

13.3.3 Lung

No EPTN survey investigating current clinical imaging protocols in lung was performed yet. The PTCOG Thoracic Subcommittee published consensus guidelines for implementing pencil beam scanning (PBS) proton therapy (Chang *et al* 2017). The necessity of 4D imaging in the lung treatment workflow was emphasized for the reduction of beam range and organ motion uncertainties. The PTCOG Thoracic Subcommittee recommended the use of 4DCT based treatment planning for estimation of tumour motion and the maximum intensity projection CT for the target contours delineation and treatment plan calculation. In case, a patient is treated in breath-hold (BH), several BH CT scans should be acquired for the evaluation of BH stability. In-room volumetric imaging, as for example CT on rails or in-beam CBCT was recommended for BH, gating or tracking treatment delivery. Alternatively, implanted fiducial markers in combination with fluoroscopic imaging might be used as gating surrogate.

Based on the POP ART PT survey (Zhang *et al* 2023), 29% and 28% of clinically operational responders use either BH or free-breathing expiration gating, respectively, as active RRMM. The most common monitoring signals were external marker (20%), surface monitoring (18%) and breathing volume (17%). The use of kV imaging either with markers or markerless was very limited (5%).

Plan adaptation was performed by 62% of the clinically operational responders of POP ART PT (Trnkova *et al* 2023). CT was the most frequently used imaging modality. The use of online imaging, either 2D x-ray or CBCT, was implemented by 45% of the clinical responders using APT for lung. It was not possible to conclude what type of imaging was available inside of the treatment room.

13.3.4 Head and neck

The EPTN survey investigating current clinical imaging protocols in head and neck was not closed at the moment of writing this chapter. The PTCOG Head and Neck Subcommittee Consensus Guidelines do not address imaging (Lin *et al* 2021). They only mention that high-quality imaging is needed for quality assurance and determination whether a plan adaptation is needed.

The POP ART PT survey indicated that head and neck is the most frequently adapted treatment site with 79% of clinically operational respondents performing the adaptation. Most commonly, a combination of several imaging modalities is used during the adaptive workflow, where 2D imaging or CBCT is used to trigger the adaptation and acquisition of additional planning CT or MR images for plan adaptation. The imaging devices were located either in the treatment room (19%), in a separate room (39%) or in both locations (24%). However, it was not possible to conclude which device is located where from the structure of the survey.

13.3.5 Breast

Results on the EPTN survey for breast treatments are currently not available. For breast treatments a significant contribution in the IGPT procedure is provided by surface imaging derived with optic scanners. Typically, surface images are combined with the acquisition of either 2D x-ray images or 3D CBCT images (Batin *et al* 2016, Liang *et al* 2020). For such tumour localisation the use of 2D images has limited value due to limitations in the image quality, therefore the use of additional marker is implemented to improve accuracy.

13.4 User satisfaction

In all surveys, the users had an opportunity to express how satisfied they are with current clinical IGPT workflows. The main issues identified in all the surveys across all the treatment sites were a lack of integrated workflows and limited resources for the implementation of new technology.

With regards to the imaging devices, the users wished to have CBCT or CT on-rails available in the treatment rooms. Currently, the most frequently used 2D x-ray imaging is not enough for daily online adaptation, and it also provides limited accuracy for daily patient setup. The integration of surface scanning or fluoroscopy into the daily clinical workflow was expected to provide a significant improvement in the management of moving tumours. Following the success of MRI-guided photon therapy, the users had high expectations from the future implementation of an MRI-guided PT workflow.

The necessity of software improvements throughout all the imaging applications was highlighted by many users: image registration software quality and accuracy of registration was identified as insufficient; the speed of image acquisition for tumour tracking and evaluation was not sufficient for online monitoring; the software for online plan adaptation is lacking in most of the institutions; the level of automation of the workflow was insufficient; the communication between different systems was rather difficult.

13.5 Research activities and future perspectives

Currently, in-beam imaging is more advanced in conventional radiation therapy than in PT. However, it has the potential of a larger impact in PT due to the relevant uncertainties during treatment planning and delivery (Engelsman *et al* 2013). Paganetti *et al* (2021) published a roadmap for future developments in PT physics and biology where improvements of imaging technology, as well as workflows were addressed.

With regards to technology, CT imaging will remain the main modality for treatment planning in the near future. As such, the CT-based range prediction uncertainty should be reduced (Paganetti *et al* 2021). DECT has the potential to reduce this range uncertainty from current 3%–3.5% (Taasti *et al* 2018) to below 2% (Wohlfahrt and Richter 2020) due to better soft-tissue differentiation (Patino *et al* 2016). Post-processing algorithms for beam hardening and scatter correction, patient size, image smoothing and de-noising might further improve the range accuracy (Paganetti *et al* 2021). The distribution of contrast agents can additionally improve the tumour visibility or can even provide information on the tumour metabolism. However, the optimal application of contrast agents has to be comprehensively investigated in future studies (Paganetti *et al* 2021). Moreover, no DECT device for widespread application in radiation oncology currently exists and, therefore, technology improvements will be needed (Wohlfahrt and Richter 2020). Alternatively, photon-counting systems are the expected next generation CT technology with multi-dimensional attenuation information, which may potentially lead to higher tissue contrast and differentiation of multiple contrast agents (Willemink *et al* 2018).

For some decades, there has been ongoing research on proton radiography (Seller Oria *et al* 2021). Proton CT would directly provide the information on the stopping power of the tissue. Its clinical implementation would, however, lead to a reduction of available treatment slots at the gantries as it has a long acquisition time (several minutes) (Johnson 2018). Moreover, as the clinical gantries usually have a maximum proton energy of approximately 230 MeV, it would be available only for few body sites. Both issues reduce the probability of wide clinical implementation. It might be used for only certain groups of patients, e.g. with metal implants where it could provide more accurate information on the material composition. The quickly developing conventional x-ray based CT systems could be clinically and economically more sufficient. With integration of range probing into proton therapy systems, an *in vivo* range prediction and verification would be possible (Parodi and Polf 2018).

With regards to improvements in workflow, the integration of especially 3D online in-beam imaging would be a major step forward. It would enable more precise position verification, online monitoring of inter- and intra-fractional changes as well as direct online treatment plan adaptation. CBCT is more frequently installed at PT facilities nowadays, similarly to photon beam therapy. The position verification and online monitoring of inter-fractional changes is already possible with current installations. Limited field-of-view and inaccuracy in HU calculations are still hindering the use of CBCT for treatment planning. Several methods are developed to solve both issues. Stitching algorithms to combine CBCT and conventional CT are explored to compensate for limited field-of-view (Shi *et al* 2017). Deformable image registration or machine-learning methods are investigated for conversion of CBCT HUs into the proton stopping power (Giacometti *et al* 2020). However, the clinical validation of dose calculation on CBCT is still missing (Paganetti *et al* 2021). For intra-fractional motion monitoring 4D CBCT is needed. However, this is currently far away from clinical implementation (Paganetti *et al* 2021).

Since MRI has gained importance in x-ray based radiation therapy for different anatomical sites thanks to its intrinsic advantages (i.e., excellent soft-tissue contrast, radiation-free modality, fast dynamic pulse sequences, and quantitative imaging), its use in PT is expected to combine the ability to visualize anatomy and biological heterogeneity with the unique dose-deposition and biological properties of PT. This brings potential novel opportunities to improve cure by biological dose escalation in specific cancer types, including pancreatic, central lung, liver, oesophagus, brain and oligometastatic cancers (Pham *et al* 2022) as well as pediatric patients, where radiation levels must be carefully controlled. The current use of MRI in the clinical routine of PT is mainly for accurate tumour and organ-at-risk delineation and to support treatment planning and verification, with near-room MRI systems installed in some of the PT facilities. The full in-beam integration of MRI is currently under investigation by several groups and a first prototype already exists (Hoffmann *et al* 2020). In photon therapy, integration of MRI into the clinical workflow was the right boost for online daily adaptive radiotherapy, for example for stereotactic body radiotherapy of prostate cancer (Kishan *et al* 2023) and liver tumours (Witt *et al* 2020). For a more detailed description of the use, role and future developments of MRI in PT, reference is made to chapter 7. Finally, quantitative MRI based on microscopic tissue properties and tissue function can be used to improve the target contouring accuracy. It also shows promise as a tool to predict treatment response for treatment regimens and hence could be used for treatment stratification, either to determine which treatment modality (x-ray vs. PT) is most promising in terms of radiation-induced side-effects (Dünger *et al* 2021) or to determine patient-specific radiation dose prescription (Gurney-Champion *et al* 2020).

References

Ajithkumar T *et al* 2018 SIOPE—brain tumor group consensus guideline on craniospinal target volume delineation for high-precision radiotherapy *Radiother. Oncol.: J. Eur. Soc. Ther. Radiol. Oncol.* **128** 192–7

Amelio D *et al* 2013 Analysis of inter- and intrafraction accuracy of a commercial thermoplastic mask system used for image-guided particle radiation therapy *J. Radiat. Res.* **54** i69–76

Andersson K M, Ahnesjö A and Vallhagen Dahlgren C 2014 Evaluation of a metal artifact reduction algorithm in CT studies used for proton radiotherapy treatment planning *J. Appl. Clin. Med. Phys.* **15** 4857

Batin E *et al* 2016 Can surface imaging improve the patient setup for proton postmastectomy chest wall irradiation? *Pract. Radiat. Oncol.* **6** e235–41

Bert C *et al* 2014 Advances in 4D treatment planning for scanned particle beam therapy—report of dedicated workshops *Technol. Cancer Res. Treat.* **13** 485–95

Bolsi A *et al* 2018 Practice patterns of image guided particle therapy in Europe: a 2016 survey of the European particle therapy network (EPTN) *Radiother. Oncol. : J. Eur. Soc. Ther. Radiol. Oncol.* **128** 4–8

Chang J Y *et al* 2017 Consensus guidelines for implementing pencil-beam scanning proton therapy for thoracic malignancies on behalf of the PTCOG Thoracic and Lymphoma subcommittee *Int. J. Radiat. Oncol., Biol., Phys.* **99** 41–50

Czerska K *et al* 2021 Clinical practice vs. state-of-the-art research and future visions: report on the 4D treatment planning workshop for particle therapy—edition 2018 and 2019 *Phys. Med.* **82** 54–63

Dünger L *et al* 2021 Reduced diffusion in white matter after radiotherapy with photons and protons *Radiother. Oncol.* **164** 66–72

Ellingson B M *et al* 2015 Consensus recommendations for a standardized brain tumor imaging protocol in clinical trials *Neuro-Oncol.* **17** 1188–98

Engelsman M, Schwarz M and Dong L 2013 Physics controversies in proton therapy *Semin. Radiat. Oncol.* **23** 88–96

Farace P *et al* 2017 Supine craniospinal irradiation in pediatric patients by proton pencil beam scanning *Radiother. Oncol.* **123** 112–8

Fattori G *et al* 2017 Monitoring of breathing motion in image-guided PBS proton therapy: comparative analysis of optical and electromagnetic technologies *Radiat. Oncol.* **12** 63

Giacometti V, Hounsell A R and McGarry C K 2020 A review of dose calculation approaches with cone beam CT in photon and proton therapy *Phys. Med.* **76** 243–76

Gurney-Champion O J *et al* 2020 Quantitative imaging for radiotherapy purposes *Radiother. Oncol.* **146** 66–75

Hoffmann A *et al* 2020 MR-guided proton therapy: a review and a preview *Radiat. Oncol.* **15** 129

Johnson R P 2018 Review of medical radiography and tomography with proton beams *Rep. Prog. Phys. Phys. Soc.* **81** 16701

Keall P J *et al* 2006 The management of respiratory motion in radiation oncology report of AAPM Task Group 76 *Med. Phys.* **33** 3874–900

Kishan A U *et al* 2023 Magnetic resonance imaging-guided vs computed tomography-guided stereotactic body radiotherapy for prostate cancer: the MIRAGE randomized clinical trial *JAMA Oncol.* **9** 365–73

Knopf A-C *et al* 2016 Required transition from research to clinical application: report on the 4D treatment planning workshops 2014 and 2015 *Phys. Med.* **32** 874–82

Knopf A-C *et al* 2022 Clinical necessity of multi-image based (4D(MIB)) optimization for targets affected by respiratory motion and treated with scanned particle therapy—a comprehensive review *Radiother. Oncol.* **169** 77–85

Knopf A *et al* 2010 Special report: workshop on 4D-treatment planning in actively scanned particle therapy—recommendations, technical challenges, and future research directions *Med. Phys.* 4608–14

Knopf A *et al* 2014 Challenges of radiotherapy: report on the 4D treatment planning workshop 2013 *Phys. Med.* **30** 809–15

Liang X *et al* 2020 Dosimetric consequences of image guidance techniques on robust optimized intensity-modulated proton therapy for treatment of breast Cancer *Radiat. Oncol.* **15** 47

Lin A *et al* 2021 PTCOG head and neck subcommittee consensus guidelines on particle therapy for the management of head and neck tumors *Int. J. Part. Ther.* **8** 84–94

Liu C *et al* 2021 Use of surface imaging in combination with IGRT for proton beam craniospinal irradiation (CSI) setup *Int. J. Radiat. Oncol. Biol. Phys.* **111** e512

Medek S *et al* 2019 Practice patterns among radiation oncologists treating pediatric patients with proton craniospinal irradiation *Pract. Radiat. Oncol.* **9** 441–7

den Otter L A *et al* 2020 Technical note: 4D cone-beam CT reconstruction from sparse-view CBCT data for daily motion assessment in pencil beam scanned proton therapy (PBS-PT) *Med. Phys.* **47** 6381–7

Paganetti H *et al* 2021 Roadmap: proton therapy physics and biology *Phys. Med. Biol.* **66** 05RM01

Parodi K and Polf J C 2018 *In vivo* range verification in particle therapy *Med. Phys.* **45** e1036–50

Patino M *et al* 2016 Material separation using dual-energy CT: current and emerging applications *Radiographics:* **36** 1087–105

Pham T T *et al* 2022 Magnetic resonance imaging (MRI) guided proton therapy: a review of the clinical challenges, potential benefits and pathway to implementation *Radiother. Oncol.: J. Eur. Soc. Ther. Radiol. Oncol.* **170** 37–47

Schneider U, Pedroni E and Lomax A 1996 The calibration of CT hounsfield units for radiotherapy treatment planning *Phys. Med. Biol.* **41** 111–24

Seller Oria C *et al* 2021 Optimizing calibration settings for accurate water equivalent path length assessment using flat panel proton radiography *Phys. Med. Biol.* **66** 21NT02

Shafai-Erfani G *et al* 2018 Effectiveness of base-of-skull immobilization system in a compact proton therapy setting *J. Appl. Clin. Med. Phys.* **19** 261–7

Shi L *et al* 2017 Fast shading correction for cone beam CT in radiation therapy via sparse sampling on planning CT *Med. Phys.* **44** 1796–808

Taasti V T *et al* 2018 Inter-centre variability of CT-based stopping-power prediction in particle therapy: survey-based evaluation *Phys. Imaging Radiat. Oncol.* **6** 25–30

Trnkova P *et al* 2023 Patterns of practice for adaptive and real-time particle therapy (POP-ART PT), part II: plan adaptation for interfractional changes *Phys. Imaging Radiat. Oncol.* **26** 100442

Trnková P *et al* 2018 Clinical implementations of 4D pencil beam scanned particle therapy: report on the 4D treatment planning workshop 2016 and 2017 *Phys. Med.* **54** 121–30

Wei J *et al* 2006 Dosimetric impact of a CT metal artefact suppression algorithm for proton, electron and photon therapies *Phys. Med. Biol.* **51** 5183–97

Willemink M J *et al* 2018 Photon-counting CT: technical principles and clinical prospects *Radiology* **289** 293–312

Witt J S, Rosenberg S A and Bassetti M F 2020 MRI-guided adaptive radiotherapy for liver tumours: visualising the future *Lancet Oncol.* **21** e74–82

Wohlfahrt P and Richter C 2020 Status and innovations in pre-treatment CT imaging for proton therapy *Br. J. Radiol.* **93** 20190590

Wood A M *et al* 2019 MRI-guided definition of cerebrospinal fluid distribution around cranial and sacral nerves: implications for brain tumors and craniospinal irradiation *Acta Oncol.* **58** 1740–4

Zechner A *et al* 2022 Evaluation of the inter- and intrafraction displacement for head patients treated at the particle therapy centre MedAustron based on the comparison of different commercial immobilisation devices *Z. Med. Phys.* **32** 39–51

Zhang Y *et al* 2023 A survey of practice patterns for real-time intrafractional motion-management in particle therapy *Phys. Imaging Radiat. Oncol.* **26** 100439

IOP Publishing

Chapter 14

Conclusions and future perspectives of imaging in particle therapy

C Paganelli, C Gianoli and A Knopf

Particle therapy (PT) is continuously growing worldwide with significant methodological and technological developments to achieve optimal geometrical selectivity and radiobiological effectiveness and, thus, improve tumour control and patient survival. In addition to the active clinical centres and those under construction with a rapid increase in the number of patients and expansion of the indications treated with PT (https://www.ptcog.site/), novel advanced treatment delivery modalities are under investigation, trying to improve the spatial and temporal dose distribution (Chang *et al* 2020, El Naqa *et al* 2022, Schneider 2022).

In the perspective of implementing very precise delivery modalities, continuous innovations must be also undertaken in image guidance for more accurate and faster patient-specific treatments. In this book, we provided insights on the technological and methodological imaging solutions currently available in clinics and under investigation at the research level, highlighting their advantages and limitations.

Among the most novel imaging technologies adopted to overcome the limitation of conventional CT in stopping power ratio (SPR) estimation, dual-energy CT (DECT) has been introduced recently in the clinical routine for reducing range uncertainty in treatment planning of proton therapy (Peters *et al* 2022). On the other side, although ion imaging could potentially match the imaging requirements for clinical applications in PT to avoid SPR calibration, no detector has been so far integrated into a treatment room. Ion imaging experiments currently suffer from important geometrical limitations, long acquisition time and high imaging dose. As most of the ion beam therapy facilities are not equipped with rotating gantries and most of the prototypes are based on bulky detectors, ion tomography experiments are currently performed by rotating the object of interest while keeping the detector aligned to the fixed beam nozzle. Except for seated treatment positions which could be considered for ocular and cranial tumours, ion imaging would be impossible for most of the patients positioned laying. This could be overcome with the future advent of upright PT treatments (Volz *et al* 2022), in which ion imaging could be particularly suited.

Additional advances in imaging technologies have been made towards the implementation of online PT workflows, which would allow one to plan, adapt and verify the treatment directly in the treatment room in a closed loop fashion, limiting inter-fraction variations and related image registration uncertainties (Paganelli *et al* 2018a). To achieve this, in-room/in-beam technologies, complemented with fast methodological solutions, need to be exploited to obtain a patient-specific image descriptive of anatomo-pathological variations between each radiotherapy fraction.

Although most of the PT clinical centres are equipped with in-room 2D x-ray projection mainly adopted for rigid alignment, the use of dedicated in-room CBCT scanners, acquiring volumetric 3D images of the day and trigger adaptation in PT is seen as mandatory for the future (Landry and Hua 2018).

Relevant advances in online (and in the future real-time) PT workflows are also expected with the development of integrated MRI-proton therapy units (Hoffmann *et al* 2020). For MRI-guidance, online adaptation has been already demonstrated with commercial MRI-linacs in conventional RT (Kishan *et al* 2023), and additional benefits are also highlighted for the treatment of moving organs with these integrated systems (Paganelli *et al* 2018b, Keall *et al* 2022). Up to now, the advantages of MRI in providing radiation-free images with good soft-tissue contrast and dynamic sequences in contrast to x-ray images, can be exploited off-line in PT, with studies successfully investigating 4DMRI as a complement of the standard 4DCT (Krieger *et al* 2020, Meschini *et al* 2020). Nevertheless, no commercial systems are yet available for PT with just few prototypes being studied up to now; thus, the real clinical benefit of online MRI for PT remains to be shown.

The necessity to implement treatment verification online to directly verify the accuracy of the delivered dose becomes specifically apparent in the context of online/real-time adaptive treatment regimes. However, there are currently no commercial systems for treatment verification based on secondary radiation imaging, although many PET imaging studies are based on commercial systems and some prompt gamma imaging prototypes rely on clinically established technologies. Fast dose accumulation procedure and dose reconstruction with log-based files can thus be adopted as alternative to verify dose deposition (Meijers *et al* 2019, Albertini *et al* 2020, Paganetti *et al* 2021).

All the above-mentioned technologies benefit from the growing interest in methodological solutions based on artificial intelligence (AI; Landry *et al* 2023), which excels at extracting features from training data and making predictions on new unseen data and is fast for online (as well as real-time) adaptation. Several works are showing that synthetic CT images can be derived from CBCT and MRI for different anatomical sites with applications in PT (Thummerer *et al* 2020a, 2020b, Parrella *et al* 2023). This allows limiting errors due to image registration procedures and SPR calibration. AI can also contribute to the management of intra-fraction variations due to respiration. The derivation of time-resolved 3D data via deep learning (Zhang *et al* 2014, Meschini *et al* 2019, 2022, Wei *et al* 2023) will push from online to real-time 4D treatments, as time-resolved 3D data provides the information needed for lateral beam adjustments and energy adaption in PT (Mori *et al* 2018). AI can also improve models for image acquisition and reconstruction as well as investigate correlations with corresponding dose distributions in in-vivo range verification or implement classification and prediction models to stratify patients and predict treatment outcome. Recently, AI has been exploited as a tool, together with radiomics (and dosiomics), to extract relevant quantitative features from images (and dose maps) for tumour aggressiveness and treatment outcome prediction (Lambin *et al* 2017, Morelli *et al* 2022). Nevertheless, although the potential of AI is very promising, its use in the clinical practice must be regulated to provide interpretable results with a quantifiable level of uncertainty.

Finally, another fundamental topic of interest in the near future and demanding for further research, is quantitative imaging (Q-imaging) (O'Connor *et al* 2017, Gurney-Champion *et al* 2020). Up to now Q-imaging is mainly limited to improve contouring in PT planning, but its potential in providing biological, microstructural and physiological features must be exploited. Q-imaging allows clinicians and researchers to account not only for tumour geometry but also for tumour biology and to better understand the biological properties at the basis of a PT treatment. Knowing and modelling the tumour characteristics and the mechanisms of PT, will help in defining optimal and individual dose schemes, as well as sculpting the dose according to each patient. In this way, the implementation of personalized and biologically-guided PT treatments will make the most of PT benefits.

Within this scenario, different working groups are currently working on the standardization of imaging protocols and on advancing imaging capabilities in PT, such as PTCOG (https://www.ptcog.site/), EPTN (Grau *et al* 2018, 2020) and AAPM (https://www.aapm.org/). These, together with the entire scientific community, also supported by dedicated conferences (MICCAI, BIGART, ICCR, 4D treatment workshop, as few examples), will continuously advance image guidance in PT towards accurate treatments and improved patient care.

References

Albertini F, Matter M, Nenoff L, Zhang Y and Lomax A 2020 Online daily adaptive proton therapy *Br. J. Radiol.* **93** 20190594

American Association of Physicists in Medicine, https://aapm.org/

Chang S, Liu G, Zhao L, Dilworth J T, Zheng W, Jawad S, Yan D, Chen P, Stevens C and Kabolizadeh P 2020 Feasibility study: spot-scanning proton arc therapy (SPArc) for left-sided whole breast radiotherapy *Radiat. Oncol.* **15** 1–11

El Naqa I, Pogue B W, Zhang R, Oraiqat I and Parodi K 2022 Image guidance for FLASH radiotherapy *Med. Phys.* **49** 4109–22

Grau C, Baumann M and Weber D C 2018 Optimizing clinical research and generating prospective high-quality data in particle therapy in Europe: introducing the European particle therapy network (EPTN) *Radiother. Oncol.* **128** 1–3

Grau C, Durante M, Georg D, Langendijk J A and Weber D C 2020 Particle therapy in Europe *Mol. Oncol.,* **14** 1492–9

Gurney-Champion O J, Mahmood F, van Schie M, Julian R, George B, Philippens M E, van der Heide U A, Thorwarth D and Redalen K R 2020 Quantitative imaging for radiotherapy purposes *Radiother. Oncol.* **146** 66–75

Hoffmann A, Oborn B, Moteabbed M, Yan S, Bortfeld T, Knopf A, Fuchs H, Georg D, Seco J and Spadea M F 2020 MR-guided proton therapy: a review and a preview *Radiat. Oncol.* **15** 1–13

Keall P J, Brighi C, Glide-Hurst C, Liney G, Liu P Z, Lydiard S, Paganelli C, Pham T, Shan S and Tree A C 2022 Integrated MRI-guided radiotherapy—opportunities and challenges *Nat. Rev. Clin. Oncol.* **19** 458–70

Kishan A U, Ma T M, Lamb J M, Casado M, Wilhalme H, Low D A, Sheng K, Sharma S, Nickols N G and Pham J 2023 Magnetic resonance imaging–guided vs computed tomography–guided stereotactic body radiotherapy for prostate cancer: the MIRAGE randomized clinical trial *JAMA Oncol.* **9** 365–73

Krieger M, Giger A, Salomir R, Bieri O, Celicanin Z, Cattin P C, Lomax A J, Weber D C and Zhang Y 2020 Impact of internal target volume definition for pencil beam scanned proton treatment planning in the presence of respiratory motion variability for lung cancer: a proof of concept *Radiother. Oncol.* **145** 154–61

Lambin P, Leijenaar R T, Deist T M, Peerlings J, De Jong E E, Van Timmeren J, Sanduleanu S, Larue R T, Even A J and Jochems A 2017 Radiomics: the bridge between medical imaging and personalized medicine *Nat. Rev. Clin. Oncol.* **14** 749–62

Landry G and Hua C h 2018 Current state and future applications of radiological image guidance for particle therapy *Med. Phys.* **45** e1086–95

Landry G, Kurz C and Traverso A 2023 The role of artificial intelligence in radiotherapy clinical practice *BJR Open* **5** 20230030

Meijers A, Jakobi A, Stützer K, Guterres Marmitt G, Both S, Langendijk J, Richter C and Knopf A 2019 Log file-based dose reconstruction and accumulation for 4D adaptive pencil beam scanned proton therapy in a clinical treatment planning system: implementation and proof-of-concept *Med. Phys.* **46** 1140–9

Meschini G, Seregni M, Molinelli S, Vai A, Phillips J, Sharp G C, Pella A, Valvo F, Ciocca M and Riboldi M 2019 Validation of a model for physical dose variations in irregularly moving targets treated with carbon ion beams *Med. Phys.* **46** 3663–73

Meschini G, Vai A, Barcellini A, Fontana G, Molinelli S, Mastella E, Pella A, Vitolo V, Imparato S and Orlandi E 2022 Time-resolved MRI for off-line treatment robustness evaluation in carbon-ion radiotherapy of pancreatic cancer *Med. Phys.* **49** 2386–95

Meschini G, Vai A, Paganelli C, Molinelli S, Fontana G, Pella A, Preda L, Vitolo V, Valvo F and Ciocca M 2020 Virtual 4DCT from 4DMRI for the management of respiratory motion in carbon ion therapy of abdominal tumors *Med. Phys.* **47** 909–16

Morelli L, Parrella G, Molinelli S, Magro G, Annunziata S, Mairani A, Chalaszczyk A, Fiore M R, Ciocca M and Paganelli C 2022 A Dosiomics analysis based on linear energy transfer and biological dose maps to predict local recurrence in Sacral Chordomas after carbon-ion radiotherapy *Cancers* **15** 33

Mori S, Knopf A C and Umegaki K 2018 Motion management in particle therapy *Med. Phys.* **45** e994–e1010

O'Connor J P, Aboagye E O, Adams J E, Aerts H J, Barrington S F, Beer A J, Boellaard R, Bohndiek S E, Brady M and Brown G 2017 Imaging biomarker roadmap for cancer studies *Nat. Rev. Clin. Oncol.* **14** 169–86

Paganelli C, Meschini G, Molinelli S, Riboldi M and Baroni G 2018a Patient-specific validation of deformable image registration in radiation therapy: overview and caveats *Med. Phys.* **45** e908–22

Paganelli C, Whelan B, Peroni M, Summers P, Fast M, Van de Lindt T, McClelland J, Eiben B, Keall P and Lomax T 2018b MRI-guidance for motion management in external beam radiotherapy: current status and future challenges *Phys. Med. Biol.* **63** 22TR03

Paganetti H, Botas P, Sharp G C and Winey B 2021 Adaptive proton therapy *Phys. Med. Biol.* **66** 22TR01

Particle Therapy Co-Operative Group, https://ptcog.site/

Parrella G, Vai A, Nakas A, Garau N, Meschini G, Camagni F, Molinelli S, Barcellini A, Pella A and Ciocca M 2023 Synthetic CT in carbon ion radiotherapy of the abdominal site *Bioengineering* **10** 250

Peters N, Wohlfahrt P, Hofmann C, Möhler C, Menkel S, Tschiche M, Krause M, Troost E G, Enghardt W and Richter C 2022 Reduction of clinical safety margins in proton therapy enabled by the clinical implementation of dual-energy CT for direct stopping-power prediction *Radiother. Oncol.* **166** 71–8

Schneider T 2022 Technical aspects of proton minibeam radiation therapy: minibeam generation and delivery *Phys. Med.* **100** 64–71

Thummerer A, De Jong B A, Zaffino P, Meijers A, Marmitt G G, Seco J, Steenbakkers R J, Langendijk J A, Both S and Spadea M F 2020a Comparison of the suitability of CBCT-and MR-based synthetic CTs for daily adaptive proton therapy in head and neck patients *Phys. Med. Biol.* **65** 235036

Thummerer A, Zaffino P, Meijers A, Marmitt G G, Seco J, Steenbakkers R J, Langendijk J A, Both S, Spadea M F and Knopf A C 2020b Comparison of CBCT based synthetic CT methods suitable for proton dose calculations in adaptive proton therapy *Phys. Med. Biol.* **65** 095002

Volz L, Sheng Y, Durante M and Graeff C 2022 Considerations for upright particle therapy patient positioning and associated image guidance *Front. Oncol.* **12** 930850

Wei R, Chen J, Liang B, Chen X, Men K and Dai J 2023 Real-time 3D MRI reconstruction from cine-MRI using unsupervised network in MRI-guided radiotherapy for liver cancer *Med. Phys.* **50** 3584–96

Zhang Y, Knopf A, Tanner C and Lomax A J 2014 Online image guided tumour tracking with scanned proton beams: a comprehensive simulation study *Phys. Med. Biol.* **59** 7793

www.ingramcontent.com/pod-product-compliance
Lightning Source LLC
Chambersburg PA
CBHW080522220326
41599CB00032B/6169